Enhancing Healthcare and Rehabilitation

Rehabilitation Science in Practice Series

Marcia J. Scherer
Institute for Matching Person & Technology, Webster, New York, USA
Dave J. Muller
Suffolk New College, UK

Neurological Rehabilitation: Spasticity and Contractures in Clinical Practice and Research
Anand D. Pandyan, Hermie J. Hermens, Bernard A. Conway

Quality of Life Technology Handbook
Richard Schulz

Computer Systems Experiences of Users with and Without Disabilities: An Evaluation Guide for Professionals
Simone Borsci, Masaaki Kurosu, Stefano Federici, Maria Laura Mele

Assistive Technology Assessment Handbook - 2nd Edition
Stefano Federici, Marcia Scherer

Ambient Assisted Living
Nuno M. Garcia, Joel Jose P.C. Rodrigues

For more information about this series, please visit: https://www.crcpress.com/Rehabilitation-Science-in-Practice-Series/book-series/CRCPRESERIN

Enhancing Healthcare and Rehabilitation

The Impact of Qualitative Research

Edited by

Christopher M. Hayre
Dave J. Muller

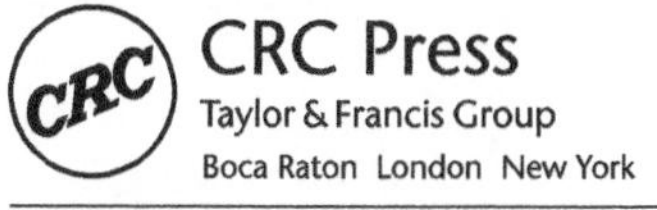

CRC Press is an imprint of the
Taylor & Francis Group, an **informa** business

CRC Press
Taylor & Francis Group
6000 Broken Sound Parkway NW, Suite 300
Boca Raton, FL 33487-2742

Printed on acid-free paper

International Standard Book Number-13: 978-0-8153-6081-0 (Hardback)

Library of Congress Cataloging-in-Publication Data

Names: Hayre, Christopher M., editor. | Muller, Dave J., editor.
Title: Enhancing healthcare and rehabilitation : the impact of qualitative research / [edited by] Dr. Christopher M. Hayre and Professor Dave J. Muller.
Other titles: Rehabilitation science in practice series. 2469-5513
Description: Boca Raton : Taylor & Francis, 2019 | Series: Rehabilitation science in practice series | Includes bibliographical references and index.
Identifiers: LCCN 2018059441| ISBN 9780815360810 (hardback : alk. paper) | ISBN 9781351116824 (ebook)
Subjects: | MESH: Rehabilitation Research | Qualitative Research
Classification: LCC RA440.85 | NLM WB 320.5 | DDC 362.1072/1--dc23
LC record available at https://lccn.loc.gov/2018059441

Visit the Taylor & Francis Web site at
http://www.taylorandfrancis.com

and the CRC Press Web site at
http://www.crcpress.com

Printed and bound by CPI Group (UK) Ltd, Croydon, CR0 4YY

Dr. Christopher M. Hayre would firstly like to dedicate this book to his wife Charlotte Hayre and his daughter Ayva Hayre. Secondly, he would like to dedicate this book to his late Grandmother, Beryl Irene Curtis. Love to all.

Professor Dave J. Muller would like to dedicate this to his extended family with love, Pam, Emily, Lucy, Tasha, Harlie, Toby, Edie, Kaya and Freya.

Contents

Preface

This book is primarily a celebration of the qualitative work undertaken internationally by a number of experienced researchers. It also focuses on developing the use of qualitative research for health and rehabilitative practitioners by recognising its value methodologically and empirically. We find that the very nature of qualitative research offers an array of opportunities for researchers in being able to understand the social world around us. Further, through experience and discussion this book identifies the multifaceted use of qualitative methods in the healthcare and rehabilitative setting. This book touches on the role of the researcher, the participants involved, and the research environment. In short, we see how these three central elements can affect the nature of qualitative work in attempts to offer originality.

This text speaks to a number of audiences. Students who are writing undergraduate dissertations and research proposals may find the myriad of examples stimulating and may support the rationale for methodological decisions in their own work. For academics, practitioners, and prospective qualitative researchers, this book also aims to demonstrate an array of opportunism in the field of qualitative research and how they may reason with arguments proffered.

This book also offers a lens that primarily focuses on the healthcare professionals perspective. As a diagnostic radiographer, the first author offers a perspective in how qualitative methods can be utilised in what has historically stemmed from positivism, but importantly recognises the value of quantitative work in his field. Further, the second author in his role as editor has a privileged insight into the emergence and development of qualitative research and its application. In short, the editors do not attempt to view qualitative research as superior to quantitative work, but merely accept the value of each.

In the introduction chapter the editors outline some key discussions for both prospective and experienced researchers. They offer a methodology that resonates with the role of a healthcare professional in light of treating and managing patients holistically. Section II offers contemporary applications of how qualitative research has enhanced the evidence base by utilising qualitative research. Section III offers two methodological chapters that address both methodological design and the researchers positionality and reflexivity.

It is anticipated that readers will find this collection of qualitative examples not only useful for informing their own research, but the editors also hope to enlighten new discussions and arguments regarding both methodological and empirical use of qualitative work internationally.

Christopher M. Hayre

Dave J. Muller

Acknowledgements

We would like to thank all contributing authors for sharing their innovative qualitative work. Your commitment to this book reflects the hard work undertaken, and it has been a pleasure for us to work with you and bring together this collection of sound works. The work of all authors demonstrates the multifaceted application of qualitative research in contemporary healthcare and rehabilitation. Further, we are grateful to have received methodological position chapters that aim to enhance the use of qualitative research for prospective researchers. Finally, we are in agreement that this has been an exciting and prosperous project, which we hope readers will enjoy.

Editors

Christopher M. Hayre, PhD, is a senior lecturer in Diagnostic Radiography and Research Lead for the School of Health Sciences, located at the University of Suffolk, United Kingdom. After 10 years working clinically as a radiographer he pursued a PhD exploring the impact of advancing technology and completed this in 2015. He has published an array of academic work in leading journals pertinent to medical imaging. In 2016, he founded the *Journal of Social Science & Allied Health Professions* and is now editor-in-chief. He is currently involved in a number of scholarly projects involving dementia, virtual reality, everyday technology, personalised medicine, dose optimisation (X-rays) and artificial intelligence.

Dave J. Muller is currently editor with Professor Marcia Scherer of the CRC series Rehabilitation Science in Practice. He was founding editor of the *Journal Aphasiology* and is currently editor in chief of the *Journal Disability and Rehabilitation.* He has published more than 40 refereed papers and has been involved either as series editor, editor or author of more than 50 books. He is a visiting professor at the University of Suffolk, United Kingdom.

Contributors

Simon Bishop
Bangor University
Bangor, United Kingdom

Shane Blackman
Cultural Students
Canterbury Christ Church University
Canterbury, United Kingdom

Barbara J. Bowers
School of Nursing
University of Wisconsin-Madison
Madison, Wisconsin

Samantha Bunzli
Allied Health Clinical Research Office
Eastern Health
Victoria, Australia

Ingela K. Carlsson
Department of Translational Medicine
Hand Surgery
Skane University Hospital
Malmö, Sweden

Anette Chemnitz
Department of Hand Surgery
Skåne University Hospital
Malmö, Sweden

Luis Columna
Department of Kinesiology
School of Education
University of Wisconsin at Madison
Madison, Wisconsin

Lars B. Dahlin
Department of Translational Medicine
Hand Surgery
Lund University
and
Department of Hand Surgery
Skåne University Hospital
Malmö, Sweden

Mary Lynn Damhorst
Department of Apparel, Events, and
Hospitality Management
Iowa State University
Ames, Iowa

Charles Edmund Degeneffe
Rehabilitation Counseling Program
San Diego State University
San Diego, California

Catherine Elson
Department of Clinical Psychology
Lancaster University
Lancaster, United Kingdom

Barbara E. Gibson
Department of Physical Therapy
Bloorview Research Institute
University of Toronto and Senior Scientist
Toronto, Canada

Christopher M. Hayre
School of Health Science
University of Suffolk
Ipswich, United Kingdom

Yani Hamdani
Department of Occupational Science and Occupational Therapy
University of Toronto
and
Azrieli Adult Neurodevelopmental Centre
Centre for Addiction and Mental Health
Toronto, Ontario, Canada

Samuel R. Hodge
Department of Human Sciences
College of Education and Human Ecology
The Ohio State University
Columbus, Ohio

Jo Jury
Department of Clinical Psychology
Lancaster University
Lancaster, United Kingdom

Shilpa Krishnan
Division of Physical Therapy
Department of Rehabilitation Medicine
Emory University
Atlanta, Georgia

Yvonne C. Learmouth
School of Psychology and Exercise Science
Murdoch University
Perth, Western Australia, Australia

Sally Lindsay
Bloorview Research Institute
Holland Bloorview Kids Rehabilitation Hospital
and
Department of Occupational Science & Occupational Therapy
University of Toronto
Toronto, Ontario, Canada

Zoey Malpus
Department of Clinical Psychology
Lancaster University
Lancaster, United Kingdom

Anne Marit Mengshoel
Department of Health Sciences
Medical Faculty
Institute of Health and Society
University of Oslo
Oslo, Norway

Victoria Molyneaux
Department of Clinical Psychology
Lancaster University
Lancaster, United Kingdom

Erika Mosor
Section for Outcomes Research
Center for Medical Statistics, Informatics, and Intelligent Systems
Medical University of Vienna
Vienna, Austria

Dave J. Muller
Department of Rehabilitation Psychology
University of Suffolk
Suffolk, United Kingdom

Craig D. Murray
Department of Health Psychologist
Lancaster University
Lancaster, United Kingdom

Kristin E. Musselman
SCI Mobility Lab
Lyndhurst Centre
Toronto Rehabilitation Institute
University Health Network
and
Department of Physical Therapy
Faculty of Medicine
University of Toronto
and
Faculty of Medicine
Rehabilitation Sciences Institute
University of Toronto
Toronto, Ontario, Canada

Beth Myers
Department of Exercise Science
School of Education
CAPE, Syracuse University
Syracuse, New York

Jennifer Paff Ogle
Department of Design and Merchandising
Center for Women's Studies and Gender Research
Colorado State University
Fort Collins, Colorado

Claudia Oppenauer
Section for Outcomes Research
Center for Medical Statistics, Informatics, and Intelligent Systems
Medical University of Vienna
Vienna, Austria

Juyeon Park
Department of Design and Merchandising
Environmental and Occupational Health (Physical Activity and Healthy Lifestyle Concentration) Colorado School of Public Health
Colorado State University
Fort Collins, Colorado

Monique R. Pappadis
Division of Rehabilitation Sciences
University of Texas Medical Branch
Galveston, Texas

Adele Phillips
Health Promotion and Public Health
School of Allied and Public Health Professions
Faculty of Health and Wellbeing
Canterbury Christ Church University
Canterbury, United Kingdom

Timothy A. Reistetter
Division of Rehabilitation Sciences
University of Texas Medical Branch
and
Department of Occupational Therapy
University of Texas Medical Branch
Galveston, Texas

Valentin Ritschl
Occupational Therapist
Section for Outcomes Research
Center for Medical Statistics, Informatics, and Intelligent Systems
Medical University of Vienna
Vienna, Austria

Anne E. Roll
Hochschule für Gesundheit
University of Applied Science (hsg)
Bochum, Germany

Rajeeb Sah
Public Health and Health Promotion
School of Allied and Public Health Professions
Faculty of Health and Wellbeing
Canterbury Christ Church University
Canterbury, United Kingdom

Merja Sallinen
Satakunta University of Applied Sciences
Pori, Finland

and

University of Oslo
Oslo, Norway

Nora Shields
Department of Physiotherapy
College of Science Health and Engineering
La Trobe University
Victoria, Australia

Jane Simpson
Lancaster University
Lancaster, United Kingdom

Hardeep Singh
SCI Mobility Lab
Lyndhurst Centre
Toronto Rehabilitation Institute
University Health Network
and
Faculty of Medicine
Rehabilitation Sciences Institute
University of Toronto
Toronto, Ontario, Canada

Tanja Stamm
Section for Outcomes Research
Center for Medical Statistics, Informatics, and Intelligent Systems
Medical University of Vienna
Vienna, Austria

Denzil A. Streete
Graduate School of Arts and Science
Yale University
New Haven, Connecticut

Nicholas F. Taylor
Department of Allied Health
College of Science Health and Engineering
La Trobe University
Allied Health Clinical Research Office Eastern Health
Victoria, Australia

Sally Thorne
School of Nursing
University of British Columbia
Vancouver, British Columbia, Canada

Janelle Unger
SCI Mobility Lab
Lyndhurst Centre
Toronto Rehabilitation Institute
University Health Network
and
Faculty of Medicine
Rehabilitation Sciences Institute
University of Toronto
Toronto, Ontario, Canada

Jason A. Wallis
Allied Health Clinical Research Office Eastern Health
Victoria, Australia

Stephen Weatherhead
Department of Clinical Psychology
Lancaster University
Lancaster, United Kingdom

David J. Wilde
Nottingham Trent University
Nottingham, United Kingdom

Linda Worrall
School of Health and Rehabilitation Sciences
The University of Queensland
Brisbane, Queensland, Australia

Section I

Introductory Perspectives

1

Qualitative Research in Contemporary Healthcare and Rehabilitative Practices

Christopher M. Hayre and Dave J. Muller

CONTENTS

Introduction

This introductory perspective discusses the value of qualitative research in the field of healthcare and rehabilitation. We begin by opening a discussion regarding qualitative research, with reflections of our own methodological and empirical experiences. This is supported with our roles as academic reviewers and editors, supported with our experiences of peer publication. On the one hand, this introductory perspective (and book) is a celebration of progressive work undertaken by researchers internationally. In addition, however, this chapter offers an opportunity to discuss the application of qualitative research, whilst also challenging commonly held perspectives, in order to drive this central research methodology forward.

We begin by emphasising how qualitative research offers practitioners unique insights to their clinical environment. This is supported by an innovative methodological strategy utilised by the first author whereby his ideology and professional practice (Hayre 2015) remained interconnected in order to uncover original phenomena. This is later deemed a 'sequentialist philosophy'. Here, we argue that all healthcare professionals utilise inductive and hypothetical-deductive reasoning in order to provide sound care for their patients and thus feel it could be an approach that resonates, but more importantly, be of use to healthcare researchers. These discussions are central because in recent years there have been many advances in the use and application of qualitative research aligned to post-modernist thinking, and here, we again aim to expand our utilisation of this important paradigmatic approach.

Next, we discuss 'trustworthiness' within the qualitative framework and how credibility, transferability, dependability, and confirmability are used to evidence rigor. For example, we provide contemporary strategies of applying these concepts methodologically within the clinical environment, but importantly reflect on our own experiences to date. In short, the purpose of this section is to explore contemporary methodological opportunities supporting and enhancing rigor in the clinical environment. This is important in order to support prospective qualitative researchers in the field.

The Value of Qualitative Research for Healthcare and Rehabilitation Practitioners

The forthcoming chapters in this book demonstrate the multi-faceted value of qualitative research within the clinical environment. Further, they demonstrate and challenge how qualitative approaches play a pivotal role in enhancing the knowledge base for healthcare and rehabilitative practitioners.

Qualitative research is generally accepted to explore phenomena juxtaposed to quantitative techniques, the latter aiming to generalise findings by statistical inference. Here, we acknowledge the value of utilising qualitative and quantitative approaches in order to support and/or refute findings, but importantly strengthen the need for qualitative work clinically. Further, it is important to affirm that we view each paradigmatic approach as 'complementary' to the other and affirm that each offers a unique perspective, depending on the research question(s), whilst seeking to understand the social world around us. We embrace these approaches because there utility resonates with the delivery of patient care clinically.

In the field of education, Maxwell (2012) asserts that qualitative research should be seen as equal to randomised control trials (RCTs). He importantly recognises how qualitative work offers causational relationships empirically claiming that scientific research in the field of education 'assumes that investigations of causation need to be quantitative, requiring randomised control trials (RCTs)'. In short, Maxwell rejects the use of RCTs as the 'only' strategy that can infer causality and accepts that qualitative approaches can be used to make causational relationships, linking these to a number of everyday circumstances. We agree and promote that qualitative research can have casual outcomes for practitioners, researchers, and policymakers alike within health and rehabilitative environments, and if appropriate, can be supported or challenged by other research approaches.

One example of this causational relationship resonates with the first author whereby equipment error led to the delivery of X-rays to a patient without any net benefit (the production of a radiograph) (Hayre et al. 2017). Here, causation was identified by means of participant observation, a generally accepted qualitative approach, thus negating the need for further quantification and generalisation by use of statistical inference. Here, it is important to argue that because this observation remained the lived experience of both the radiographer and the patient (with potential risks associated with X-rays) it should be seen as equal to RCTs in terms of advancing knowledge and impacting clinical decisions. One example of this is the rationale for ensuring that patients (and staff) are kept safe whilst receiving medical treatment and/or care. For example, if a patient (or staff member) is observed to be at risk or in immediate danger, we are morally, ethically, and legally obliged to intervene in order to prevent undue harm. Thus, by means of observation we can detect causality which may (or may not, if prevented) lead to poor outcomes.

Put simply, we do not observe poor healthcare delivery and decided to run an RCT or survey to support whether findings are 'generalisable'. Our point is that qualitative research should not be seen as inferior in terms of empirical importance because of its inability to infer outcomes statistically. Observation and communication remain pertinent tools for healthcare professionals in order to assess clinical and patient outcomes. Here, then, we also feel that RCTs should offer a qualitative lens in order to inform research directions and/or to reflect on the patient's journey of the trial itself in order to provide a holistic picture of the clinical setting.

The argument that qualitative work can inform quantitative methods is reflected in the PhD work by the first author. For example, participant observation remained the tool of choice, primarily observing diagnostic radiographers within the clinical environment. This generation of theory and new knowledge was then later explored by utilising semi-structured interviews and undertaking X-ray experiments. Here, Hayre (2015) argued the need for inductive approaches (by means of participant observation), enabling him to not only develop an interview schedule, but also hypothetically deduce X-ray experimentation based on 'what had been seen' of diagnostic radiographers. In short, because X-rays cannot be seen, felt, heard, nor touched, abutting the human senses, the author remained acutely aware of the importance of quantifying radiation dose in order to learn and understand the optimisation of X-rays within the clinical environment, but affirm that without the use of qualitative causality, these experiments would have been based on the author's own biases.

In diagnostic radiography, a plethora of quantitative evidence exists documenting the optimisation of ionising radiation to patients within the clinical environment. Yet, recent qualitative research by the author identified a 'disconnect' between the evidence base and clinical practice (Hayre 2016), something, which Snaith comments as 'practice drift', whereby historical evidence may not always be adhered (Snaith 2016). In short, recent developments, and the utility of qualitative enquiries, have critiqued the theory practice gap in diagnostic radiography by challenging the application of evidence-based research. Not only does this re-emphasise the value of qualitative work in order to support/refute quantitative enquiry, it further recognises how as healthcare professionals we can utilise qualitative methods in order to critically reflect on quantitative empiricism.

Our argument that qualitative research can inform quantitative enquiries within the healthcare environment offers an opportunity to discuss its philosophical application for prospective researchers. Originally, the first author felt juxtaposed in the early stages of his research following the utilisation of observational and experimental methods. Initial assumptions led the author to align his research lens to pragmatism, an approach that evaluates theories or beliefs in terms of their practical evaluation. However, upon reflection, this was later challenged because the methods utilised alone were not seen as 'practical', but more advocated by my own ideological and professional role as a diagnostic radiographer. For example, whilst a 'mixed method' approach was initially seen to be utilised by means of polarisation of the paradigmatic approaches, this was later rejected by adopting a sequentialist strategy whereby the methods utilised were required to be undertaken 'in order', reflected by his [Hayre] own professional practices. This is depicted in Figure 1.1 (Hayre 2015, p. 74).

The rationale for this sequentialist philosophy was grounded by the author's role as a diagnostic radiographer. As healthcare practitioners, we observe and interact with our patients prior to making clinical decisions about the healthcare we deliver. For diagnostic

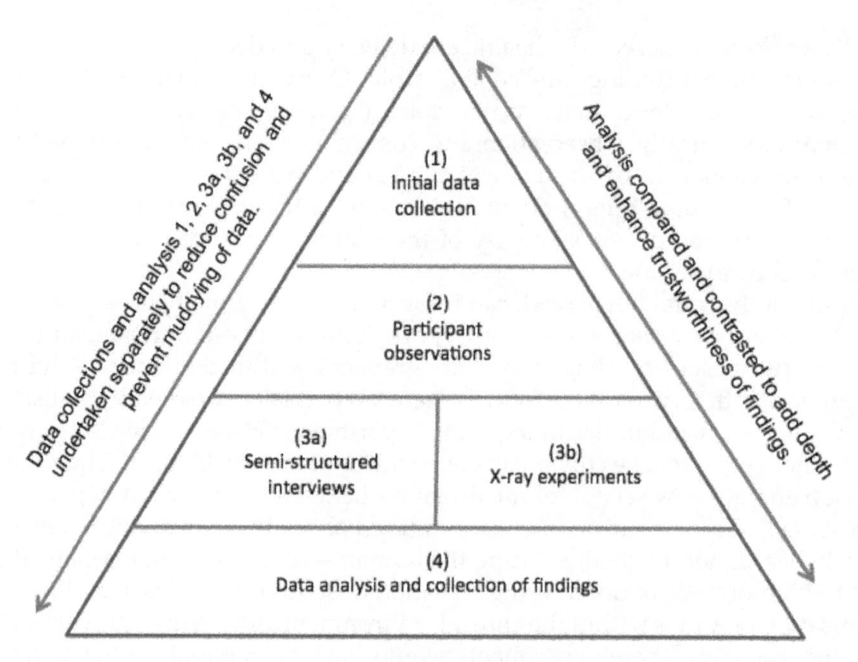

FIGURE 1.1
Sequentialism philosophy used as part of an overarching ethnographic methodology.

radiographers, this is primarily aligned to selecting an appropriate X-ray exposure and imaging parameters that will enable sound image quality – the formation of an X-ray image in order to detect pathology. By observing and communicating with a patient, this reflects on the use of inductive reasoning by radiographers in order to hypothetically deduce an appropriate X-ray exposure based on the type of examination, pathology, and size of the patient. This 'sequential' approach of delivering care within the X-ray room is not typically seen as polar opposites, but rather as 'holistic' when delivering optimum patient care.

On reflection, then, the utilisation of both inductive and hypothetical-deductive reasoning remains part of all healthcare professionals day-to-day practices whereby observation, communication, and treatment/management remain at the centre of an individual's care. In response, we offer 'sequentialism' as a methodological strategy that reflects the role of health and rehabilitative practitioners clinical work in order to enhance a body of knowledge. Further, this utilitarian philosophy offers healthcare professionals a methodological approach that critically reflects on our day-to-day practices whereby research tools are incorporated into what Hayre (2015) termed in his work 'an ethnographic sphere'. This strategy was later termed 'an umbrella approach' which encompassed an array of methods in order to answer the healthcare professionals research question(s). This strategy was supported by Holliday (2016) in a recent monograph:

> My personal conclusion to this [Hayre's] discussion is that there does need to be an 'umbrella' strategy of investigation or methodology within any research project that drives whatever methods of data collection and analysis are used whether they are quantitative or qualitative. This means that within a post modern paradigm the

> understanding that both the social phenomena being investigated and the methodology for investigating them are socially and ideologically constructed will apply also to quantitative methods.

Accepting this approach implies a post-modern sequentialist philosophy that is not mixed methods, but complementary, and one that is used to better understand the social world of health and rehabilitative environments. This leads to affirm that the value of qualitative research can not only inform quantitative approaches within the healthcare environment, but also be seen as a 'sequentialist methodology'. In short, whilst this sequentialist strategy remained central to the author's ethnographic work, we argue that this philosophical lens can be utilised in other methodological contexts in order for researchers to reflect and engage in original phenomena around them.

Credibility, Transferability, Dependability, and Confirmability: Reflections in Practice

Ensuring methodological rigor in qualitative research remains paramount. It is important to note that whilst we accept the importance of rigor, which we will now term 'trustworthiness' hereafter, we do not offer a prescriptive model. This is important to recognise, as different researchers will have different experiences with participants within their unique research environment(s). We do, however, accept the four generally accepted terms, credibility, transferability, dependability, and confirmability and feel that these remain central to ensuring that qualitative research remains 'trustworthy' in healthcare and rehabilitative environments.

We begin by highlighting the importance of the methodological approach in all qualitative research. We affirm that a methodological approach adopted by a researcher should be informed by the research question(s) and existing gaps within the evidence base. As academics, we agree that a research methodology is analogous to a 'car engine', enabling a researcher to reach their destination [by answering the initial research question(s)]. This analogy is also relevant when discussing data saturation and accepting when researchers should 'leave the field'. One way of limiting this is by critically evaluating one's own biography. To date, we have seen the value of researchers providing critical auto/biographical contextualisation of 'self' in order to critically examine the context of the researcher and his/her participants (West 2014). In short, we feel that researchers should offer auto/biographical accounts in order to help situate the researcher within the context of his/her research. This will enable outsiders to gain a perspective from the researcher's standpoint, a rationale for exploring the topic of interest and outline any inherent biases.

It is generally accepted that researchers need to outline how they have ensured their research remains 'trustworthy' by describing how credibility, transferability, dependability, and confirmability have been met. Whilst these are generally accepted, we feel that the representation of these four terms in peer-reviewed journals can often be omitted, and as academic reviewers we also appreciate that reviewers may differ in their opinion on the level of detail required in order to ensure the study remains 'trustworthy'. The first author has direct experience of the level of detail required by academic reviewers whereby his own publications have no discussion (Hayre 2016), little discussion

(Hayre et al. 2018), or detailed discussion (Hayre et al. In Press) of these four terms. Again, whilst we do not propose a linear model, on reflection, we feel that authors and reviewers should offer sufficient detail that reflects the researchers approach to ensuring rigor in their qualitative work.

In the classic work of Lincoln and Guba (1985, p. 290), they explain the basic question of ensuring qualitative rigor:

> How can an inquirer persuade his or her audiences (including self) that the findings or an inquiry are worth paying attention to, worth taking account of?

This statement illustrates the importance of being able to ensure that researchers offer descriptive accounts that will resonate with peers of that professional community. We will now discuss the four generally accepted terms, whilst importantly reflecting on our own research experiences.

Credibility ensures whether a reader can 'trust' the work of the researcher. For example, it refers to researchers ability to check the truth of the data of his/her participants, commonly termed 'member checking'. Lincoln and Guba (1985) assert this to be of primary importance for assessing trustworthiness whereby a researcher follows up with participants to verify that the findings reflect the intended meaning(s). In our view, member checking remains an important tool for qualitative researchers whereby participants can verify interview/focus group transcripts and observational data. In addition to participant verification, Holliday (2016) recommends that qualitative researchers enhance the credibility of their work by engaging in ongoing discussions with peers during and post-data analysis. This offers an alternate form of triangulation whereby the findings are continually discussed with colleagues, enabling the researcher to continuously reflect on the empirical findings. We agree and utilise both member checking and peer-debriefing in our work, whereby discussions held with PhD supervisors, colleagues (healthcare practitioners/academics), and students (in seminar led discussions) enhanced the credibility of the qualitative work. In short, we agree that credibility moves beyond member checking and into the researchers community.

Another facet enhancing credibility is prolonged engagement with participants in the field. In the author's ethnographic work, prolonged engagement remained paramount, enabling the researcher to become familiar with both the environment and his participants. Whilst prolonged engagement may arise from a 'researcher position', we argue that there may be other elements that enhance prolonged engagement. For example, the author reflects on his clinical experiences as a radiographer and interactions with peers. On reflection, the author already knew *some* of the participants prior to becoming 'the researcher' and thus influencing the research context. These historical experiences provided greater understanding of the clinical environment. Here, however, the balance of remaining objective was often problematic with some participants, but through critical reflection, the researcher was often required to balance 'friendship' with 'becoming a stranger' in order to provide a balanced and honest approach.

Transferability within the qualitative context is seen as a tool that enables other healthcare practitioners to be able to resonate with the empirical work presented. More specifically, Lincoln and Guba (1985, p. 290) assert that transferability 'determines the extent to which the findings of a particular inquiry have applicability in other contexts or with other subjects/participants' and is equivalent to external validity in quantitative research. Transferability can be achieved if researchers provide thorough description(s) of the research context in order for readers to judge and transfer the findings into their clinical environments. We feel this is achieved when researchers offer comprehensive description of the informants partaking in the research, supported with contextual information about the environment. This, then, enables a reader to judge the extent to which the findings resonate with the lived experience. This is important because whilst it has been argued that qualitative findings cannot be generalised, we argue that qualitative work can be generalised, as it remains the lived [potential] reality of others. We affirm that generalisation of qualitative work can be achieved (as discussed above), but not by conventional numerism. In short, whilst qualitative work is not typically quantified, it does not mean that it fails to be generalised by healthcare professionals either nationally and/or internationally and inform their clinical decisions.

Attempts of enhancing the transferability can also be supported by undertaking multi-sited research. In the field of diagnostic radiography techniques vary amongst practitioners, which is dependent on both protocols and workplace cultures. In the author's (Hayre 2015) work, he undertook research at multiple sites in order to provide a holistic perspective of behaviours and actions of practitioners. In this multi-sited ethnographic work, the author aimed to 'build a more transferable picture' of the clinical setting to his readers. Thus, whilst we feel that the lived experience of an individual can be generalised, the practice of multi-sited work can also help convince readers of an overarching perspective to the research questions posed.

Transferability can also be enhanced in light of socio-technological advances. For example, social media adds an alternate lens to understanding the transferability of empiricism by means of digital dialogue internationally. The evolution of social media, supported with metric data adds and alternate lens by supporting the 'transferable nature' of qualitative work via 'online discussions'. In short, social media offers 'digital conversations' of research from healthcare practitioners around the world. For example, some of the authors' own work has been discussed by peers from the United Kingdom, Australia, and New Zealand in the form of 'tweets' on the social media platform 'Twitter'. The following tweets are readily available in the public domain and are presented verbatim below:

> Radiographers: Want to find out if general practices adhere to person-centred care?
>
> *MIT's* Good insight into patient-centred care in x-ray dept's. DR = ↓ time with pt's = ↓ in care?? I can see how it happens!
>
> Gr8 point. ↓ in time should = ↑ time for care. Our 2 min with patient is 2 min more than reporting radiologist.

This demonstrates the extent in which individuals find qualitative research impactful in their clinical environment via a digital platform. As technology continues to impact on how we interact with others, this will arguably impact on our 'measures' of assessing the transferability of empirical work. To surmise, we feel that the use of social media can be used as a tool to ascertain and enhance transferable attributes of qualitative work in order to provide a holistic view of supporting the trustworthiness of qualitative findings internationally.

Dependability is generally achieved when the research questions are clearly connected to the research methodology. In our discussions above, we have already asserted that the initial research questions should drive the methodology and that researchers should avoid being 'methodologically led'. Whilst this demonstrates linearity in terms of basing a methodological approach on existing literature and original research questions, we also suggest that researchers remain reflexive as a study progresses. For example, in author's own experiences, the use of inductive reasoning enabled him [Hayre] to 'explore the unknown' within the clinical setting. This is important to recognise in the research environment because as a researcher progresses through data collection, analysis, and write up, inherent discussions and thought processes naturally impact on the interpretation by the researcher. In response, then, for research question(s) to remain 'rigid', this may suggest a lack of critical reflexivity pre and post-data analysis. In short, we accept that whilst the research questions should initially inform data collection methods, researchers may find themselves 'moving back and forth' (as depicted in Figure 1.1), whereby they remain impacted by data analysis, empirical outcomes, ongoing discussions with peers, and during the 'write up' phase. In the authors' experience, these have all led to amendments to the initial research questions, and whilst this does not propose that qualitative work is in danger of losing its 'scientific finesse', it merely accepts that a researchers' positionality and reflexive journey may impact on pre-emptive conjectures, which may then need to be refined.

One approach of ensuring dependability is maintained by the representation of an audit trail. Because qualitative researchers interpret the social around him/her impacting on any final assertions made, critical reflective accounts need to be traceable by the reader(s). For example, the researcher's 'position' and 'presence' in the clinical environment will impact on relations with his/her participants (Hayre et al. 2017). In the author's work, Hayre (2015) reflects on the impact of being asked to wear a white doctors coat in the X-ray room, leading participants to challenge his attire. In addition, the author reflects on how the layout of multiple medical imaging environment(s) both facilitated and hindered data collection in his PhD work. For example, on the one hand, some environments were conducive whereby the researcher had 'space' to record interactions and communicate effectively with participants. On the other hand, the author reports of a single occasion where he was asked to leave the clinical environment because he was 'in the way'. These open and honest reflections detail the researchers journey within the research environment whereby repetition by others elicit similar responses. Marcus (1998, p. 98) reminds us that when conducting multi-sited research, researchers may become 'the research activist', renegotiating identities in different situations. In short, we recognise the importance of reflecting on experiences that both hinder and facilitate the research process in order to create a sound audit trail for prospective researchers.

Lastly, confirmability refers to the adequacy of information reported from the research question(s). It is generally accepted that different researchers might produce different constructions with the same data (Glaser and Strauss 1967), yet it should be possible to trace constructions and assertions to their original sources and make them available to outside reviewers of the study (Lincoln and Guba 1985). Further, the data should represent the participant's responses and not the researcher's biases or viewpoint. In the authors' view, the participants can achieve this by offering dichotomous verbatim quotes of particular phenomena. This will prevent any underlying assertions of researcher bias whereby a balanced analysis and discussion has taken place.

In addition, we claim that qualitative researchers have a responsibility of critically evaluating their role in the field. We recommend that researchers utilise a reflexive lens in order to continually assess their relationships with participants (and patients) with the intended research outcomes. One way of being 'ethically mindful' is identifying when a researcher should 'leave the field'. There have been numerous papers highlighting 'when to stop' and 'whether one more interview is enough' when qualitative researchers may find themselves discussing sensitive topics and uncovering rich data (National Centre for Research Methods 2013). Our analogy is, again, reflected in the role of the diagnostic radiographer (and other healthcare professionals) whereby he/she has a duty of care in the X-ray environment to take as fewer radiographs as possible to answer 'the clinical question(s)'. This is analogous to having a moral duty as qualitative researchers whereby researchers remain mindful of obtaining data saturation in order to recognise if/when the researcher should leave the field. Discussions concerning 'leaving the field' by researchers are important, but rarely discussed in accepted manuscripts. This is important because a central element of all qualitative research is the people who are involved and thus should be reflected upon (Hayre 2016). Further, where a number of gatekeepers have played central roles in allowing a researcher to observe and/or access their everyday lives is also another importance facet to consider. Looking back, upon leaving the field, special thanks were made to all staff. This was coincided with the feeling of 'sadness', whereby friendships had been established in professional and social contexts. Further, we remind readers that leaving the field is not too dissimilar from discharging and/or transferring a patient in the hospital setting. For example, as a diagnostic radiographer, we ensure that patients are aware of the next steps, signposted to key information, and offer opportunities for patients to reflect on experiences of receiving care via a short questionnaire. In brief, qualitative researchers should remain mindful of leaving the field, and ensure that it is reflected as part of the methodological process, as this will help convince readers of sound ethical conduct by completing the audit trail of the research process.

It remains generally accepted that qualitative researchers should abide to these principles in order to enhance the trustworthiness of qualitative research. Here, we have not only offered approaches, but provided insight into how this can be achieved in the clinical environment. We accept that all qualitative researchers will encounter unique challenges, and the examples outlined here may not resonate with peers. It does, however, aim to extend our understanding of ensuring trustworthiness in qualitative research within the healthcare and rehabilitation environment, which can be utilised by researchers.

Summary

Here, we have discussed the value of qualitative work within the health and rehabilitative environment. First, we outlined the growing acceptance of qualitative work and how it remains central to understanding the lived reality of key participants. We have further championed the importance of qualitative approaches by offering a methodological approach that may be utilised by prospective researchers in healthcare and rehabilitation. Healthcare professionals are reminded of our need to understand both social and scientific phenomena, whereby qualitative and quantitative approaches are typically used. In response to this, we argue that 'sequentialisim' can be used to strategically complement our ontology and epistemology. In short, whilst the authors have published quantitative and qualitative work, we do not see ourselves as 'mixed method researchers', but as a healthcare professional and psychologist utilising techniques to holistically inform and enhance patient outcomes.

Next, we discussed the importance of ensuring the trustworthiness of research findings. The generally accepted terms credibility, transferability, dependability, and confirmability are outlined with examples linking to the author's experiences. We discuss contemporary approaches to achieving trustworthiness in an attempt to aid prospective qualitative researchers. Further, we offer original discussions of maintaining trustworthiness within the clinical environment with discussions pertinent to the healthcare and/or rehabilitative environment.

The forthcoming chapters not only demonstrate the versatility of qualitative approaches in the health and rehabilitative settings, but also celebrate the novel and ambitious approaches utilised by researchers in the contemporary setting.

References

Glaser, B. and Strauss, A. (1967) *The Discovery of Grounded Theory: Strategies for Qualitative Research.* New York: Aldine De Gruyter.

Hayre, C.M. (2015) *Radiography Observed: An Ethnographic Study Exploring Contemporary Radiographic Practice.* PhD Thesis, Canterbury Christ Church University.

Hayre, C.M. (2016) 'Cranking up, whacking up and bumping up: X-ray exposures in contemporary radiographic practices'. *Radiography* 22 (2), pp. 194–198.

Hayre, C.M., Blackman, S., Carlton, K., and Eyden, A. (2018) 'Attitudes and perceptions of radiographers applying lead (Pb) protection in general radiography: An ethnographic study'. *Radiography* 24 (1), pp. e13–e18.

Hayre, C.M., Blackman, S., Carlton, K., and Eyden, A. (In Press) 'The use of digital side markers and cropping in digital radiography'. *Journal of Medical Imaging and Radiation Sciences,* doi:10.1016/j.jmir.2018.11.001.

Hayre, C.M., Eyden, A., Blackman, S., and Carlton, K. (2017) 'Image acquisition in general radiography: The utilisation of DDR'. *Radiography* 23 (2), pp. 147–152.

Holliday, A. (2016) *Doing and Writing Qualitative Research.* Los Angeles, CA: Sage.

Lincoln, Y. and Guba, E. (1985) *Naturalistic Inquiry.* London, UK: Sage.

Marcus, G.E. (1998) *Ethnography through Thick and Thin.* Princeton, NJ: Princeton University Press.

Maxwell, J.A. (2012) 'The importance of qualitative research for causal explanation in education'. *Qualitative Enquiry* 18 (8), pp. 655–661.

National Centre for Research Methods Review Paper (NCRM). (2013) *How Many Qualitative Interviews Is Enough?* [Online] Available at: http://eprints.ncrm.ac.uk/2273/ (Accessed 30 October 2018).

Snaith, B. (2016) 'Evidence based radiography: Is it happening or are we experiencing *practice creep* and practice drift'. *Radiography* 22 (4), pp. 267–268.

West, L. (2014) 'Transformative learning and the form that transforms'. *Journal of Transformative Education* 12 (2), pp. 164–179.

2

The Role of Qualitative Research in Adapted Physical Activity

Samuel R. Hodge, Luis Columna, Beth Myers and Denzil A. Streete

CONTENTS

Introduction

From early traditional research methodologies to current expanded conceptualisations of scientific research in education, conducting research in adapted physical activity settings has been, at times, a complex endeavour. These complexities necessitate the identification of qualitative research methodologies and quality indicators that represent rigorous application of methodology to questions of interest in adapted physical activity research.

In this chapter, we discuss the role of qualitative research in adapted physical activity and how qualitative research enhances our learning about and involving individuals with disabilities and their caregivers. Further, we identify and discuss quality indicators (criteria) for qualitative research that represent rigorous application of methodology to questions of interest in adapted physical activity research. Moreover, we discuss transforming qualitative research into practice and its impact on stakeholders (e.g., families, educators). Lastly, we articulate how qualitative research might enhance the future of our profession.

Origins of Adapted Physical Activity

In the United States, physical education is defined within special education under the Individuals with Disabilities Education Improvement Act. Specifically, Public Law 108-446, Individuals with Disabilities Education Improvement Act (2004) defines special education as 'specially designed instruction, at no cost to parents, to meet the unique needs of a child with a disability, including (a) instruction conducted in the classroom, in the home, in hospitals and institutions, and in other settings; and (b) instruction in physical education' (p. 118). This is important because it means in essence that all students being served in special education must receive physical education instruction with one exception. The exception under the Individuals with Disabilities Education Improvement Act is that public schools 'must make physical education available to children and youth with disabilities unless the school does not offer it to students without disabilities in the same grades' (U.S. Government Accountability Office, 2010, p. 8). Adapted physical education specialists and physical education generalists are among those who work with individuals with special needs in schools.

In 1973, leaders from Canada and Belgium more broadly conceptualised the scope of adapted physical education to adapted physical activity and founded the International Federation of Adapted Physical Activity (IFAPA, 2009) in Quebec, Canada.

IFAPA is an international cross-disciplinary professional organisation of individuals, institutions, and agencies supporting, promoting, and disseminating knowledge and information about adapted physical activity, disability sport, and all aspects of sport, movement, and exercise science for the benefit of persons who require adaptations to enable their participation (IFAPA n.d.).

According to the By-laws of the IFAPA

Adapted physical activity is a cross-disciplinary body of knowledge directed towards the identification and solution of individual differences in physical activity. It is a service-delivery profession and academic field of study that supports an attitude of acceptance of individual differences, advocates access to active lifestyles and sport, and promotes innovation and cooperative service delivery programs and empowerment systems. Adapted physical activity includes, but is not limited to, physical education, sport, recreation, dance and creative arts, nutrition, medicine, and rehabilitation (IFAPA n.d.).

IFAPA's former presidents Hutzler and Sherrill (2007) explained that in some countries adapted physical activity is not the preferred verbiage, instead such terms as sports for the disabled, sport therapy, and psychomotor therapy are similar in meaning. Hutzler and Sherrill (2007) called for more communication and collaboration internationally across these areas in research and information sharing. Scholarly journals are an important medium for communication, research collaboration, and information sharing. In 1984, founded by Geoffrey D. Broadhead, the Adapted Physical Activity Quarterly (APAQ) was first published. APAQ is now considered the primary international academic journal that focuses specifically on adapted physical activity research and is considered a main source of published research in the field (Haegele, Lee, & Porretta, 2015). It is the official publication of IFAPA and is published by Human Kinetics.

Qualitative Research in Adapted Physical Activity

In examining the efficacy of adapted physical activity, particularly for school-aged children, much of what is involved is the question of impact. While other research methodologies specifically treat with cause and effect, qualitative research offers the field an approach which is descriptive and examines the processes involved (Odom et al., 2005). Brantlinger, Jimenez, Klingner, Pugach, and Richardson (2005) in highlighting the value of qualitative studies to special education defined qualitative research as 'a systematic approach to understanding qualities, or the essential nature, of a phenomenon within a particular context' (p. 195).

Qualitative research, with no disciplinary allegiance, has made valuable contributions to adapted physical activity and is believed to have been introduced to the field in Maureen Connolly's 1994 article in APAQ 'Practicum Experiences and Journal Writing in Adapted Physical Education: Implications for Teacher Education' (Zitomer & Goodwin, 2014). As in Connolly (1994), qualitative research seeks to understand 'insiders' experiences' (p. 307), and in an interactive field such as adapted physical activity, understanding that knowledge is co-constructed, with facilitators and participants both worthy of having their contributions acknowledged and worthy of study is to be valued. As opposed to quantitative research, qualitative research differs in the following ways: '(1) the distinction between explanation and understanding as the purpose of inquiry; (2) the distinction between a personal and impersonal role for the researcher; and (3) a distinction between knowledge discovered and knowledge constructed' (Stake, 1995, p. 37).

Qualitative Research Methodologies and Quality Indicators

In 2014, Zitomer and Goodwin reviewed and synthesised criteria for evaluating the quality of qualitative research, particularly in adapted physical activity as well as identified strategies towards their achievement. In their words, Zitomer and Goodwin (2014) sought to articulate 'a flexible and parsimonious framework that may facilitate researchers, readers, and reviewers of qualitative inquiry to constructively evaluate research quality' (p. 193). They identified six criteria that may be applicable to evaluating the quality of qualitative research conducted in adapted physical activity. The six criteria are: (a) reflexivity, (b) credibility, (c) resonance, (d) ethics, (e) contribution, and (f) coherence.

Table 2.1 presents the six criteria and common terms that coincide with these criteria based on Zitomer and Goodwin's review of published qualitative studies. Further, the quality criteria and accompanying strategies for qualitative research are presented in Table 2.2. Noteworthy, the editorial board of the APAQ recommended that

TABLE 2.1

Quality Criteria and Coinciding Terms from Published Qualitative Studies

Reflexivity	Credibility	Resonance	Ethics	Contribution	Coherence
Audibility	Adequacy	Aesthetic Aesthetic merit	Caring	Actualisation	Achieve purpose
Balance	Authenticity	A story that moves	Dialogic	Advocacy	Adequacy
Criticality	Commitment	Clarity	Engagement	Community	Clarity
Engagement	Concreteness	Craftsmanship	Empathetic	Construction of further Questions	Coherence
Explicitness	Contextual sensitivity	Creativity	Empowered	Contribution:	Congruence
Honesty	Credibility	Divergent Reactions	Ethical Self-Consciousness	Heuristic, Methodological, Practical, Theoretical	Delimitation
Impact	Critical interpretation	Fittingness	Ethics: Procedural	Impact	Integration
Openness	Data sufficiency	Formulation	Ethics: Situational	Importance	Internal consistency
Positionality	Dependability	Generalisation	Ethics: Relational	Originality	Interpretation
Positioning	Explication	Naturalistic	Ethics: Exiting	Outcome	Meaningful coherence
Process	Express a reality	Presentation	Reciprocity	Persuasive	Transparency
Researcher Presuppositions	Plausibility	Relevance	Sacredness	Rational	Understandability
Self/Social Critique	Reliability	Resonates	Sensitivity	Relevance	
Sincerity	Trustworthiness	Responsiveness		Scope and Purpose	
Subjectivity	Validity	Social Context		Social Validity	
Transparency	Verification	Transferability		Substantive Contribution	
Vulnerability	Verisimilitude	Typicality		Usefulness	
	Voice	Vividness		Value	
		Writing		Worth/Worthy Topic	

Source: Zitomer, M.R., and Goodwin, D., *Adapt. Phys. Activ. Q.*, 31, 193–218, 2014.

TABLE 2.2

Quality Criteria and Accompanying Strategies for Qualitative Research

Reflexivity	Credibility	Resonance	Ethics	Contribution	Coherence
Articulate theoretical position	Abundant detail	Aesthetic	Collaboration	Future research suggested	Appropriate research aims
Audit trail	Adequate data	Attention to context	Confidentiality	Implications for practice	Coherence across aim, purpose, question, sampling method, and data collection
Bracketing	Analysis described	Evocative	Data safeguarded	Influences multiple audiences	
Disclose researcher bias	Code checking	Presentation	Ethics approval	Moves reader to action	Methodological congruence
Reflexivity	Complex narratives	Sample situated	Informed consent	New methodological approach	
Self-reflective journaling	External audits	Thick description	Legend of cautions	Question and interpretation grounded in current research	
	Grounded in examples		Multivocality		
Transparency	Member checks		Participant welfare		
	Negative cases		Promises to participants kept	Theory applied in new context	
	Peer debriefing		Reflexivity		
	Prolonged engagement		Researcher and participant hierarchy challenged		
	Reciprocity				
	Sampling				
	Triangulation				

Source: Zitomer, M.R., and Goodwin, D., *Adapt. Phys. Activ. Q.*, 31, 193–218, 2014.

APAQ contributing authors should consider these criteria in their qualitative research. Specifically, a new set of instructions to APAQ's contributing authors includes the criteria that Zitomer and Goodwin (2014) articulated along with brief explanations (Table 2.3). Further, APAQ's editorial board explains,

TABLE 2.3

APAQ Recommendations for Authors of Qualitative Research

Quality Indicator	Considerations
Reflexivity is the means by which researcher background and theoretical assumptions impacting study process and findings becomes apparent. The extent to which reflexivity would be evident in qualitative papers depends on the paradigmatic approach with which you align.	• Identify your background as a researcher/practitioner in the field. • Identify your personal bias that may impact the research process and findings and how it was addressed (distancing one-self or incorporate it into your study).
Credibility encompasses the extent to which findings represent experiences shared by participants or observed by researcher.	• Clearly identify the strategies you used throughout your data collection process in order to demonstrate the credibility of your work. • Explain how your chosen strategies align with your paradigmatic perspective.
Resonance is the impact a study has on readers and its ability to meaningfully reverberate with them. Depending on the paradigmatic approach with which you align, resonance can be achieved by the adjacent considerations.	• **Writing style**. Is the writing aesthetic and evocative in a way that can make readers feel like they are present in the context with the researcher? • **Transferability**. Are context and findings described in depth allowing readers to consider other situations to which they may be relevant?
Contribution addresses ways in which research contributes to deeper understanding, clarifying confusion, extending knowledge, and generating insights.	• Do the introduction and review of literature clearly demonstrate the need for the study? • How do the study findings contribute to professional practice in the field? • How do the study findings contribute to enhancing theoretical knowledge and thought in the field? • How do study findings enhance other research findings in the field? • Is future research suggested based on the study findings?
Ethics addresses the importance of carrying out research in a respectful, humane, honest, and empathic way. Ethical considerations are imperative in all stages of a research process, but may differ in their relevance and interpretation based on the paradigmatic approach.	• Was ethical approval obtained from a university ethics review board or other form of ethics review board? • What was the nature of the relationship between researcher and participants during the research process? • How did your relationship with participants impact your findings? • What procedures did you follow for leaving the field and sharing your findings?
Coherence. A coherent study follows a consistent, clear, and concise epistemological perspective from its introduction through to its conclusions.	• Is there a clear line of thought from the introduction throughout to the conclusions? • Do your methods align with your methodology and stated paradigmatic approach? • Do the strategies you chose align with your stated research purpose? • Did your study achieve its stated purpose?

It is important to note that not all the above mentioned six criteria would necessarily be equally important or evident in all qualitative studies. Therefore, we recommend the following:

- Be aware of and indicate the paradigm under which you are working.
- Indicate the criteria of importance to your work based on your paradigmatic perspective and criteria that can be broken without impacting the quality of your work.
- Demonstrate evidence that your criteria of importance were achieved.
- Demonstrate evidence that your chosen criteria and strategies are consistent with the overall intent and value of your study. Moreover, APAQ's guidelines for judging studies in conducting literature reviews asks several questions for contributing authors' consideration (APAQ, 2015).
- How did you assess methodological quality?
- Did you use guidelines or a rubric for systemic review?
- Did you have quality summary scores to distinguish between high- and low-quality studies?
- Did you exclude studies of low methodological quality?

Zitomer and Goodwin's suggestions for qualitative studies are quite useful for those conducting literature reviews, examining the extant literature in preparing theses and dissertations, as well as useful for both emerging and advanced scholars conducting adapted physical activity research. In addition to those articulated by Zitomer and Goodwin, researchers should consider such quality indicators as those articulated by Brantlinger et al. (2005) for example, which are relevant to common data collection and analysis methods in qualitative studies (Table 2.4).

TABLE 2.4

Quality Indicators for Qualitative Research

Interview Studies (or Interview Components of Comprehensive Studies)

- Appropriate participants are selected (purposefully identified, effectively recruited, adequate number, representative of population of interest).
- Interview questions are reasonable (clearly worded, not leading, appropriate, and sufficient for exploring domains of interest).
- Adequate mechanisms are used to record and transcribe interviews.
- Participants are represented sensitively and fairly in the report.
- Sound measures are used to ensure confidentiality.

Observation Studied (or Observation Components of Comprehensive Studies)

- Appropriate setting(s) and/or people are selected for observation.
- Sufficient time is spent in the field (number and duration of observations, study time span).
- Researcher fits into the site (accepted, respected, unobtrusive).
- Research has minimal impact on setting (except for action research, which is purposely designed to have an impact).
- Field notes systematically collected (videotaped, audiotaped, written during or soon after observations).
- Sound measures are used to ensure confidentiality of participants and settings.

Document Analysis

- Meaningful documents (texts, artefacts, objects, pictures) are found and their relevance is established.
- Documents are obtained and stored in a careful manner.
- Documents are sufficiently described and cited.
- Sound measures are used to ensure confidentiality of private documents.

(Continued)

TABLE 2.4 (*Continued*)

Quality Indicators for Qualitative Research

Data Analysis

- Results are sorted and coded in a systematic and meaningful way.
- Sufficient rationale is provided for what was (or was not) included in the report.
- Documentation of methods used to establish trustworthiness and credibility are clear.
- Reflection about researchers' personal position/perspectives are provided.
- Conclusions are substantiated by sufficient quotations from participants, field notes of observations, and evidence of documentation inspection.
- Connections are made with related research.

Source: Brantlinger, E. et al., *Exceptional Children*, 71, 202, 2005.

TABLE 2.5

Comparison of Criteria for Judging Quality in Quantitative and Qualitative Research

Quantitative	Qualitative	Description	Strategies
Objectivity or neutrality	Confirmability	The extent to which the findings are the product of the inquiry and not the bias of the researcher	Audit trail of the process of data analysis
			Triangulation
			Member checking
			Reflexive research journal
Reliability	Dependability (consistency, auditability)	The extent to which the study could be repeated and variations understood	Audit trail of procedures and processes
			Triangulation
			Reflexive research journal
Internal validity	Credibility (truth value)	The degree to which the findings can be trusted or believed by the participants of the study	Prolonged engagement Persistent observation
			Referential adequacy materials
			Peer debriefing
			Member checking
			Triangulation
			Negative case analysis
			Reflexive research journal
External validity	Transferability (applicability, fittingness)	The extent to which the findings can be applied in other contexts or with other participants	Thick description Purposive sampling
			Reflexive research journal

Source: Petty, N.J. et al., *Man. Ther.*, 17, 382, 2012.

Petty, Thomson, and Stew (2012) compared criteria for judging quality (or rigor) in quantitative research and qualitative research with accompanying strategies (Table 2.5). In general, quantitative researchers rely on research questions and hypothesis testing, design controls, and statistical manipulation and interpretation (i.e., deductive reasoning and reductionistic logic) using carefully selected research designs in making sample to population generalisations. In contrast, qualitative methodologies have relied on the conception that meaning-making endeavours constitute forms of realities as meaningful, or more meaningful, to study than physical realities when dealing with phenomena associated with the human experience. Qualitative studies are situated by inductive reasoning strategies used to explore, describe, understand, explain, change, or evaluate phenomena with no effort to control variables.

Relevant to this issue, Carano (2014) developed taxonomies useful in evaluating the strength of quality of research in adapted physical activity from strong to weak. In other words, she developed matrixes which present a set of quality indicators (criteria) for judging the rigor of experimental (true and quasi), correlational, single-subject, and qualitative research designs, respectively (Carano, 2014). Each matrix presents three levels of strength of quality: level 1 represents strong evidence of rigor (quality), level 2 represents moderate evidence of quality, and level 3 indicates weak evidence of rigor (Carano, 2014; Carano, Silliman-French, French, Nichols, & Rose 2015). In using the taxonomies, the user first selects the taxonomy that matches the research design (e.g., single-subject design) and then completes the review. Next, the user determines the level of recommendation (Sharon L. Carano, personal communication, 28 July 2015). Established scholars as well as emerging professionals such as early career faculty and graduate students interested in research pertaining to physical education for individuals with disabilities should use quality indicators such as those appearing in these matrixes in planning, conducting, and analysing research within the quantitative and qualitative paradigms. The reader is encouraged to consult Carano's (2014) work to learn more about this comprehensive process.

Learning about and Individuals with Disabilities through Qualitative Research

In recent years, Columna and his research teams have led an emergent line of research involving parents and their children with visual impairments (Columna, Lepore-Stevens, & Work, 2017; Columna, Rocco-Dillon, Norris, Dolphin, & McCabe, 2017; Columna et al., in press, a, b). Columna and colleagues' scholarly work is positioned in both quantitative (e.g., survey method) and qualitative (descriptive-qualitative using an interview approach) research paradigms. Whereas the research teams used quantitative methods to examine the efficacy of training interventions on treatment groups, they used qualitative methods to glean valuable understandings of the impact of such interventions from a more in depth analysis of participants lived experiences and beliefs. The inclusion of observation reports and extended interviews of the parents involved allowed for the researchers to explore the lived experiences of the participants and through analysis facilitated a thorough understanding of the impact of adapted physical activity on research participants and their families.

Disability research has been largely dominated by the medical model of disability, focusing on disability as internal to the person and a trait to be fixed, cured, or rehabilitated (Haegele & Hodge, 2016). Traditionally, research in this domain has been largely quantitative in methodology (Allender, Cowburn, & Foster, 2006). Large-scale quantitative studies can capture data trends, but are often unable to reflect issues that underlie the data such as participant motivation or contextual factors. Methodological positivism, a core tenant of quantitative research, strives for 'value-free' (Neuman, 2011) knowledge creation. Disability studies scholars, on the other hand, argue that neutral knowledge about disability cannot exist in an ableist world. A positivist approach misses the underlying social influences that create and maintain disability.

Qualitative methods, however, can provide that deeper look that research sometimes needs. In adapted physical activity research, instead of solely informing where or when physical activity increases, qualitative research allows us to more deeply examine the why or how. In situating research in the qualitative research paradigm, adapted physical activity scholars, for example, can explore, explain, and interpret barriers to physical activity and motives for change. In addition, qualitative researchers can delve into the individual stories that make up the larger data sets. As Creswell (2013) explains, the use of a 'disability interpretive lens' views the research in the context of disability as human variation. This philosophical framework can influence all aspects of the study. Therefore, qualitative research is often a recursive process, leading to unanticipated mid-study changes that bring a more complete understanding of the issues studied (Creswell, 2016; Leiter, 2015).

When disability policy and practice are informed almost entirely by quantitative research, the individual and their experience becomes diminished. In an area so critically important as public health and so determined by motivational factors, qualitative research becomes essential (Allender et al., 2006). Another advantage of qualitative inquiry is the focus on inductive, rather than deductive, logic, beginning with observations instead of hypotheses (Leiter, 2015). This allows for revelations that might not have been anticipated rather than confirming or failing to confirm a sub-theory (i.e., hypothesis). Qualitative inquiry also works in contrast to quantitative research's focus on statistical techniques, which reduces participants to quantifiable data, whereas, qualitative inquiry embraces each participant's role and reality in the research endeavour. For example, in the United States, the Fit Families Program (Columna, 2017) have been a fruitful site for both quantitative and qualitative research (to be described in a later section) and on the qualitative side focuses on empowering research participants to create change. The relationship between researchers and participants is critical to the success of the project, rather than striving for some neutral positivism. This work is enhanced by the qualitative lens. Participants not only have voice in this research, but are enfranchised as co-collaborators or research informants (Allender et al., 2006; Berger & Lorenz, 2015; Creswell, 2013; Leiter, 2015).

As the implications of studies in adapted physical activity are relevant to public health, this body of research is critical to healthcare professionals, parents, teachers, policymakers, and many other constituent groups. Policy documents, in particular, tend to focus on quantitative studies despite the need to look at underpinning motivational factors. Ongoing research in adapted physical activity must prioritise the identification of motivation and barriers to inform the promotion of health and physical activity for individuals with disabilities. Additionally, it is essential that this research, as it affects individuals with disability, their families, and their teachers, be accessible to these constituents. Qualitative methods, as Agger (1991) explains, help to democratise science, providing analysis that is more easily understood outside of academia.

Exemplars of Scholarly Rigor in Qualitative Research

In qualitative research, the 'process of data collection involves a dynamic interaction between the researcher and the participants and context under investigation' (Gerdes & Conn, 2001, p. 186). Common data collection strategies used in qualitative work include: interviewing, observing, documenting (artefacts), and researcher immersion (Patton, 2002; Petty, Thomson, & Stew, 2012). Through the data collection process, the researcher seeks 'to develop a "thick" description of the context, the participants, and the dynamic processes that occur between and among them' (Gerdes & Conn, 2001, p. 186). Most often researchers in adapted physical activity use interviewing as the primary or only data source in their qualitative studies. In those studies, however, multiple sources of data are used in order to establish trustworthiness. Trustworthiness is one of various criteria used for judging the rigor, credibility, and quality of qualitative inquiry (Gerdes & Conn, 2001; Zitomer & Goodwin, 2014). Establishing trustworthiness refers to the techniques used to confirm the credibility of the research and maintain academic and scholarly rigor (Gerdes & Conn, 2001). There are numerous techniques used in establishing a study's trustworthiness such as audit trails, prolonged engagement, persistent observation, triangulation, referential adequacy, member checking, and peer debriefing (Gerdes & Conn, 2001).

Over the years, scholars of adapted physical activity research have used multiple data sources (e.g., artefacts, photographs, and documents; researcher's observations and field notes; individual and focus group interviews; reflective journaling) to ensure trustworthiness in their studies using multiple techniques as indicators of scholarly rigor (An & Goodwin, 2007; An & Hodge, 2013; Grenier, 2011; Grenier, Collins, Wright & Kearns, 2014; Leo & Goodwin, 2014, 2016; Wynnyk & Spencer-Cavaliere, 2013). Exemplars of techniques used to ensure scholarly rigor in adapted physical activity research situated in the qualitative paradigm include multiple data sources and data saturation (An & Goodwin, 2007; An & Hodge, 2013; Grenier, 2011; Grenier et al., 2014; Wynnyk & Spencer-Cavaliere, 2013); audit trails (An & Hodge, 2013; Wynnyk & Spencer-Cavaliere, 2013); field notes (Grenier, 2011; Leo & Goodwin, 2014, 2016; Wynnyk & Spencer-Cavaliere, 2013); data triangulation (An & Goodwin, 2007; An & Hodge, 2013; Grenier, 2011; Grenier et al., 2014; Wynnyk & Spencer-Cavaliere, 2013); investigator triangulation (An & Goodwin, 2007; An & Hodge, 2013); method triangulation (An & Goodwin, 2007; An & Hodge, 2013); member checks (An & Goodwin, 2007; An & Hodge, 2013; Grenier, 2011; Leo & Goodwin, 2014, 2016; Wynnyk & Spencer-Cavaliere, 2013); participant or non-participant observations (Grenier, 2011; Grenier et al., 2014; Leo & Goodwin, 2014, 2016; Wynnyk & Spencer-Cavaliere, 2013); peer debriefs (An & Goodwin, 2007; An & Hodge, 2013; Grenier, 2011); and reflective researcher's and/or participants' journals (An & Hodge, 2013; Leo & Goodwin, 2014, 2016). In their study, as a noteworthy example, Leo and Goodwin (2016) explored the meaning three men and four women who experience disability ascribed to disability simulations as a pedagogical strategy. In the extensive quote below, Leo and Goodwin explained the criteria they used for judging the quality of their work.

> Criteria for judging the quality of IPA [interpretative phenomenological analysis] research include sensitivity to context, commitment and rigor, transparency and coherence, and impact and importance *perspective on disability simulations.* (p. 164)

These criteria are also known as reflexivity, credibility, coherence, and contribution, respectively (Zitomer & Goodwin, 2014). Sensitivity to context was addressed by awareness of researcher positionality and biases. The researchers possess backgrounds in adapted physical activity as well as expertise in qualitative inquiry and disability simulation use. They acknowledge that they do not have impairments, are financially independent, and are white.

Commitment requires attentiveness to the participants and care in the analysis of each case. The themes and a descriptive summary were shared with the participants by e-mail, all of whom responded that their thoughts were reflected. The first author established initial rapport with the participants through e-mail correspondence before the interviews. Participants' questions were answered in advance of the interviews. Rigor was established by piloting the interview guide and completing a thorough ideographic analysis of the data.

Coherence, or adherence to the underlying principles of IPA, was achieved through transparent accounting of researcher position and bias and the methods used throughout the research process (e.g., description of the participants, data collection, phases used in the analysis). Impact and importance are satisfied if the reader is left with a new perspective, one that is interesting, useful, or important. The impact and importance of our work lies in the effort to bring seldom-heard disability voices to the debate of simulation use and provide the reader with a new perspective on disability simulations (p. 164).

Clearly there are many techniques used and an increasing number of scholars using multiple strategies in their work, which are essential to scholarly rigor in adapted physical activity research.

Computer Aided Qualitative Data Analysis Software

The reliability and objectivity of quantitative research are often heralded in their promotion. To address these concerns in the subjective environment of qualitative research, trustworthiness is of primary concern (Marshall & Rossman, 2017). The use of computer software, particularly in the analysis of interview data and other artefacts, has revolutionised the trustworthiness of qualitative data – especially when analysis of said data is being made sense of by a group of researchers. Computer Aided Qualitative Data Analysis Software (CAQDAS) has assisted in not only data management of the voluminous data collected as part of the process, but also brings rigor to the analysis of the data (Wickham & Woods, 2005). In recent qualitative studies, NVivo has been used to organise, code, and analyse qualitative data with particular usefulness by teams of researchers (Columna et al., 2018, 2019). Wickham and Woods (2005) further argued that 'much of the criticism directed at qualitative research stems from a perception that the process is not always demonstrated to be transparent or rigorous in the same ways that quantitative research can be' (p. 699), and that the use of CAQDAS provides for transparency and significantly improves the quality of the qualitative research.

In fact, the rigor espoused by qualitative research is made transparent by the processes involved in using CAQDAS for analysis in adapted physical activity. In research conducted by the researchers (see studies by Columna et al., 2018, 2019), the process using CAQDAS has insured that the findings of the analysis have produced findings that consolidate the lived experiences of adapted physical activity participants. More important, the use of CAQDAS facilitated an expansive view of the data since the codes developed in NVivo were linked directly to the corresponding transcript passages, allowing for the easy retrieval of relevant quotes. Additionally, working as a collaborative research team provided its own organisational challenges. NVivo facilitated the proper organisation of the data, provided a tool to verify intercoder reliability using Cohen's kappa coefficient. Researchers were also able to develop descriptions for each code and write linked memos and notes to interview transcripts – allowing for the simpler identification of themes and production of the final manuscript. Moreover, the use of computer software has enhanced the data analysis process in qualitative studies.

Transforming Qualitative Research into Practice

Scholars in adapted physical activity are calling for the utilisation of evidence-base practice when developing interventions for underserved populations, such as individuals with disabilities. Quantitative methodologies have demonstrated that individuals with disabilities faced multiple barriers to participate and have limited access to physical activity settings (Columna, Fernandez-Vivo, Lieberman, & Arndt, 2015). This lack of access and participation contributes to individuals adopting sedentary lifestyles (Pan, Frey, Bar-Or, & Longmuir, 2005). Consequently, due to inactivity, individuals with disabilities are prone to secondary conditions such as obesity and other health related issues (Augestad & Jiang, 2015). Quantitative research has a significant role in the field of adapted physical activity. One such role is the identification of areas of need or concern. Through quantitative studies, we know that there is a need for physical activity interventions that address the barriers for individuals with disabilities and their families. We believe that qualitative research can support the evidence gained from quantitative research and vice versa. As such, we advocate for the utilisation of mixed-methods designs when designing and implementing interventions for individuals with disabilities. Through the utilisation of both approaches, professionals may have the tools to transform research into practice. Similarly, practice or interventions can help shape research. One such example is the Fit Families Program (Columna, 2017).

The Fit Families Program (FFP) is a physical activity program designed to maximise physical activity opportunities for children with visual impairments (Columna, 2017) and for children with autism and their families (Davis et al., 2017). Prior to the delivery of the first FFP program, our research team conducted a series of semi-structured interviews to: (a) understand parents' perceptions regarding physical activity (PA) experiences for their family and children with visual impairments (VI) (Columna, Rocco-Dillon, et al., 2017), (b) explore why families with children with VI seek out and participate in PA, and (c) describe the strategies and supports (Columna et al., in press, a, b). The findings of these research studies provided us with an opportunity to identify what areas we needed to focus our intervention on and provided us an opportunity in regard to what type of information we needed to share with the families. In essence, prior to their participation in the FFP, parents identified multiple barriers they faced when trying to engage in physical activity and voiced the need for a PA program that meets their needs and the needs of their children.

Based on the parental feedback, Columna and his colleagues and graduate students have designed the structure of the program with the ultimate aim of maximising the physical activity opportunities of the participants. This initial program consisted of four one-day workshops focusing on the areas of: (1) orientation and mobility, (2) physical activity and motor development, (3) aquatics, and (4) sports. Each workshop had three main components: (1) individual workshop for parents, (2) separated physical activities and games for the children, and (3) joined interaction between parents and their children. This interaction provided parents an opportunity for them to practice the skills learned with their children. This also provided an opportunity for the children to display to their parents the skills they acquired during the different activities.

After the first year of the program was concluded, the researchers conducted a series of post program interviews to explore the impact of the program on the intentions to participate in physical activity among the participants. The results of these studies are published elsewhere (Columna et al. in press, a, b). In short, the findings of these studies highlighted multiple benefits that accrued from the families' participation in the physical activity program. For several of the participating parents, being able to take part in FFP was an 'eye-opening' experience. This program allows parents to gain a deeper understanding of their children's ability level and allow them to learn more about a variety of physical activities they can perform as a family. Furthermore, the interventions provided their children with opportunities to socialise with other children with visual impairments.

Using Qualitative Methodologies to Inform Future Program Directions

Qualitative research has been the foundation of FFP-based research. Whilst the research teams highly value the contributions of quantitative methodologies, it is through qualitative methodologies that they have been able to identify what areas are in need of improvement in order to develop programs that meet the physical activity needs of the participants. As such, and motivated to explore the impact of the FFP on other populations, Columna and colleagues designed an intervention for children with autism spectrum disorders (ASD) and their families. Similar to the previous version of the FFP for children with visual impairments and their parents, we conducted a series of interviews to explore parents' perceptions to physical activity, barriers, and facilitators. Preliminary findings indicated that these families had difficulty motivating their children to take part in PA. In addition, parents indicated that they lacked the teaching skills to teach and promote PA for their children (Columna et al., in press, a, b).

As a result of the pre-program interviews, the FFP team designed five workshops: (1) sensory motor activities, (2) communication, (3) physical activity, (4) aquatic, and (5) sports. Each of these workshops was carefully designed to address the needs of the children and their parents (Columna, 2017; Columna, Lepore-Stevens, et al., 2018; Norris et al., 2018). According to the Diagnostic and Statistical Manual of Mental Disorders-5, hallmarks of the ASD are sensory processing and communication disorders (American Psychiatric Association, 2013), thus, the team focused on these issues for the first two workshops. The present literature related to physical activity among children with ASD indicate that these children are not meeting national guidelines related to physical activity (Lee & Hodge, 2017). Therefore, the intent of the third workshop was to address this issue. Further, drowning is the number one cause of death among children with ASD, leading us to the inclusion of an aquatic program. Lastly, children with ASD tend to participate in solitary activities. The team intended to address this through the final workshop focused on sports.

At the culmination of the program, the families are to be interviewed to explore the impact of the program on their intentions to engage in physical activity with their children with ASD and their entire family.

Qualitative Research and Its Role in the Future of Adapted Physical Activity

Qualitative research in adapted physical activity can make academic work more accessible to relevant practitioners, parents, and other stakeholders. As professionals seek to find utility in practical terms for their work, including practitioners, parents, and other stakeholders in the research endeavour is essential. The purpose of research should not be limited to generating new knowledge or confirming existing knowledge or even answering isolated questions with little or no practical use, but instead effecting change. Qualitative research in adapted physical activity can inform policy in crucial and practical ways.

Qualitative research provides a lens on data outside of a positivist model, a critical stance when considering the centuries of marginalisation of individuals with disabilities. This kind of research can honour the experiences of individuals, their families, and communities. By gaining an understanding of their life experiences, the needs, wants, and expectations of these groups can be met. Furthermore, qualitative research is essential to the empowerment of research participants, including individuals, families, educators, and professionals, to create change (Patton, 2002). They become enfranchised in the work. The researcher, too, takes on a critical role in the intervention with an emphasis on built relationships (Creswell, 2016). In the adapted physical activity field, this means listening to and interacting with the population of interest. It is well known that individuals with disabilities are constantly facing barriers that negatively affect their participation in physical activity. By listening to their experiences, some of these barriers can be diminished.

Similarly, research has shown that practitioners often lack the skills to effectively include individuals with disabilities and their families into physical activity programs. As such, through qualitative research, their attitudes, expectations, and level of comfort in working and interacting with individuals with disabilities can be identified.

Qualitative research can help us examine complex and nuanced phenomena such as the motivation of parents of children with disabilities or complex social issues. Adapted physical activity researchers are engaging qualitative research endeavours to shed light on the ways in which phenomena occur, exposing participants' realities, and effecting in change.

Summary and Conclusions

Over the years, various educational scholars as well as organisations (e.g., National Research Council) have asserted that the enterprise of research is shaped by different types of questions and that different methodologies are needed to address these questions (Haegele & Hodge, 2015a, 2015b; Haegele & Sutherland, 2015; O'Sullivan, 2007;

Shavelson & Towne, 2002). On the other hand, other entities (e.g., Coalition for Evidence-Based Policy, 2003) and 'research clearinghouses' (e.g., the What Works Clearinghouse) have focused mostly on the question of "whether a practice is effective and proposed that the 'gold standard' for addressing this question is a single type of research methodology – randomised experimental group designs (also called randomised clinical trials; What Works Clearinghouse, 2003)" (Odom et al., 2005, p. 138). Our view is broad, in that, we also believe the enterprise of research is shaped by different types of questions and that different methodologies are needed to address these questions. In this chapter, however, we identified and discussed quality indicators specific to qualitative research that represent rigorous application of methodology to questions of interest in adapted physical activity research. Established scholars and emerging professionals interested in research pertaining to physical education for individuals with disabilities should use quality indicators such as those appearing in this chapter in evaluating theirs and others' research.

References

Adapted Physical Activity Quarterly. (2015). Guidelines for a review paper for APAQ. Retrieved from http://journals.humankinetics.com/guidelines-for-a-review-paper-for-apaq.

Agger, B. (1991). Critical theory, poststructuralism, postmodernism: Their sociological relevance. *Annual Review of Sociology, 17*, 105–131.

Allender, S., Cowburn, G., & Foster, C. (2006). Understanding participation in sport and physical activity among children and adults: A review of qualitative studies. *Health Education Research, 21*, 826–835.

American Psychiatric Association. (2013). *Diagnostic and statistical manual of mental disorders* (5th ed.). Washington, DC: Author.

An, J., & Goodwin, D. L. (2007). Physical education for students with spina bifida: Mother's perspectives. *Adapted Physical Activity Quarterly, 24*, 38–58.

An, J., & Hodge, S. R. (2013). Exploring the meaning of parental involvement in physical education for students with developmental disabilities. *Adapted Physical Activity Quarterly, 29*, 147–163.

Augestad, L. B., & Jiang, L. (2015). Physical activity, physical fitness, and body composition among children and young adults with visual impairments: A systematic review. *British Journal of Visual Impairments, 33*(3), 167–182. doi:10.1177/0264619615599813.

Berger, R. J., & Lorenz, L. S. (2015). *Disability and qualitative inquiry: Methods for rethinking an ableist world*. New York: Routledge.

Brantlinger, E., Jimenez, R., Klingner, J., Pugach, M., & Richardson, V. (2005). Qualitative studies in special education. *Exceptional Children, 71*(2), 195–207.

Broadhead, G. D. (1984). Birth of a journal. *Adapted Physical Activity Quarterly, 1*, 1–2.

Carano, S. L. (2014). Development of a research taxonomy for adapted physical activity (Order No. 3672826). Available from ProQuest Dissertations & Theses A&I.

Carano, S. L., Silliman-French, L., French, R., Nichols, D., & Rose, K. (2015). *Development of a research taxonomy for adapted physical activity*. Paper presented at the annual meeting of the National Consortium for Physical Education for Individuals with Disabilities, McLean, VA.

Coalition for Evidence-Based Policy. (2003). *Identifying and implementing educational practices supported by rigorous evidence: A user friendly guide*. Washington, DC: U.S. Department of Education Institute of Education Sciences, National Center for Education Evaluation and Regional Assistance. Retrieved from http://coalition4evidence.org/468-2/publications/.

Columna, L. (2017). Syracuse University's Fit Families Program: Physical activity program for families of children with visual impairments. *Palaestra, 31*(1), 32–39.

Columna, L., Fernandez-Vivo, M., Lieberman, L., & Arndt, K. (2015). Recreational physical activity experiences among Guatemalan families with children with visual impairments. *Journal of Physical Activity and Health, 12*(8), 1119–1127.

Columna, L., Lepore-Stevens, M., & Work, E. (2017) Orientation and mobility skills for families of children with visual impairments and blindness in physical activity environments. *British Journal of Visual Impairments, 35*(2), 165–177.

Columna, L., Rocco-Dillon, S., Norris, M. L., Dolphin, M., & McCabe, L. (2017). Parents' perceptions of physical activity experiences for their families and children with visual impairments. *British Journal of Visual Impairments, 35*(2), 88–102. doi:10.1177/0264619617691081.

Columna, L., Streete, D. A., Dillon, S., Hodge, S. R., Prieto, L., Myers, B. A., Barreira, T., & Heffernan, K. (2019). Parents' intentions toward including their children with visual impairments in physical activities. *Disability and Rehabilitation*. doi:10.1080/09638288.2018.1505969.

Columna, L., Streete, D. A., Hodge, S. R., Dillon, S. R., Myers, B., Norris, M. L., Barreira, T., & Heffernan, K. S. (2018). Parents' beliefs about physical activity for their children with visual impairments. *Adapted Physical Activity Quarterly*. https://doi.org/10.1123/apaq.2017-0084.

Connolly, M. (1994). Practicum experiences and journal writing in adapted physical education: Implications for teacher education. *Adapted Physical Activity Quarterly, 11*(3), 306–328.

Creswell, J. W. (2013). *Qualitative inquiry & research design: Choosing among five approaches* (3rd ed.). Thousand Oaks, CA: Sage.

Creswell, J. W. (2016). *30 essential skills for the qualitative researcher*. Thousand Oaks, CA: Sage Publications.

Davis, T., Columna, L., Abdo, A., Russo, N., Toole, K., & Norris, M. (2017). Sensory motor activities training for families of children with autism spectrum disorders. *PALAESTRA, 31*(3), 35–40.

Gerdes, D. A., & Conn, J. H. (2001, Early Winter). A user-friendly look at qualitative research methods. *The Physical Educator*, 183–190.

Grenier, M. A. (2011). Coteaching in physical education: A strategy for inclusive practice. *Adapted Physical Activity Quarterly, 28*, 95–112.

Grenier, M., Collins, K., Wright, S., & Kearns, C. (2014). Perceptions of a disability sport unit in general physical education. *Adapted Physical Activity Quarterly, 31*, 49–66. doi:10.1123/apaq.2013-0006.

Haegele, J., & Hodge, S. R. (2015a). Applied behavior analysis research paradigm and single-subject designs in adapted physical activity research. *Adapted Physical Activity Quarterly, 32*, 285–301.

Haegele, J., & Hodge, S. R. (2015b). Quantitative methodology: A guide for emerging physical education and adapted physical education researchers. *The Physical Educator, 72*, 59–75.

Haegele, J., & Hodge, S. R. (2016). Disability discourse: Overview and critiques of the medical and social models. *Quest, 68*(2), 193–206. doi:10.1080/00336297.2016.1143849.

Haegele, J. A., Lee, J., & Porretta, D. L. (2015). Research trends in Adapted Physical Activity Quarterly from 2004 to 2013. *Adapted Physical Activity Quarterly, 32*(3), 187–205. doi:10.1123/APAQ.2014-0211.

Haegele, J. A., & Sutherland, S. (2015). Perspectives of students with disabilities toward physical education: A qualitative inquiry review. *Quest, 67*(3), 255–273.

Hutzler, Y., & Sherrill, C. (2007). Defining adapted physical activity: International perspectives. *Adapted Physical Activity Quarterly, 24*, 1–20.

Individuals with Disabilities Education Act of 2004, Pub. L. No. 108-446, Sec. 602, 118 Stat. 2657.

International Federation of Adapted Physical Activity. (n.d.). Retrieved from http://www.ifapa.biz/.

International Federation of Adapted Physical Activity. (2009). Countries. Retrieved from http://www.ifapa.biz/.

Lee, S. H., & Hodge, S. R. (2017). Children with autism spectrum disorder and physical activity: A review of literature. *Journal of Physical Education and Sport Management, 8*(1), 1–23.

Leiter, V. (2015). A bricolage of urban sidewalks: Observing locations of inequality. In R. J. Berger, & L. S. Lorenz (Eds.), *Disability and qualitative inquiry: Methods for rethinking an ableist world*. New York: Routledge.

Leo, J., & Goodwin, D. (2014). Negotiated meanings of disability simulations in an adapted physical activity course: Learning from student reflections. *Adapted Physical Activity Quarterly, 31*, 144–161. doi:10.1123/apaq.2013-0099.

Leo, J., & Goodwin, D. (2016). Simulating others' realities: Insiders reflect on disability simulations. *Adapted Physical Activity Quarterly, 33*, 156–175. doi:10.1123/APAQ.2015-0031.

Marshall, C., & Rossman, G. B. (2017). *Designing qualitative research*. Newbury Park, CA: Sage publications.

Neuman, W. L. (2011). *Social research methods: Qualitative and quantitative approaches*. New York: Pearson.

Norris, M., Toole, K. & Columna, L. (2018). Educating parents in aquatic activities for children with visual impairments. *British Journal of Visual Impairments, 36*(3), 262–273.

Odom, S. L., Brantlinger, E., Gersten, R., Horner, R. H., Thompson, B., & Harris, K. R. (2005). Research in special education: Scientific methods and evidence-based practices. *Exceptional Children, 71*(2), 137–148.

O'Sullivan, M. (2007). Research quality in physical education and sport pedagogy. *Sport, Education and Society, 12*(3), 245–260. doi:10.1080/13573320701463962.

Pan, C.-Y., Frey, G. C., Bar-Or, O., & Longmuir, P. (2005). Concordance of physical activity among parents and youth with physical disabilities. *Journal of Developmental and Physical Disabilities, 17*(4), 395–407. doi:10.1007/s10882-005-6622-7.

Patton, M. Q. (2002). *Qualitative research and evaluation methods* (3rd ed.). Thousand Oaks, CA: Sage.

Petty, N. J., Thomson, O. P., & Stew, G. (2012). Ready for a paradigm shift? Part 2: Introducing qualitative research methodologies and methods. *Manual Therapy, 17*, 378–384.

Shavelson, R. J., & Tbwne, L (Eds.). (2002). *Scientific research in education*. Washington. DC: National Academy Press.

Stake, R. (1995). *The art of case study research*. Thousand Oaks, CA: Sage.

U.S. Government Accountability Office, Report to Congressional Requesters. (2010, June). *Students with disabilities: More information and guidance could improve opportunities in physical education and athletics* (*GAO-10-519*). Washington, DC: USGAO.

What Works Clearinghouse. (2003). *Standards*. Washington, DC: Author. Retrieved from http://www.w-w-c.org/.

Wickham, M., & Woods, M. (2005). Reflecting on the strategic use of CAQDAS to manage and report on the qualitative research process. *The Qualitative Report, 10*(4), 687–702.

Wynnyk, K., & Spencer-Cavaliere, N. (2013). Children's social relationships and motivation in sledge hockey. *Adapted Physical Activity Quarterly, 30*, 299–316.

Zitomer, M. R., & Goodwin, D. (2014). Gauging the quality of qualitative research in adapted physical activity. *Adapted Physical Activity Quarterly, 31*, 193–218. doi:10.1123/apaq.2013-0084.

Section II

Enhancing Healthcare and Rehabilitation

Contemporary Applications of Qualitative Research

3

Exploring the Value of Qualitative Comparison Groups in Rehabilitation Research: Lessons from Youth with Disabilities Transitioning into Work

Sally Lindsay

CONTENTS

Introduction

The growing qualitative literature within rehabilitation is helping to inform evidence-based practice and clinical decision-making (Gibson & Martin 2002; Grypdonck 2018; O'Day & Killeen 2002; Vanderkaay et al. 2018). Qualitative research sheds light on the in-depth experiences and perspectives of patients, which can facilitate improvements to the rehabilitation services they receive (Vanderkaay et al. 2018). A benefit of this type of research is that it can address the increasing focus on patient-centred care – referring to the needs, values, and preferences of individual patients who should be viewed as informed decision-makers in their care (Hammell 2004; Institute of Medicine 2001; Rathert et al. 2012). Understanding patient's perspectives can enhance their satisfaction with the services they receive and their outcomes (Rathert et al. 2012). Further, qualitative research can provide explanations about why certain outcomes occurred (e.g., employed, unemployed), the perceived impact of a program or intervention, and shed light on complex processes such as self-care at work or disclosure of a condition to employers (Grypdonk 2006). Applying qualitative methodology encourages us to look beyond the condition or disability and to consider the whole person, their needs, and experiences in an effort to facilitate their integration into their community (Gibson & Martin 2002).

Given that the aim of rehabilitation is to help patients to participate in the community whilst improving their quality of life, it is critical to understand their lived experiences through qualitative approaches (Gibson & Martin 2002). We can do this by considering the unique circumstances, goals, values, and challenges that people with disabilities may encounter. For example, qualitative research can enhance our knowledge of occupational rehabilitation by exploring such things as meaning, lived experience, and process of enabling occupational engagement (Gewurtz et al. 2008). In this chapter, I draw on examples from my qualitative research exploring youth with disabilities transitioning into work.

Youth with Disabilities Transitioning into Work – The Importance of Qualitative Research

Qualitative researchers increasingly recognise the importance of exploring youth's experiences (Garth & Aroni 2003; Kramer et al. 2012; Lindsay & Cancelliere 2018). Until recently most research on youth with disabilities focused on the perspectives of healthcare providers, or their parents, whilst little was known about youth's first-hand experiences (Darbyshire 2000; Lindsay et al. 2013, 2015a, 2015b, 2015c). Research examining youth's perspectives, particularly on the topic of transition to employment, is relatively sparse (Foley et al. 2012; Lindsay et al. 2013, 2015a, 2015b, 2015c). Most research on transitions amongst youth with disabilities concentrates on their healthcare needs, even though youth frequently mention wanting more assistance with vocational and employment goals (Lindsay 2014; Lindsay et al. 2015a, 2015b, 2015c, 2018a, 2018b). Drawing attention to youth with disabilities is salient because they are at a critical stage in their development and may need additional support, particularly with social development and role functioning (Lindsay et al. 2016a, 2016b, 2016c, 2016d). For example, disadvantages are often compounded for youth who start life with a disability (Lustig & Strauser 2003), therefore, gaining early employment experience is critical for enhancing their future employment outcomes (Lindsay et al. 2013).

Understanding youth's perspectives is essential because there are often discrepancies between parent and clinician reports of their functioning and well-being (Lindsay et al. 2017a, 2017b, 2017c; Schiariti et al. 2014). Further, listening to youth's experiences about transitioning to work can help to highlight potential gaps and areas for improvement in the programs and services they receive. Therefore, drawing on qualitative research can add to our knowledge about how youth with disabilities transition into work by providing rich descriptions of their lived experiences regarding how their condition affects their participation in everyday life.

Enhancing employment opportunities of youth with disabilities is important given that their employment rate for those aged 20 years old–24 years old is 63.7% and 81.5% for those without disabilities (Statistics Canada 2006). Employment rates are even lower for youth aged 15 years old–19 years old (i.e., 40.1% for those with disabilities vs 51.4% for those without disabilities) (Statistics Canada 2006). Using qualitative methodology can help to uncover the experiences behind these trends and show us where youth may need further support. This type of research can help us to move beyond focusing only on employment outcomes (i.e., employed, not employed) and to explore in further depth how youth seek and maintain employment and other meaningful occupations during their transition to adult life.

Most transitions to employment programs for youth with disabilities are often a one-size-fits-all and do not account for the varying needs that youth with specific types of disabilities have (i.e., accessibility, accommodations, self-care, and personal support needs) (Foley et al. 2012; Lindsay et al. 2013). Further, little is known about what supports are required to assist youth in their decisions about transitioning to employment and when they should receive such supports (Lindsay et al. 2018a, 2018b). Research shows that transition programs for youth with disabilities have had little impact on improving post-high school transition experiences (Foley et al. 2012). Therefore, more work is needed to consider youth's experiences of transitioning to work so we can support them in optimising successful outcomes.

Personal Reflections

My inspiration for using qualitative comparison groups stemmed from my social location of having my office and lab physically located within a paediatric rehabilitation hospital. Here, researchers are encouraged to have patients, and in my case youth with disabilities, actively involved in all stages of their research. Our hospital has been leading the way in regards to patient-engaged research (Anderson et al. 2018). Most of my projects involve youth as advisors, mentors, or facilitators. I have hired 10 youth and young adults with disabilities in paid positions within my lab over the past 9 years. At first, my motivation was to help them gain valuable employment experience and skills, but now, I find that their insight into project design and implementation is invaluable. I have learned so much from working with these youth – not only in my day-to-day projects, but I have the opportunity to see the abilities and future potential of these young people. In working closely with them I have learned that we (as researchers, employers, and clinicians) often have many incorrect assumptions about their capabilities and particularly how they compare to youth without disabilities. As such, I started to build comparison groups into my qualitative studies, not only to further my own understanding, but also to showcase to others that we often have many biases and inappropriate assumptions about people with disabilities.

The objective of this chapter is to provide an overview of why it is important to have qualitative comparison groups and examples of how to do this within the context of youth with disabilities transitioning into employment. Next, I describe why we should use qualitative comparison groups and highlight three different types of comparison groups that I have used within the context of transitioning to work amongst youth with disabilities.

Qualitative Comparison Groups

Control and comparison groups are often used in quantitative research, but rarely in qualitative. In quantitative studies, control groups can help to assess the effect of an intervention (e.g., Horder et al. 2013; Le et al. 2013; Lindsay et al. 2009;

Thomas et al. 2004). Although some studies have a qualitative component alongside a randomised controlled trial, there are surprisingly few qualitatively driven studies that use a comparison group. Having comparison groups embedded within a qualitative design can benefit our understanding of lived experiences, and processes, whilst highlighting how phenomena vary between groups (Lindsay et al. 2015a, 2015b, 2015c, 2017a, 2017b, 2017c; Ritchie et al. 2014; Lindsay 2019). For example, within rehabilitation research, a comparison group could support us in exploring the similarities and differences between those who have a particular condition and those who do not (Lindsay et al. 2015a, 2015b, 2015c).

Qualitative research that uses comparison groups in their design often cite it as a strength of their study (e.g., Dickie et al. 2009; Lindsay et al. 2015a, 2015b, 2015c, 2017a, 2017b, 2017c). Meanwhile, others note that lacking one is considered a limitation (e.g., Deitrick et al. 2010; Heugten 2004; Rodriquez 2013). For example, one qualitative researcher said, '…we have no comparison group. As a result, we cannot draw any conclusions about differences and similarities' (Davey et al. 2012, p. 1267). Not having a comparison group makes it is challenging to determine whether any differences exist between those with and without a particular characteristic (i.e., health condition). Further, lacking a comparison group could potentially introduce bias into your study. For instance, researchers often make assumptions about their participants by adding their own interpretations about how they think their sample compares to others. Some have noted this as 'pink elephant bias', where researchers tend to see what is anticipated (Morse & Mitcham 2002; Spiers 2016). Having a comparison group could help to address some of the biases common within qualitative research by enhancing rigour and credibility (i.e., internal validity) of the findings through persistent observation and negative case analysis (Morse 2015). Further, comparison groups can enhance the dependability (i.e., reliability) of the findings through a splitting of the data and duplicating the analysis (see example 2 below) (Guba & Lincoln 1989; Morse 2015).

Applying comparison groups in qualitative research could also facilitate the incorporation of varying perspectives from people who have different social positions (e.g., youth with and without disabilities, clinician, and parent perspectives). Further, having qualitative comparison groups can help to advance rehabilitation science (e.g., opportunities and challenges) by adding to the rigour, quality, and credibility whilst potentially enhancing the uptake of research by clinicians to improve clinical practice (Vanderkaay et al. 2018).

I argue that qualitative health researchers should consider using qualitative comparison groups to enhance the rigour of their work and to develop a better understanding of how their sample compares with healthy controls. Using a comparison group encourages researchers to think of other possibilities and also negative cases. Through using qualitative comparison groups in my own work, I have often found several surprising similarities and differences between groups with and without a particular condition (Lindsay et al. 2015a, 2015b, 2015c, 2017a, 2017b, 2017c). In the next section, I provide examples of three different types of comparison groups: (1) with and without a condition; (2) split sample comparison; and (3) multiple perspectives comparison group (see Table 3.1 for overview).

TABLE 3.1

Overview of Characteristics of Qualitative Comparison Groups

	Healthy Comparison	Split Sample Comparison	Multiple Perspectives Comparison
When to use	• When you want to understand differences between those who have the condition and those who do not	• When you want to understand differences based on 1 characteristic among a similar group (e.g., gender)	• When you want to understand perspectives of different groups on the same issue (e.g., patients, caregivers, health providers)
Sample	• Both groups should be homogeneous (similar ages, gender, and other aspects associated with the inclusion criteria) • Have at least 10–15 participants per group or until thematic saturation achieved (within and between groups)	• Homogenous sample (all inclusion criteria as similar as possible with the exception of the 1 factor that the sample is being spilt by (e.g., gender) • Have a large enough sample (e.g., 20–30) to ensure that thematic saturation is reached (within and between groups)	• All groups should be homogeneous as possible with sufficient sample sizes to reach saturation within each group • Have at least 10–15 participants per group or until thematic saturation (within and between groups) is reached
Recruitment	• Both groups recruited in the same way (e.g., mailed, emailed, phoned), from the same or very similar location • Group with the condition should be recruited first so that the sample can be matched to those without the condition • Closely monitor recruitment to ensure that the comparison group is closely matched to the group with the condition	• Recruit both sets of participants in the same way, from the same location • Monitor recruitment to ensure that the groups are evenly matched as possible	• All groups should be recruited from the same or very similar location using the same recruitment procedures
Data collection	• Same method of data collection (e.g., interviews) and same questions for both groups; same interviewer(s) • Same place and mode of data collection (e.g., face-to-face over-the phone)	• Same method of data collection and same questions for both groups; same interviewer(s) • Same place and mode of data collection (e.g., face-to-face over-the phone)	• Same method of data collection and same or very similar questions for all groups; same interviewer(s) • Same place and mode of data collection (e.g., face-to-face over-the phone)

(*Continued*)

TABLE 3.1 (*Continued*)

Overview of Characteristics of Qualitative Comparison Groups

	Healthy Comparison	Split Sample Comparison	Multiple Perspectives Comparison
Analysis	• Same method of analysis for each group (within group themes) • At least 2 researchers reading all transcripts and compile list of preliminary themes • Compare within and between groups • Overview table of themes comparing by group	• Same method of analysis for each group (within group themes) • At least 2 researchers reading all transcripts and compile list of preliminary themes • Compare within and between groups • Overview table of themes comparing by group	• Same method of analysis for each group (within group themes) • At least 2 researchers reading all transcripts and compile list of preliminary themes • Compare within and between groups • Overview table of themes comparing by group
Benefits	• Helps us to understand similarities and differences between those who have the condition and those who do not • Can highlight areas where those with a condition need further or different types of support • Can help to reduce bias	• Helps to understand the role of how one characteristic influences the experiences of living with the condition • Can highlight areas where further or different supports may be needed	• Highlights the areas that are important to the patient and any gaps that might exist within and between other perspectives (e.g., parent or clinician)
Challenges	• Matching participants for the comparison group • Added time and cost	• Recruiting a large enough sample size to make the comparison	• Difficulty balancing a similar number of interviews across the groups • Feasibility of the same mode of data collection for all groups
Advice	• Carefully document any ways in which the sampling, recruitment, analysis differed between each group and consider how this may have influenced your findings • Have an overview table of themes comparing by group • Recruit sample with disabilities first then recruit sample without for optimal matching • Pilot test the interview guide to ensure it addresses key issues for both groups	• Recruit both characteristics of the sample at the same time, but continually monitor during the recruitment phase to ensure that the sample is evenly matched (by age and other characteristics) • Pilot test the interview guide to ensure it addresses key issues for both groups	• Have an overview table of themes comparing by group • Pilot test the interview guide to ensure it addresses key issues for all groups

Example 3.1: Healthy Comparison Group

In three studies, we compared youth with and without disabilities as they transition to employment (see Figure 3.1) (Lindsay & Depape 2015; Lindsay et al. 2014a, 2015a, 2015b, 2015c). For example, we compared differences in job interview content between youth with and without a physical disability. Doing so is important because people with disabilities often encounter barriers based on employer's stigma and discriminatory attitudes about the abilities of people with disabilities (Lindsay & Depape 2015). Thus, we wanted to understand how experiences compare between the two groups.

Although studies regularly show that youth with disabilities experience worse employment rates compared to youth without disabilities (Lindsay et al. 2014a, 2014b), we know little about how they perform in a job interview. By exploring the content of job interviews, we can foster an understanding about how youth with disabilities may vary in their performance compared to those without disabilities. Understanding such differences can help to inform occupational rehabilitation interventions and also areas where we can further educate employers about their potential unconscious biases during the hiring process (Lindsay et al. 2015a, 2015b, 2015c).

For this study, we drew a purposive sample of 31 youth (15 with a disability and 16 without). Each youth took part in a mock job interview where the questions asked about their skills, experiences, actions taken during workplace problem-based scenarios, and areas for improvement (Lindsay et al. 2014). Our inclusion criteria involved: youth with a diagnosed physical disability (without a cognitive impairment); currently enrolled in grade 11 or 12 of an academic/applied university stream within high school; and currently attending an integrated high school (Lindsay et al. 2014). Our comparison group also met the above criteria with the exception of not having a disability (Lindsay et al. 2014).

We developed job interviews that were based on discussions with a sample of job counsellors and employers (Lindsay et al. 2014) from industries where youth commonly work (e.g., retail, entertainment and recreation, hospitality and food services, arts, education services) (Marshall 2010). This allowed us to learn about skills that employers look for when hiring youth (Lindsay et al. 2014a, 2014b). Each youth had the same questions that were given by a professional actor in the role of a human resource position.

We used a content analysis approach to analyse our data (Lindsay et al. 2015a, 2015b, 2015c). First, we immersed ourselves in the interview transcripts to understand the context and developed the themes (Elo & Kyngäs 2008; Vaismoradi et al. 2013). Second, we applied an open coding process where we read and coded each transcript whilst noting themes. We compared and contrasted our themes (within and between the two groups – see Figure 3.1) and grouped them under higher order headings, then generated

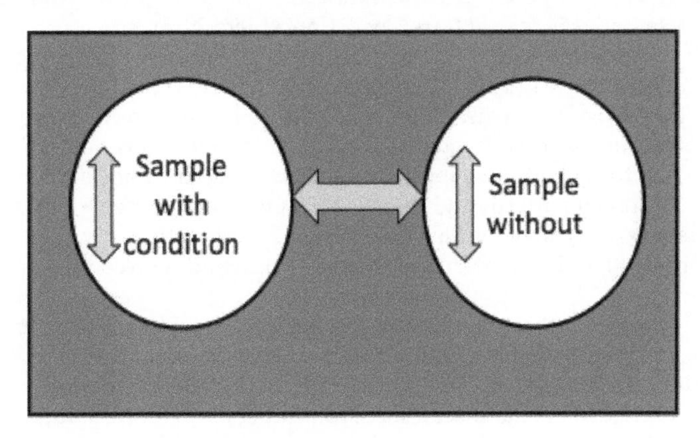

FIGURE 3.1
Healthy comparison.

categories and sub-categories whilst abstracting representative quotes (Elo & Kyngäs 2008; Vaismoradi et al. 2013). Then, we organised the themes by type of participant (youth with or without a disability) (Lindsay et al. 2014).

Our results highlighted several similarities and differences between youth with and without disabilities regarding their job interview content (Lindsay & Depape 2015). Similarities included youth providing examples based on their experiences from school, emphasising their soft skills, (i.e., people and communication skills) and relevant experience (Lindsay & Depape 2015). Although both groups of youth shared comparable examples of things they were proud of, fewer youth with disabilities gave examples for this question. Variations in their answers between the two groups included youth with disabilities disclosing their condition, giving fewer examples related to customer service and teamwork, and challenges with responding to scenario-based problem-solving questions (Lindsay & Depape 2015). Youth with disabilities also had difficulties drawing on examples from past experiences (e.g., work, volunteer, and extracurricular activities) (Lindsay & Depape 2015).

Our results indicate how clinicians should help educate youth on the timing and process for disability disclosure and how to showcase their marketable skills in an interview (Lindsay & Depape 2015). Doing this is important because employers expect workers to have good interview skills, which includes being able to sell their transferable skills (Lindsay et al. 2012, 2014). Further, employers should consider that the experiences of youth with disabilities may differ from youth without disabilities. Our results help to inform occupational rehabilitation programs and interventions by underscoring areas where youth with disabilities may need extra support compared to youth without disabilities (Lindsay & Depape 2015).

Occupational therapists and rehabilitation counsellors should help youth to understand employers' interest in transferable skills related to the position they are applying for. Although many youths with disabilities have limited work experience, they could still highlight the relevant and valuable skills they have acquired through schooling or volunteer experience. Clinicians and educators should provide youth with opportunities to practice their interview skills so they can optimise their chances of success in an employment interview (Lindsay & Depape 2015; Lindsay et al. 2012).

In a second example of using this type of qualitative comparison groups, we focused on how disability confidence develops during volunteer placements amongst youth with and without disabilities. Disability confidence refers to having comfort with, and inclusion of people with disabilities (Lindsay & Cancelliere 2018). Lacking knowledge about people with disabilities can adversely affect them through stigma/discrimination, social exclusion, and poor self-image (Lindsay & Edwards 2013; Morgan & Lo 2013). Therefore, developing a better understanding of how to improve attitudes towards people with disabilities is critical (Lindsay & Cancelliere 2018).

A strength of our study is that we compared two perspectives including youth with and without disabilities (Lindsay & Cancelliere 2018). In this study, we conducted 30 in-depth interviews (16 without a disability; 14 with disabilities) with youth aged 15–25. Our analysis involved an interpretive, qualitative, thematic approach (Lindsay & Cancelliere 2018). We read all transcripts and applied an open coding, thematic approach (Braun & Clarke 2006). We noted patterns and themes about the development of disability confidence. We first analysed all of the data together (i.e., youth with and without disabilities) before we compared and contrasted the themes within and between the groups of participants (see Figure 3.1) (Lindsay & Cancelliere 2018).

Our findings showed that youth with and without disabilities both had a similar process of developing disability confidence, but there were nuances between the two groups (Lindsay & Cancelliere 2018). For example, both groups (those with and without disabilities) experienced some discomfort around people with disabilities and lacked disability confidence to a certain extent. For those without disabilities, this may have resulted from lacking exposure to people with disabilities in general. Meanwhile, for youth with disabilities, lacking confidence may have resulted from having disability-specific related experience. For youth without disabilities, reaching beyond their comfort zone referred to being around and developing a sense of ease with people who have a disability (Lindsay & Cancelliere 2018). Meanwhile, for youth with disabilities, this involved having exposure to people with different types of disabilities (Lindsay & Cancelliere 2018).

Our results highlighted that another stage in developing disability confidence involved broadening perspectives, which included youth having social contact with people who have a disability and challenging common misperceptions about them (Lindsay & Cancelliere 2018). Our findings show that the development of disability confidence is critical for enhancing the social inclusion of people with disabilities. For example, volunteering with people who have a disability, or a disability different from their own, can help develop disability confidence (i.e., positive attitudes, empathy, and appropriate communication skills). The implications of our findings included that youth, clinicians, and employers should consider working with people who have a disability through employment, volunteering, or service learning to develop their disability confidence (Lindsay & Cancelliere 2018).

Benefits and Challenges of Healthy Comparison Groups

The benefits of having this type of comparison group includes that it helps us to understand the similarities and differences between those who have a condition and those who do not. It can highlight areas where those with a condition may need further support. Further, having a comparison group can help to add rigour and reduce bias within your study (Tomlin & Borgetto 2011). When a comparison group is not used, researchers often implicitly use their own socio-cultural comparative perspectives (Morse 2004). Therefore, researchers should consider using this type of comparison group when they want to understand differences between those who have the condition and those who do not (see Table 3.1).

It is important to design your study with a comparison group in mind and not simply add it in after the data has been collected (see Table 3.1 and Figure 3.1). Indeed, a more structured approach to data collection is needed so that similar issues are explored in similar ways (Ritchie et al. 2014). For instance, the sample for both groups should be homogenous as possible (e.g., similar ages, gender, and other aspects related to the inclusion criteria). Further, each comparison group should be large enough to reflect the diversity of the population so that you can look for patterns within and between comparison groups (Ritchie et al. 2014).

Researchers should aim to have a sample size that is typical for qualitative research (e.g., 10–15 participants) for each group or until researchers feel that they have reached thematic saturation (within and between the groups). Researchers should ensure that they have a similar number of participants for each variable of interest (for both groups). The same recruitment, data collection, and analysis process should be used for both groups. I recommended recruiting the sample that has the health condition first so that a matching technique can be used for the comparison group (see Table 3.1). Matching techniques are particularly useful in studies that have small numbers of participants and can help to add rigour for enhancing the comparability of the groups (Cook et al. 2008).

If you are recruiting for both groups at the same time, your comparison sample may end up being uneven (in number and matched characteristics), making it difficult to know whether any differences are a result of having the condition or other factors. I recommend having some checkpoints along the way to assess where you may need to target more specific recruitment (e.g., more males of a particular age range). Some challenges to keep in mind include that the matching participants for the comparison group can be challenging and time consuming.

Example 3.2: Split Sample Comparison Group

A second type of comparison group involves splitting the sample by one characteristic (e.g., gender) (see Table 3.1 and Figure 3.2). For example, in our Lindsay et al. (2018a, 2018b) study, we compared the role of gender in transitioning to employment amongst youth with physical disabilities. Exploring this topic is important because employment rates vary considerably for young females with disabilities (i.e., 1%–27%) compared to 50%–75% of males with disabilities (i.e., 50%–75%) (Lindsay et al. 2018a, 2018b).

Understanding the role of gender in youths' transition to employment is salient because young women with disabilities often fall behind their male counterparts on several health and social outcomes (Hogansen et al. 2008; Lindsay et al. 2018a, 2018b). Gender shapes career aspirations, engagement in vocational training, and employment status (Lindsay et al. 2018a, 2018b). Socio-environmental factors (e.g., domestic work and caregiving) can also influence gender roles in a way that can impact employment outcomes (Livingstone et al. 2016; Mattingly & Blanchi 2003). Some research shows that women with disabilities often lack career development opportunities compared to men, which can impact their ability to engage in paid work (Doren et al. 2011; Lindsay et al. 2018a, 2018b).

Although some research highlights the need for gender specific vocational supports for youth with disabilities (Blackorby & Wagner 1996; Lindsay et al. 2018a, 2018b; Sung et al. 2015), surprisingly few studies consider how gender influences employment for young people with disabilities (Hanif et al. 2017). A recent systematic review on transitioning to employment for people with disabilities showed that gender was largely absent (Lindsay et al. 2018a, 2018b). Of the limited research focusing on gender and employment amongst youth with disabilities, the attention was mostly on employment outcomes and pay differences. Therefore, there is an important need for more research to unravel the multi-faceted relationships between gender and employment amongst youth with disabilities (Lindsay et al. 2018a, 2018b; Magill-Evans et al. 2008), particularly from a qualitative perspective. Understanding this intersection is imperative because inequitable employment outcomes are significant for both men and women with disabilities, compared to people without disabilities (Roebroeck et al. 2009). In addition, investigating the role of gender is important for decision-making, communication, stakeholder engagement, and implementation of interventions (Tannenbaum et al. 2016).

In the study that we draw on for this example, we had a purposive sample of 23 youth involving 13 females (mean age 22.9) and 10 males (mean age 21.3) (Lindsay et al. 2018a, 2018b). We also compared youth's perspectives to 10 clinicians that we interviewed who

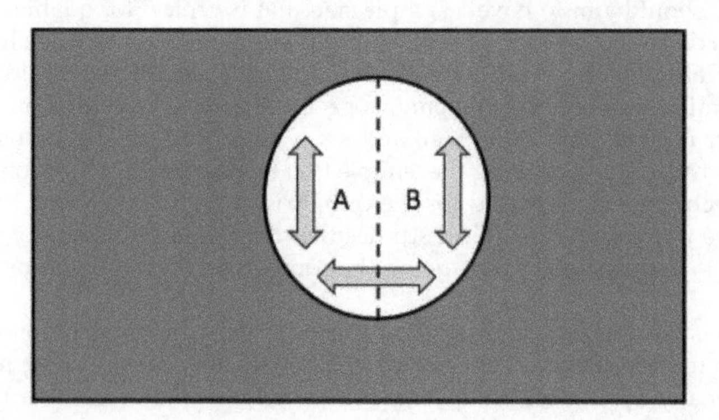

FIGURE 3.2
Split sample comparison.

are involved in the transition care of youth whilst also having a multiple perspectives comparison group (described further in example 3) (Lindsay et al. 2018a, 2018b).

Our results showed several similarities and some difference between young males and females with physical disabilities as they transition to employment (Lindsay et al. 2018a, 2018b). Our findings indicate that both groups of youth should be realistic about their abilities and often made some career adjustments based on their condition (e.g., self-care, fatigue, etc.). We found that males and females encountered transportation challenges which they mentioned affected their ability to find employment. Some females in particular reported problems with travelling independently, mostly due to unease about safety and parental overprotection (Lindsay et al. 2018a, 2018b). Further, both males and females received social support from their parents, however, there were gendered patterns within the types of support they received. For example, females mentioned that their mothers were often a primary source of support, whilst for males it was often both parents or their father (Lindsay et al. 2018a, 2018b). Males told us about contrasting experiences regarding the extent of support they received from their family. For example, some males received support and others did not. Meanwhile, females often drew on a more extensive social support network, which is particularly useful when looking for a job (Lindsay et al. 2018a, 2018b). Gender differences between males and females with disabilities were also noted in terms of requesting workplace accommodations and asking for assistance. Specifically, females were often at ease with requesting help, whilst most males were not. In fact, some males hid their condition altogether (Lindsay et al. 2018a, 2018b).

Our results emphasise that youth's decision to discuss their disability with others was influenced by the visibility of their condition, their comfort level in disclosing, and their inclination to ask for help (Lindsay et al. 2018a, 2018b). Males and females contrasted in regards to their comfort level with disclosing to employers, asking for help, and requesting accommodations. Females articulated how they needed to feel at ease with their supervisor before disclosing their condition and requesting accommodations (Lindsay et al. 2018a, 2018b).

Further, we noted that although most clinicians described gender differences amongst their clients they were helping to transition, many reported that they did not tailor their approach based on gender (Lindsay et al. 2018a, 2018b). By comparing youth (i.e., splitting the sample by gender), as well as comparing with clinicians, we identified where youth need further assistance, and importantly, where clinicians should revise their practice and/or programming to be more patient-centred (Lindsay et al. 2018a, 2018b). Using a comparative approach helped us to realise that clinicians should tailor their vocational rehabilitation practices to the gender-specific needs of youth with disabilities to best support their transition into employment (Lindsay et al. 2018a, 2018b).

Benefits and Challenges of This Approach

The benefits of having this type of comparison group includes that it helps us to understand the role of how one characteristic influences the experiences of living with a condition along with the similarities and differences between the two groups based on this characteristic (see Table 3.1). This type of comparison group can also highlight areas where further support, different types of support, or interventions may be needed. The design, data collection, and analysis should be the same for both groups. Researchers should aim for a homogenous sample and match as much as possible by the characteristic that they are exploring (e.g., gender – aim to have a similar number of males and females). Further, researchers should ensure that the sample size is large enough to reach saturation to be able to look for thematic comparisons within and between the groups. Finally, it is also important to give a rationale why this type of comparison is needed and what it will add to the literature.

Example 3.3: Multiple Perspectives Comparison Group

Another example of a comparison group involves having multiple perspectives (see Table 3.1, Figure 3.3). Having comparison groups are important because considerable evidence shows that patients often do not share the same priorities or perceptions of problems as clinicians or parents (Lindsay et al. 2017a, 2017b, 2017c). Our team has conducted studies focusing on transition to employment for youth with disabilities whilst comparing different perspectives (e.g., parents, clinicians, and youth). For example, in our study on school-to-work transitions amongst youth with spina bifida, we explored three different perspectives (i.e., youth, parents, and clinicians) (Lindsay et al. 2017a, 2017b, 2017c). Supporting youth with disabilities to transition to employment is salient because the impact of having limited job experience at a young age on their longer-term employment outcomes is profound (Lindsay et al. 2015a, 2015b, 2015c; Liptak et al. 2010). Amongst youth without disabilities, being employed is often seen as an indicator of thriving transition to adulthood (Lindsay 2014; Lindsay et al. 2015a, 2015b, 2015c). Employment is an important and meaningful activity that offers income, social relationships, social inclusion, and enhanced quality of life (Lindsay 2014; Lindsay et al. 2015a, 2015b, 2015c). Youth with spina bifida have unique needs as they transition to adulthood and are susceptible to unemployment (Zukerman et al. 2010). They may also encounter challenges in caring for the medical aspects of their condition at work and the associated stigma and discrimination that often accompanies it (Zukerman et al. 2010). Unemployment rates are high amongst youth with spina bifida. For example, more than half of those who finish school do not have a regular job (van Mechelen et al. 2008). Although such unemployment trends are consistent amongst youth with disabilities, we know very little about the experiences and perspectives of school-work transitions amongst youth with spina bifida and their caregivers (Cohen et al. 2003; Lindsay et al. 2017a, 2017b, 2017c). Therefore, developing a better comprehension of school-work transitions amongst youth with spina bifida is helpful for informing approaches to assist their entrance to college and work.

Until recently, most studies on employment amongst people with disabilities focussed on adults who are returning to work after injury or illness (Paniccia et al. 2018). Much less is known about youth with disabilities, especially those who are looking for their first job (Lindsay 2014). Second, there is little research on the work experiences of youth with physical disabilities and even less so on spina bifida in particular (Lindsay 2014; Lindsay et al. 2015a, 2015b, 2015c). The relatively sparse literature on this topic tends to focus on youth with various types of disabilities, without discerning the diverse needs related to specific disabilities (Lindsay et al. 2017a, 2017b, 2017c).

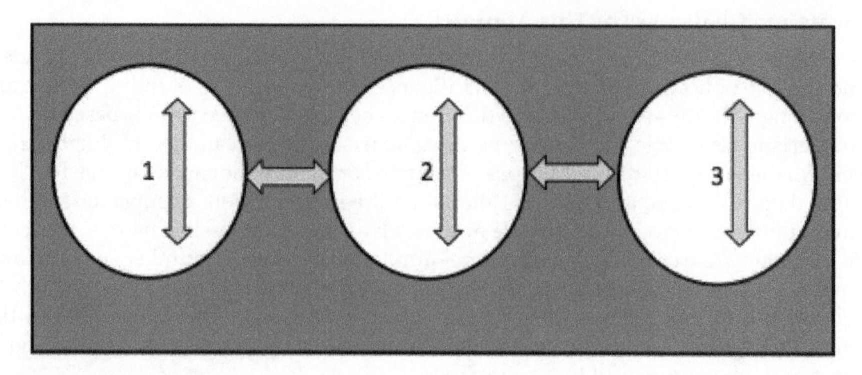

FIGURE 3.3
Multiple perspectives comparison.

Exploring youth with spina bifida is important because most youth with this condition do not live independently, are less likely to be employed (34% vs 75%), and to go to college than youth without disabilities (49% vs 66%) (Cohen et al. 2003; Zukerman et al. 2010). Although youth with spina bifida are often aware of the benefits of working, they often lack goal-oriented plans to achieve this outcome (Lindsay et al. 2017a, 2017b, 2017c). Further, some research shows that youth with spina bifida are often delayed in transitioning to adulthood and may need further support in pursuing education and finding employment (Lindsay et al. 2017a, 2017b, 2017c; Ridosh et al. 2011). Of the few studies that explore youth with spina bifida, they are quantitative and focus on employment outcomes. Thus, having a more qualitative approach is relevant for revealing the barriers and enablers to realising vocational milestones (Lindsay 2014). Further, few comparisons have been made between varying perspectives (e.g., youth, parents, and clinicians) on school-work transitions amongst youth with disabilities. By drawing such comparisons, we aim to unearth further understandings of the complexities of school-work transitions amongst youth with spina bifida (Lindsay et al. 2014).

Within this comparison study, we investigated the enablers, barriers, and experiences of employment and post-secondary education amongst youth with spina bifida, and how perspectives on these issues vary between youth with spina bifida, their parents, and healthcare providers (Lindsay et al. 2017a, 2017b, 2017c). We led in-depth interviews with 44 participants (21 youth, 11 parents, 12 clinicians). We used purposive sampling procedures to recruit all participants from one paediatric rehabilitation hospital (Lindsay et al. 2017a, 2017b, 2017c).

We used a qualitative content analysis approach to investigate the data, which is useful for capturing key themes across a large qualitative dataset (Graneheim & Lundman 2004; Sawin et al. 2009). First, we used NVivo to extract all relevant quotes from the transcripts, based on the words 'school', 'employment', and related synonyms (e.g., job, work, high school, post-secondary, college, university, co-op, internship, volunteer, scholarship, accommodation). We also read all the interview transcripts to ensure this stage of analysis was comprehensive and captured all relevant quotes related to school and employment (Lindsay et al. 2017a, 2017b, 2017c). Next, we extracted quotes and organised them into logical categories through an iterative process (Graneheim & Lundman 2004). We reviewed all of the extracted quotes several times, whilst observing themes and patterns within and between the groups of participants (i.e., youth, parents, and clinicians) (see Figure 3.1).

Our results indicated similarities and differences across the groups. For example, clinicians wanted to help youth understand the life skills that are needed to support their employment goals (Lindsay et al. 2017a, 2017b, 2017c). They also underscored that youth should be capable of managing the medical aspects of their condition at work. Clinicians described that more assistance is needed to help youth with spina bifida to connect to employment training. Although many clinicians stressed the value of volunteering for youth, they were often unaware of the potential benefits it can offer for transitioning to employment. Some youth who completed high school often saw the advantages of volunteering for acquiring work-related skills, developing social networks, and exploring career options (Lindsay et al. 2017a, 2017b, 2017c).

Youth shared their worries about transitioning to college and work, struggled to gain independence skills, which were often due to a lack of resources and/or overprotective parents (Lindsay et al. 2017a, 2017b, 2017c). Meanwhile, parents also reporting needing support on how to let go and encourage their youth to develop skills that would help them with their transition to adulthood. Both groups (parents and youth) found it challenging to manage the ongoing care of their condition (Lindsay et al. 2017a, 2017b, 2017c).

Many youth and parents recognised the barriers involved in obtaining a job or volunteer placement that matched their interests and abilities (Lindsay et al. 2017a, 2017b, 2017c). Although some supports are available, youth with spina bifida face barriers in transitioning to work including a discrimination and stigma; challenges coping with their condition; and lack of information on finances, housing, and transportation.

Our findings highlight that clinicians should assist youth with preparing for their transition to employment by connecting them to appropriate information and resources. Starting from a young age, parents and clinicians should help youth prepare for work transitions by promoting their career goals, independence, life skills, and self-care of their condition (Lindsay et al. 2017a, 2017b, 2017c).

Another example of multiple perspectives comparison groups included our study that explored the barriers to employment for youth with disabilities compared to youth without disabilities whilst also considering the views of employers and job counsellors (Lindsay et al. 2015a, 2015b, 2015c). Exploring this is important because there have been very few comparisons of how employment barriers encountered by youth with disabilities differ from youth without disabilities. Understanding these similarities will contribute to the further development of job training and life skills interventions and help to direct efforts to support for work environments (Lindsay 2011; Lindsay et al. 2012). Focusing on youth with disabilities is salient because early job experience during adolescence is critical to obtaining future employment and income (Carter & Lunsford 2005; Lindsay et al. 2012). Most previous research focuses on individual level challenges, whilst a gap exists regarding other socio-structural factors influencing work. Comparing multiple perspectives is useful for uncovering the multi-faceted barriers to employment for youth with disabilities (Lindsay et al. 2015a, 2015b, 2015c).

Our study drew on 50 qualitative in-depth interviews with a purposive sample of 31 youth (16 without a disability and 15 with a disability) and youth employers and job counsellors knowledgeable about employment readiness amongst adolescents (n = 19) (Lindsay et al. 2015a, 2015b, 2015c). We analysed the data by reading each transcript several times to uncover themes about factors influencing work for youth with and without disabilities. We first analysed all groups of participants separately (i.e., youth with and without disabilities and employers) before we compared and contrasted themes between the two groups. After developing a list of themes, we compared and contrasted using a constant comparative method within and between the groups (Lindsay et al. 2015a, 2015b, 2015c).

Our findings showed that only half of youth with a disability were working or looking for work compared to youth without disabilities (Lindsay et al. 2015a, 2015b, 2015c). The results indicate that this was a result of different attitudes towards youth with disabilities. For many youths with a disability, their peers, family, and social networks often posed a barrier to them getting a job. Many youths lacked independence and life skills that are needed to get a job (i.e., self-care and navigating public transportation) compared to their peers (Lindsay et al. 2015a, 2015b, 2015c). Job counsellors focused on linking youth to employers and mediating parental concerns. Meanwhile, employers appeared to have weaker connections to youth with disabilities. System level barriers included lack of funding and policies to enhance disability awareness amongst employers (Lindsay et al. 2015a, 2015b, 2015c). Youth with physical disabilities experience some similar barriers to finding work compared to youth without disabilities, but to a greater extent. The results highlight that although there are several challenges in finding work for youth at the individual level, they are linked with larger social and environmental barriers (Lindsay et al. 2015a, 2015b, 2015c). Job counsellors focused on linking youth to employers and mediating parental concerns. Employers appeared to have weaker connections to youth with disabilities (Lindsay et al. 2015a, 2015b, 2015c).

We found several similarities and differences in the type and extent of barriers encountered for youth with disabilities compared to youth without disabilities, however, disadvantages may be compounded for youth with disabilities (i.e., discrimination and inaccessible environments) (Lindsay et al. 2015a, 2015b, 2015c). There are fewer youth with a disability who are working or looking for work and may need more help and encouragement with life skills to help them achieve independence. It is important to remember that finding employment is not simply about individuals preparing for work, it is also about society, employers, and work environments accommodating and being inclusive of people with disabilities (Lindsay et al. 2015a, 2015b, 2015c).

The implications of our findings include that clinicians should help develop skills that can lead to improved self-confidence and communication skills for youth. They should encourage youth to engage in extracurricular activities and social networking to build these skills and to help make connections for finding work (Lindsay et al. 2015a, 2015b, 2015c). Clinicians should support youth and their parents in practicing independence skills (i.e., self-care, self-advocacy, and navigating public transportation) that they need prior to looking for employment. Occupational therapists and rehabilitation clinicians should educate youth about disclosing their condition to potential employers, how to ask for ask for accommodations, and how to market their abilities (Lindsay et al. 2015a, 2015b, 2015c).

Benefits and Challenges of Multiple Perspectives Comparison Group

Multiple perspectives comparison groups should be used when researchers want to understand viewpoints of different groups (e.g., patients, caregivers, healthcare providers) on the same issue (see Table 3.1 and Figure 3.3). Benefits of this type of comparison group include that it can highlight the areas that are important to the patient (and enhance patient-centred care) and also any gaps that might exist within and between other groups (e.g., parent or clinician). When using this method, researchers should ensure that all groups are as homogeneous as possible with sufficient sample sizes to reach saturation (within and between groups). All groups should be recruited in the same or very similar location using the same methods (e.g., interviews for all groups, interviewed separately) and data collection procedures. It is also helpful to have an overview table of themes comparing by the different groups. Challenges in using this type of comparison group include that it is sometimes difficult to balance a similar number of interviews across the different groups.

Summary

Qualitative research can help to inform the development and refinement of rehabilitation services (i.e., clinician-patient interactions, lived experiences, clinical decision-making, program, and intervention development). Having a patient-centred approach involves focusing on the values, priorities, and goals of the patient rather than those of the therapist. It can help clinicians to understand how to adapt processes and programs and clinical decision-making (Grypdonck 2018). Further, developing a better understanding of the lived experiences and perspectives of youth with disabilities can help to inform health and social programs and interventions, particularly those that can help with their transition to adulthood (Lindsay et al. 2017a, 2017b, 2017c). Qualitative research can contribute to the development of theory, practice, and service delivery (Hammell 2004). It can also help to reaffirm or further develop theoretical frameworks, expose limitations in current theories, or identify previously unrecognised relationships of a phenomenon (Hammell 2004). This type of research also helps to contextualise research by considering the larger socio-cultural and environmental structures that affect people's lives (Hammell 2004).

In considering the use of qualitative comparison groups, it is important that qualitative researchers do not make comparisons to healthy controls within their results and discussion sections if they have not used a comparison group in their study. When qualitative researchers use a comparison group, they should be clear about their methods and analysis involving comparison groups (i.e., what they are doing, why, and how).

Although comparison groups may add a bit more time and cost to the study, they can also add rigour by addressing potential bias, and help us to understand how a group compares to another. To conclude, qualitative researchers should consider adding comparison groups to their design because they can offer a valuable approach to enriching their data and understanding patient experience.

References

Anderson, J., Williams, L., Karmali, A., Beesley, B., Tanel, N., Doyle-Thomas, K., Sheps, K. & Chau, T. (2018). Client and family engagement in rehabilitation research: A framework for health care organizations. *Disability and Rehabilitation*, 40(7), 859–863.

Blackorby, J. & Wagner, M. (1996). Longitudinal postschool outcomes of youth with disabilities: Findings from the National Longitudinal Transition Study. *Exceptional Child*, 62, 399–413.

Braun, V. & Clark, V. (2006). Using thematic analysis in psychology. *Qualitative Research in Psychology*, 3, 77–101.

Carter, E. & Lunsford, L. (2005). Meaningful work: Improving employment outcomes for transition-age youth with emotional and behavioural disorders. *Prevention of School Failure*, 49, 63–69.

Cohen, P., Kasen, S., Chen, H. et al. (2003). Variations in patterns of developmental transitions in the emerging adulthood period. *Developmental Psychology*, 39, 657–669.

Cook, L., Cook, B., Landrum, T. & Tankersley, M. (2008). Examining the role of group experimental research in establishing evidence-based practices. *Intervention in School and Clinic*, 44(2), 76–82.

Darbyshire, P. (2000). Guest editorial: From research on children to research with children. *Neonatal, Paediatric and Child Health Nursing*, 3(1), 2–3.

Davey, M., Nino, A., Kissil, K. & Ingram, M. (2012). African American parent's experiences navigating breast cancer while caring for their children. *Qualitative Health Research*, 22(9), 1260–1270.

Deitrick, L., Paxton, H., Rivera, A., Gertner, E., Biery, N., Letcher, A., Lahoz, L., Maldonado, E. & Salas-Lopez, D. (2010). Understanding the role of the promotora in a Latino diabetes education program. *Qualitative Health Research*, 20, 386–399.

Dickie, V., Baranek, G., Schultz, B., Watson, L. & McComish, C. (2009). Parent reports of sensory experiences of preschool children with and without autism: A qualitative study. *American Journal of Occupational Therapy*, 63(2), 172–281.

Doren, B., Gau, J. & Lindstrom, L. (2011). The role of gender in the long-term employment outcomes of young adults with disabilities. *Journal of Vocational Rehabilitation*, 34(1), 35–42.

Elo, S. & Kyngäs, H. (2008). The qualitative content analysis process. *Journal of Advanced Nursing*, 62, 107–115.

Foley, K., Dyke, P., Girdler, S. et al. (2012). Young adults with intellectual disability transitioning from school to post-school: A literature review framed within the ICF. *Disability &Rehabilitation*, 34, 1747–1764.

Garth, B. & Aroni, R. (2003). 'I value what you have to say': Seeking the perspective of children with a disability, not just their parents. *Disability & Society*, 18, 561–576.

Gewurtz, R., Stergiou-Kita, M., Shaw, L., Kirsh, B. & Rappolt, S. (2008). Qualitative meta-synthesis: Reflections on the utility and challenges in occupational therapy. *Canadian Journal of Occupational Therapy*, 75(5), 301–307.

Gibson, B. & Martin, D. (2002). Qualitative research and evidence-based physiotherapy practice. *Physiotherapy*, 89(6), 350–358.

Graneheim, U. & Lundman, B. (2004). Qualitative content analysis in nursing research: concepts, procedures and measures to achieve trustworthiness. *Nursing Education*, 24, 105–112.

Grypdonck, M. (2018). Qualitative health research in the era of evidence-based practice. *Qualitative Health Research*, 16(10), 1371–1385.

Guba, E. & Lincoln, Y. (1989). *Fourth Generation Evaluation*. Newbury Park, CA: Sage.

Hammell, K. (2004). Using qualitative evidence as a basis for evidence-based practice. In: *Qualitative Research in Evidence-Based Rehabilitation*. London, UK: Elsevier, pp. 129–143.

Hanif, S., McDougall, C. & Lindsay, S. (2017). A systematic review of vocational interventions for youth with disabilities. In: B. Altman, Editor. *Factors in Studying Employment for Persons with Disability*. Bingley, UK: Emerald Publishing Limited, pp. 181–202.

Heugten, K. (2004). Managing insider research. *Qualitative Social Work*, 3(2), 203–219.

Hogansen, J., Powers, K., Geenen, S. et al. (2008). Transition goals and experiences of females with disabilities: Youth, parents, and professionals. *Exceptional Child*, 74, 215–234.

Horder, H., Frandin, K. & Larsson, M. (2013). Self-respect through ability to keep fear of frailty at a distance: Successful ageing from the perspective of community-dwelling of older people. *International Journal of Qualitative Studies in Health and Well-Being*, 8, 1–10.

Institute of Medicine. (2001). *Crossing the Quality Chasm: A New Health System for the 21st Century*. Washington, DC: National Academy Press.

Kramer, J., Olsen, S., Mermelstein, M., Balcells, A. & Liljenquist, K. (2012). Youth with disabilities' perspectives of the environment and participation: A qualitative meta-synthesis. *Child, Care, Health & Development*, 38(6), 763–777.

Le, H., Perry, D., Genovez, M. & Cardeli, E. (2013). In their own voices: Experiences with a randomized controlled trial. *Qualitative Health Research*, 23, 834–846.

Lindsay, S. (2011). Employment status and work characteristics of adolescents with disabilities. *Disability & Rehabilitation*, 30(10), 843–854.

Lindsay, S. (2014). A qualitative synthesis of adolescents' experiences of living with spina bifida. *Qualitative Health Research*, 24(9), 1298–1309.

Lindsay, S. (2019). Five approaches to qualitative comparison groups in health research: A scoping review. *Qualitative Health Research*, 29(3), 455–468.

Lindsay, S., Adams, T., McDougall, C. & Sanford, R. (2012). Skill development in an employment training program for adolescents with disabilities. *Disability & Rehabilitation*, 34(3), 228–237.

Lindsay, S., Adams, T., Sanford, R., McDougall, C., Kingsnorth, S. & Menna-Dack, D. (2014a). Employers' and employment counselors' perceptions of desirable skills for entry-level positions for adolescents: How does it differ for youth with disabilities? *Disability & Society*, 29(6), 953–967.

Lindsay, S. & Cancelliere, S. (2018). A model for developing disability confidence. *Disability & Rehabilitation*, 40, 2122–2130.

Lindsay, S., Cagliostro, E., Albarico, M., Mortaji, N. & Srikathan, D. (2018a). Gender matters in the transition to employment for young adults with physical disabilities. *Disability & Rehabilitation* (in press).

Lindsay, S., Cagliostro, E., Albarico, M., Srikathan, D. & Mortaji, N. (2018b). Systematic review of the role of gender in finding and maintaining employment among youth and young adults with disabilities. *Journal of Occupational Rehabilitation*, 28, 634–685.

Lindsay, S., Cruickshank, H., McPherson, A. & Maxwell J. (2016a). Implementation of an inter-agency transition model for youth with spina bifida. *Child: Care, Health & Development*, 42(2), 203–212.

Lindsay, S. & Depape, A. (2015). Exploring differences in the content of job interviews between youth with and without a physical disability. *PlosOne*. http://journals.plos.org/plosone/article?id=10.1371/journal.pone.0122084.

Lindsay, S., Duncanson, M., Niles-Campbell, N., McDougall, C., Diederichs, S. & Menna-Dack, D. (2017a). Applying an ecological framework to understand transition pathways to post-secondary education for youth with disabilities. *Disability & Rehabilitation*, 40(3), 277–286.

Lindsay, S. & Edwards, A. (2013) A systematic review of disability awareness interventions for school-aged children. *Disability and Rehabilitation*, 35(8), 623–646.

Lindsay, S., Fellin, M., Cruickshank, H., McPherson, A. & Maxwell, J. (2016b). Youth and parent's experiences of an inter-agency transition model for spina bifida. *Disability & Health*, 9(4), 705–712.

Lindsay, S., Hartman, L. & Fellin, M. (2016c). A systematic review of mentorship interventions to improve school and work outcomes for youth with disabilities. *Disability & Rehabilitation*, 38, 1329–1349.

Lindsay, S., McAdam, L. & Mahenderin, T. (2017b). Enablers and barriers of men with Duchenne muscular dystrophy transitioning from an adult clinic within a pediatric hospital. *Disability & Health*, 10(1), 73–79.

Lindsay, S., McDougall, C., Menna-Dack, D., Sanford, R. & Adams, T. (2015a). An ecological approach to understanding barriers to employment for youth with disabilities compared to their typically developing peers: Views of youth, employers and job counselors. *Disability & Rehabilitation*, 37(8), 701–711.

Lindsay, S., McDougall, C. & Sanford, R. (2013). Disclosure, accommodations and self-care at work among people with disabilities. *Disability & Rehabilitation*, 35(26), 2227–2236.

Lindsay, S., McDougall, C. & Sanford, R. (2014b). Exploring supervisor's attitudes of working with youth engaged in an inclusive employment training program. *Journal of Human Development, Disability and Social Change*, 20(3), 12–20.

Lindsay, S., McDougall, C., Sanford, R., Menna-Dack, D., Kingsnorth, S. & Adams, T. (2015b). Exploring employment readiness through mock job interview and role-play exercises: Comparing youth with physical disabilities to their typically developing peers. *Disability and Rehabilitation*, 37(18), 1651–1663.

Lindsay, S., McPherson, A. & Maxwell, J. (2017c). Perspectives of school-work transitions among youth with spina bifida, their parents and health care providers. *Disability & Rehabilitation*, 39(7), 647–652.

Lindsay, S., Morales, E., Yantzi, N., Vincent C., Howell, L. & Edwards, G. (2015c). The experiences of participating in winter among youths with a physical disability compared to typically developing peers. *Child: Care, Health and Development*, 41(6), 980–988.

Lindsay, S., Proulx, M., Maxwell, J., Hamdani, Y., Bayley, M., Macarthur, C. & Colantonio, A. (2016d). Gender, transition from pediatric to adult health care among youth with acquired brain injury: Experiences in a transition model. *Archives of Physical Medicine and Rehabilitation*, 92(2), S33–S39.

Lindsay, S., Smith, S., Baker, R. & Bellaby, P. (2009). The health impact of an online heart disease support group: A comparison of moderated vs. unmoderated support. *Health Education Research*, 24(4), 646–654.

Liptak, G., Kennedy, J. & Nienke, D. (2010). Youth with spina bifida and transitions: Health and social participation in a nationally represented sample. *Journal of Pediatrics*, 157, 584–588.

Livingstone, D., Pollock, K. & Raykov, M. (2016). Family binds and glass ceilings: Women managers' promotion limits in a 'knowledge economy'. *Critical Sociology*, 42, 145–166.

Lustig, D. & Strauser, D. (2003). An empirical typology of career thoughts of individuals with disabilities. *Rehabilitation Counselling Bulletin*, 46, 98–107.

Magill-Evans, J., Galambos, N., Darrah, J. et al. (2008). Predictors of employment for young adults with developmental motor disabilities. *Work*, 31, 433–442.

Marshall, K. (2010). Employment patterns of postsecondary students. *Perspectives*. Statistics Canada. (75-001-X), 5–17.

Mattingly, M. & Blanchi, S. (2003). Gender differences in the quantity and quality of free time: The US experience. *Social Forces*, 81, 999–1030.

Morgan, P. & Lo, K. (2013). Enhancing positive attitudes towards disability: Evaluation of an integrated physiotherapy program. *Disability & Rehabilitation*, 35, 300–305.

Morse, J. (2004). Qualitative comparison: Appropriateness, equivalence and fit. *Qualitative Health Research*, 14(10), 1323–1325.

Morse, J. (2015). Critical analysis of strategies for determining rigor in qualitative inquiry. *Qualitative Health Research*, 25(9), 1212–1222.

Morse, J. M. & Mitcham, C. (2002). Exploring qualitatively-derived concepts: Inductive-deductive pitfalls. *International Journal of Qualitative Methods*, 1(4), 9.

O'Day, B. & Killeen, M. (2002). Research on the lives of persons with disabilities: The emerging importance of qualitative research methodologies. *Journal of Disability Policy Studies*, 13, 9–15.

Paniccia, A., Colquohoun, H., Kirsh, B. & Lindsay, S. (2018). Youth and young adults with acquired brain injury transition towards work-related roles: A qualitative study. *Disability & Rehabilitation*, 1–8.

Rathert, C., Wyrwich, M. & Boren, S. (2012). Patient-centered care and outcomes: A systematic review of the literature. *Medical Care Research and Review*, 70(4), 351–379.

Ridosh, M., Braun, P., Roux, G., Bellin, M. & Sawin, K. (2011). Transition in young adults with spina bifida: a qualitative study. *Child: Care, Health & Development*, 37(6), 866–874.

Ritchie, J., Lewis, J., McNaughton Nicolls, C. & Ormstrom, R. (2014). *Qualitative Research Practice.* London, UK: Sage.

Rodriquez, J. (2013). Narrating dementia: Self and community in an online forum. *Qualitative Health Research*, 23, 1215–1229.

Roebroeck, M., Jahnsen, R., Carona, C. et al. (2009). Adult outcomes and lifespan issues for people with childhood-onset physical disability. *Developmental Medicine & Child Neurology*, 51, 670.

Sawin, K., Bellin, M. & Roux, G. (2009). The experience of self-management in adolescent women with spina bifida. *Rehabilitation Nursing*, 34, 26–39.

Schiariti, V., Sauve, K., Klassen, A., O'Donnell, M., Cieza, A. & Masse, L. (2014). He does not see himself as being different: The perspectives of children and caregivers on relevant areas functioning in cerebral palsy. *Developmental Medicine & Child Neurology*, 56, 853–861.

Spiers, J. (2016). The pink elephant paradox (or, avoiding the misattribution of data). In: J. Morse, Editor. *Analyzing and Constructing the Conceptual and Theoretical Foundations of Nursing.* Philadelphia, PA: F. A. Davis.

Statistics Canada. (2006). Disability in Canada: A 2006 profile. Ottawa, Statistics Canada.

Sung, C., Sanchez, J., Kuo, H. et al. (2015). Gender differences in vocational rehabilitation service predictors of successful competitive employment for transition-aged individuals with autism. *Journal of Autism and Developmental Disorders*, 45, 3204–3218.

Tannenbaum, C., Greaves, L. & Graham, I. (2016). Why sex and gender matter in implementation research. *BMC Medicine Research Methodology*, 16, 145.

Thomas, J., Harden, A., Oakley, A., Oliver, S., Sutcliffe, K., Rees, R., Brunton, G. & Kavanagh, J. (2004). Integrating qualitative research with trials in systematic reviews. *British Medical Journal*, 328(7446), 1010–1012.

Tomlin, G. & Borgetto, B. (2011). Research pyramid: A new evidence-based model for occupational therapy. *American Journal of Occupational Therapy*, 65, 189–196.

Vaismoradi, M., Turunen, H. & Bondas, T. (2013). Content analysis and thematic analysis: Implications for conducting a qualitative descriptive study. *Nursing and Health Sciences*, 15, 398–405.

VanderKaay, S., Moll, S., Gewurtz, R., Jindal, P., Loyola-Sanchez, A., Packham, T. & Chun, Y. (2018). Qualitative research in rehabilitation science: Opportunities, challenges, and future directions. *Disability and Rehabilitation*, 40, 705–713.

van Mechelen, M., Verhoef, M., Van Asbeck, F. et al. (2008). Work participation among young adults with spina bifida in the Netherlands. *Developmental Medicine & Child Neurology*, 50, 772–777.

Zukerman, J., Devine, K. & Holmbeck, G. (2010). Adolescent predictors of emerging adulthood milestones in youth with spina bifida. *Journal of Pediatric Psychology*, 36, 265–276.

4

Unravelling the Irrational – Addressing the Subjective Nature of Sexual Risk-Taking through Qualitative Research

Simon Bishop

CONTENTS

Sex as a Risk Behaviour

Sex is something that most people engage in, particularly during the middle years of life. Although commonly a facet of long-term, romantic relationships, not all sex takes place within this context, some sex is casual, whilst yet more is distinctly commercial. The results of the 2010 British National Survey of Sexual Attitudes and Lifestyles suggest that, on average, 3.6% of British men and 0.1% of British women regularly choose to pay for sex (Mercer et al. 2007). Yet, whether practiced for procreation, recreation, or another social or economic purpose entirely, throughout recorded history this activity, a blissful pastime for so many, has walked hand-in-hand with disease and death (Taithe 2001).

Whenever we cross the street, get on our bicycle, or drive our car to work we are taking a risk. Yet most of us give little thought at all to these sorts of risks because they are familiar to us, lessened in their perceived danger because of their ubiquity (Thompson et al. 1990; Tansey and O'Riordan 1999). At apparent odds with logic, such contradiction between objectively real risk and subjectively perceived risk is present everywhere in our lives. From road travel, what we choose to eat, and with whom and how we choose to have sex, there is often a dissonance between what the numbers say about the risks that we take and how we understand and engage with these risks in practice. This is not to downplay the importance of numbers, of quantitative data, as they provide an excellent way to represent risk as a statistical probability and the only way to make robust inferences within and between populations (Bryman 2008). The problem is that quantitative data can only ever illuminate part of the picture, informed as they are by an epistemology that seeks to explain complex systems by reduction to their fundamental parts. Whilst of great utility in identifying at-risk groups, or particularly risky activities or behaviours, this approach is not well-equipped to engage with people's subjective understandings of risk, their motivations for taking risks, or the ways in which they might seek to mitigate such risks in their own mind. In seeking to grapple with this dissonance, this chapter engages with a very particular type of sexual risk (unprotected sex with commercial sex workers), practiced by a very particular group of people (Western male sex tourists to Thailand).

Sexually transmitted infections (STIs) represent an especially important challenge to good sexual health, collectively taking a substantial toll on the well-being of the world's population. The WHO (2016) suggests that more than a million new cases of sexually transmitted infections are contracted globally every day. A large proportion of these are bacterial infections, including syphilis, gonorrhoea, and chlamydia, all of which are usually curable with the use of antibiotics. Additionally, there are also a number of viral infections that can be transmitted sexually, such as genital herpes, human papilloma virus, and hepatitis B and C that are more difficult to manage clinically (Colson and Raoult 2016). However, it is the human immunodeficiency virus (HIV) that has had the greatest public health impact globally in recent years (Fairchild and Bayer 2011; Mykhalovskiy 2015), as it can lead, if untreated, to acquired immune deficiency syndrome and a premature death (Cooper et al., 2013). For those fortunate enough to be able to access it, the advent of highly active anti-retroviral therapy has meant that HIV has become a chronic disease, unlikely to significantly shorten life (Delpech 2013). However, infection, whilst not necessarily life-limiting anymore can still be life-changing, impacting on many of the psychological, physical, and social needs of those with the virus (Webel et al. 2014; Monteiro et al. 2016). The correct and consistent use of condoms has been shown to be highly effective at reducing the transmission of STIs, including HIV (Regan and Morisky 2013). Yet despite this, and for a variety of reasons, many people still do not use condoms, even when they have sex with multiple partners. Mercer et al. (2013) report that in 2010 in Britain, 7.6% of men and 4.9% of women had sex with two or more partners without using a condom – rates that were particularly high (up to 16.4%) amongst younger men. Since the emergence of the HIV pandemic in the 1980s, the United Kingdom (UK) government's attempts to protect the population from the threat of HIV/acquired immune deficiency syndrome have focused predominantly on promoting safer-sex through the use of condoms (Kippax and Race 2003). Yet despite these efforts, the prevalence of HIV has continued to rise amongst heterosexuals (Public Health England 2017). Through an analysis of the UK national HIV database, Rice et al. (2012) identified that roughly 15% of new HIV diagnoses in UK-born persons between 2002 and 2010 were acquired outside the UK, the highest number of these were found amongst men who had been infected in Thailand.

Sex Tourism, Risk and Rationalisation in Thailand

Thailand is located at the centre of the Indochina peninsula in Southeast Asia and is an important tourist hotspot in the region, attracting in excess of 35 million visitors each year (Reuters 2018). Most come to enjoy the vibrant cultural heritage and outstanding natural beauty that the country has to offer, however, Thailand also holds the rather unenviable reputation of being one of the most important global destinations for sex tourism (Williams 2002; Singh and Hart 2007). The term 'sex tourism' refers to the usually, although not exclusively, male practice of travelling overseas in order to participate in paid-for sexual activity with commercial sex workers (Mercer et al. 2007; Manieri et al. 2013). Although prostitution is technically illegal in Thailand (Khruakham and Lawton 2012), it contributes significantly to the economy and so remains widespread and highly visible.

Patpong and Soi Cowboy in Bangkok throng with go-go bars and massage parlours, as does Patong on the island of Phuket, and much of the city of Pattaya (Garrick 2005; Hobbs et al. 2011). In addition to this type of venue-based sex work, there are also large numbers of women working directly from the street in most towns and cities (Singh and Hart 2007). Of itself, this represents an important social problem for Thailand through the exploitation of largely poor, frequently disempowered Thai women who come from areas such as Isaan in the rural heart of the country (Crawford 2006). However, this situation is made worse because much of the paid-for sex that these women find themselves supplying takes place without the use of a condom, placing both themselves and their customers at risk of acquiring sexually transmitted infections, including HIV. During their study, Manieri et al. (2013) identified inconsistent condom use amongst groups of Swedish male sex tourists to Thailand, with 20% of those interviewed reporting their planned intention to engage in unprotected sex with female sex workers there. The study authors reported that, because of their average age (over 40), these men should have been exposed to the peak of government safer-sex messages during the 1990s, and yet no explanation for their contrary risk-taking behaviour was suggested.

Motivated by the absence of an explanation for a behaviour that appeared to suggest abject recklessness, in 2014, we participated in a piece of qualitative research designed to try to get a better understanding of the nature of sexual risk-taking by Western male sex tourists to Thailand (Bishop and Limmer 2017). Whilst some qualitative evidence already existed around exploring condom avoidance by men, most of this focused on men who have sex with men (Greene et al. 2014; Goldenberg et al. 2015) or men from economically or socially deprived backgrounds (Peterson et al. 2010; Bowleg et al. 2011; Limmer 2014). Yet limited attention had been given to understanding non-condom use amongst heterosexual men from less disadvantaged backgrounds, with sufficient affluence to be able to travel overseas and who were likely to be well-educated enough to be aware of the risks that they were taking. However, it was not just about the men, it was about the women too. The majority of safer sex interventions in Thailand to date have been geared towards trying to encourage female sex workers to use condoms with their clients (Wariki et al. 2012) and moderate success has been achieved through a combination of targeted health promotion advice and the distribution of free condoms (Treerutkuarkul 2010). However, the perennial problem is that in most commercial sexual transactions of this type, the power lies firmly with the demand-side of the arrangement, which is the men (Okal et al. 2011; Urada et al. 2012). Additionally, as many female sex workers in Thailand are trafficked for sex by a third-party with a vested interest in them, they are often subject to intimidation or violence should they fail to earn sufficient money (Decker et al. 2011). As a result, although some negotiation may be possible, there is a tremendous amount of pressure on these women to give in to demands for unprotected sex. Yet, whilst this may explain why some Thai female sex workers participate in unprotected sex with male sex tourists, it does not explain why any Western man would want to take the risk in the first place. Ironically, it emerged that many of the men in our study did not think that they were taking any real risk at all.

The study analysed data from two different sources, in-depth face-to-face interviews with Western men in Pattaya, Thailand and online discussion boards used by male sex tourists to share ideas and experiences between each other virtually. Across both these sources, men frequently reported engaging in unprotected sex with female sex workers in Thailand, primarily because they enjoyed the experience more without a condom. The most common arguments for not using condoms were that they numbed the pleasure, a view often expressed by men in other settings (Dove et al. 2006; Calabrese et al. 2012;

Geter and Crosby 2014), and that they stripped away the authenticity of having 'real' sex. Whilst men often sought to engage in unprotected sex with female sex workers, they were not ignorant of the fact that every time they did so they ran the risk of acquiring an STI. Collectively, this placed them between the 'rock' of not wanting to use a condom and the 'hard-place' of not wanting to contract an STI either. Whilst the majority of men acknowledged that engaging in unprotected sex with sex workers potentially carried some health risks, the perceived relevance and significance of these risks varied substantially. Oral sex was widely considered not to be a risk behaviour at all, and something that could be engaged in with impunity. Unprotected vaginal sex (referred to as 'barebacking') with sex workers was more contested, but there was an inescapable tension. Whilst most men considered participating in vaginal sex without the use of a condom to be a higher risk for STI transmission than oral sex, the fact remained that condoms were viewed very negatively, not as a source of protection, but as a barrier to pleasure. This tension between risk and pleasure underpinned negotiations around condoms that were driven by two broad considerations – firstly, the likelihood of contracting an STI from a sex worker as a result of participating in an unprotected sexual act, and, secondly, if this occurred, what impact the STI would have on their lives. Overall, although few men underplayed the seriousness of HIV as an STI, it was largely viewed as being a homosexual disease, which heterosexual men need not really fear. This made HIV a high consequence, but low probability infection for many of these men, they were aware that the disease could be devastating if contracted, but felt that there was very little risk of that actually happening to them.

Having largely rationalised themselves out of harm's way with regard to HIV, the men still had other STIs to deal with. Other viral infections, such as herpes or hepatitis B, did not figure within their narratives. Bacterial STIs such as gonorrhoea, however, were well known and the consequences familiar, with men frequently reporting having contracted one of these infections at some point in the past. In response to this threat, there were a number of protective strategies employed that were felt to be able to lower the odds of contracting an infection whilst still avoiding the need to use condoms. One of the simplest risk reduction strategies involved visual appraisal, either based on a woman's age (younger was considered safer) or else a subjective evaluation of their physical condition, with excessive thinness being associated with potential disease and something to be avoided. Beyond this physical appraisal, there was also a general sense of a geography of risk whereby sex workers from different venues were felt to have different degrees of sexual risk attached to them. Women who worked in bars and massage parlours were considered to pose the least risk as the belief was that they were subject to regular sexual health testing, although this was never evidenced beyond anecdote. There was sometimes an even more nuanced approach to this whereby some bars, particularly those with a Western owner, were considered to be safer than others by only employing sexually healthy women. The rationalisation here was that Western bar owners were particularly keen on ensuring that the sex workers operating from their venues were free of STIs in order to maintain a good reputation with their customers. In contrast, non-venue-based sex workers, typically those who worked from the street, were considered to be much higher risk than women from bars, they were not subject to the same sexual health checks that men believed venue-based sex workers were and, as such, represented an unknown, an uncontrolled, risk. Further, it was argued that as all sex workers would probably prefer to work in venues rather than being out on the street, the only logical reason why they were not doing so was that they were already carrying an STI and would fail the required sexual health checks. In Pattaya, the majority of non-venue-based sex workers congregate on Beach Road, a busy road along the Pattaya shoreline that was frequently referred to as the 'Coconut Bar' by interviewees due to the stands of coconut trees that frame its margins. Amongst most of the men interviewed, having sex with a sex worker from Beach Road was considered to present an unreasonably high-risk, and one which none openly admitted to taking.

Aware that their homebrewed screening systems remained fallible, there were additional steps that some men felt they could take in order to seek to mitigate their risks of contracting a bacterial infection once an appropriate partner had been selected. Washing of the genitals with vinegar or antiseptic, both prior to and following the sexual act, was one strategy believed to kill potentially harmful bacteria and allow for safer sex, as was the use of coconut oil as an antibacterial lubricant. The prophylactic use of the antibiotic azithromycin (Zithromax), available from pharmacists without prescription in Thailand, was also employed by men to permit planned unprotected sex with sex workers without fear of (bacterial) consequence. However, the most frequently reported method of reducing the risk of acquiring an STI was arguably the least scientifically credible and hinged solely on relabelling a sex worker to a girlfriend, and so recategorising them from high-risk to effectively no-risk. Across the data, but almost ubiquitously within the interviews in Pattaya, men argued that they were not really in Thailand for sex, but rather to find romantic love. They often recounted how they had met their present Thai 'girlfriend' or how long they had been together, occasionally sharing photographs carried around in their wallets. So common was the phenomenon of the Thai girlfriend amongst these men, that finding a sex tourist in Pattaya who did not profess to be, or to have been, in such a relationship represented a notable exception.

Across all of the data, it was clear that many of the Western male sex tourists in this study were relying on a complex and overlapping system of risk control strategies – some practical, others conceptual – that they felt reduced the health risks of engaging in unprotected sex. The question then arose as to where men acquired these beliefs, contrary as they were to all conventional health promotion messages that highlight risk and advocate condom use. In the end, it turned out that it was the views of other sex tourists, co-constructed and distributed internally, that were the primary source of risk information for these men. In addition to being social venues, bars also operated as informal centres of learning for systems of peer knowledge and practice (outside of Thailand the discussion boards fulfilled this purpose). Male sex tourists in Pattaya tended to spend much of the day drinking with each other in small, gender-homogenous groups, and it is in these settings that beliefs were reconstructed as knowledge and shared. The men privileged information acquired from peers over all other sources because it was considered to have been tried and tested, and so was demonstrably reliable. Of course they were aware of external health information and advice that warned them about the risks of having unprotected sex and advised them to use condoms, the problem was that these messages did not tally with their own experiences or with those of their peers (insider information). Several even considered government sexual health advice to be a way of trying to control their behaviour and stop them from doing what they wanted to. Consequently, information that came to them via mainstream media (outsider information), whether it was part of a health promotion campaign or simply a news story, was subordinated, distrusted as having ulterior motives.

There are a number of take-home messages to come from this study that may be usefully applied in attempting to increase condom usage amongst this, and perhaps other similar groups of men. To begin with, HIV needs to be reframed more clearly, not only as a homosexual disease, but as an infection that can be contracted by any sexually active person. Although this may appear obvious to many people, and has long been the central message of the majority of safer-sex campaigns (Kaye and Field 1997; Treerutkuarkul 2010), it was strongly contested here. Secondly, other STIs need to take more of a centre stage in the health promotion arena, emphasising perhaps the potential consequences of acquiring one of the emerging drug-resistant strains of gonorrhoea (WHO 2016), since this was a disease that these men felt more vulnerable to as heterosexuals. However, if this is the educational 'payload', more thought also needs to be given to the 'delivery system', as traditional lines of health communication were insufficient. Overall, very little weight was given by men to external health promotion messages, which were largely distrusted and so disregarded. A similar study conducted in Finland on men who engaged in paid-for sex with female sex workers (Regushevskaya and Tuormaa 2014) also found that condom use was not at all a concern among many there. As with the men in Thailand, wider health promotion messages that should have informed their behaviour were subverted by personal experience, and this subversion was then shared with other men via online discussion boards. For groups like these, where internally generated knowledge is valued far more highly than external knowledge, it seems clear that health promotion information needs to come from inside the community in order to be accepted within existing internal constructions of risk. Without this paradigm shift, the wider public health community may shout as loudly as it wants and still not be heard.

The Value of Qualitative Approaches in Sex Research

It is an empiricist fallacy (Roberts 1997) to suggest that only quantitative research conducted on participants, rather than qualitative research conducted with participants is the only way, or even the best way, to understand human behaviour. By its very nature, qualitative research seeks to explore and explain the world through an understanding of the subjective experiences of social actors. A qualitative approach is far better equipped to help us to unpick and begin to address sexual risk-taking behaviours, informed as it is directly by evidence from those taking the risks and not solely on assumptions made by others. It interrogates the relationship between knowledge, experience, and action, exploring the social factors that influence these interactions. Its pre-eminent strength, particularly when dealing with the subjective nature of social reality, stems from its premise that there is no single truth in terms of what and how we experience and understand our social world (Bryman 2008). Even the use of questionnaires, which often promise some degree of deeper understanding, are a poor tool for interrogating populations as the questions asked, and the language used, largely depends on the (potentially flawed) assumptions of the researcher. Whilst these may be mitigated to some extent by attempts at validation, they will always be born of the researcher and never of the subject. However, contrary to popular opinion, qualitative research is not the opposite of quantitative research, the concept of 'measurement' is not necessarily absent in the qualitative (Popay and Williams 1998). Qualitative methods may still measure things, albeit in a different way to quantitative approaches, with concepts often being identified as being more or less prominent within data. Ideas, concepts, or themes may even be physically counted in order to work out their relative importance within the overarching narrative, words such as 'more', 'less', 'better', or 'worse' may also crop up in qualitative data as measurements of the subjective. A perceived lack of generalisability has frequently been a concern, but although qualitative research may not be 'probabilistically generalisable', it is often 'logically generalisable' (Popay and Williams 1998), and it has been argued that one of the key measures for good qualitative research is that its findings should be transferable between similar populations

(Hammersley 1992). In terms of Western male sex tourists at least, this appears to be largely true, with condom avoidance, risk rationalisation, and the romanticisation of essentially commercial relationships being found across a variety of settings not just in Thailand, but as far apart as the Dominican Republic (Murray et al. 2007), Mexico (Syvertsen et al. 2015), and the Philippines (Regan and Morisky 2013). Qualitative approaches have also shown themselves to be particularly well suited to conducting studies on hard-to-reach at-risk populations, as well as being a way of identifying and understanding risk behaviours, because they typically seek to draw out embedded meanings rather than just collect 'facts' (Faugier and Sargeant 1997; Peterson et al. 2008; Dhalla and Poole 2011), focusing on the 'how' and the 'why' rather than merely on the 'what'. By exploring not just what people do, but also why they do what they do, allows such subjective and personal concepts to be interrogated and hopefully understood (Ailinger 2003). Only through this deeper understanding may robust health promotion interventions be tailored specifically to best fit the needs of the target group. Research into HIV, in particular, has highlighted the role of qualitative research in both understanding the social context of risk behaviours and for developing pragmatic recommendations for appropriate interventions (Rhodes 2000, Dowson et al. 2012; Rosen et al. 2018).

Qualitative evidence has been used effectively in several settings in order to guide and underpin sexual health interventions. The Women's CoOp HIV intervention described by Rosen et al. (2018) was designed to address the sexual risk behaviour of women prisoners who had experienced interpersonal violence. A qualitative approach was used in order to identify the attitudes, beliefs, and motivations of women – which included difficulty trusting, poor self-esteem, and poor self-care – and then used this information to develop an intervention designed to support women to make healthy choices. From their qualitative study on women in Iran, Khalesi et al. (2016) identified a variety of factors underpinning sexual risk, including issues around stigma and power, specifically the relative lack of power, including economic power, for women in sexual relationships with men. However, there were additional factors too more specific to the setting, such as the role of religion and fears that the legal system was not capable of protecting them against sexual abuse. Addressing a more specific aspect of sexual health, Evans et al. (2016) conducted a successful intervention designed to reduce HIV transmission by increasing the uptake of HIV testing that was underpinned by a community-based participatory social marketing design. The intervention was derived from evidence around social and structural barriers to HIV testing that was qualitative in nature and suggested a lack of trust and a fear of stigma, evidence that would have been extremely difficult to obtain quantitatively. Although each of these interventions was different, both in terms of their target populations and their subsequent approaches, they were all underpinned by qualitative research that allowed them to be tailored to precisely fit the needs of those that they sought to help. Simply telling these groups that they should use condoms, or be tested for HIV, because the epidemiological evidence demonstrated an objective benefit would not necessarily have been sufficient to change their behaviours. This is because these behaviours were also informed by structures, meanings, and interpretations that sat outside objective, external 'truths', and occasionally in direct opposition to them. Similarly, the men in our Thai study were well aware that they were supposed to use condoms, and in this sense were by no means ignorant, they just did not want to and were able to rationalise their way around the problem of STIs. This highlights the necessity of incorporating qualitative research into practice. In terms of the highly personal, private, and often hidden world of human sexuality, each different population that sits within the cross-hairs of a safer-sex intervention, whether they be Western male sex tourists to Thailand or female prisoners in the United States, will be different, although the overarching problem of sexual risk remains the same. Although an effective intervention may exist for one population, applying the same approach to a different population without really understanding and then adapting that intervention risks setting oneself up for failure, unique characteristics of a population, such as ethnicity, gender, age, language, or simply geography may change a situation entirely.

Conclusion

It is clear that we cannot understand the extent and scope of the problem of sexual risk-taking without good quantitative data, we need to know which populations are at risk and whether things are getting better or worse. However, only qualitative approaches have the power to get under the skin of the data, to explore the social worlds in which sexual risk-taking takes place, and really understand what is going on, and why. Any intervention aimed at tackling the problem of sexual risk taking, or arguably any other aspect of human behaviour, without a complete understanding of the ways in which behaviours and practices are constructed, understood, and performed risks being limited from the outset. As a consequence, qualitative research has much to offer the study of sexual risk-taking behaviour that can both complement quantitative approaches, as well as provide unique insights into the complex world of human sexuality in order to develop and refine future interventions. Ultimately, the devil is in the detail, and the detail, at least in terms of human behaviour, is only truly revealed in the qualitative. Without a rich and thorough understanding of those on the receiving end of our well-meaning health promotion efforts, we may develop interventions that risk being ineffective because they were based upon how we, rather than our target population, understand and engage with the world. What is necessary going forward is closer cooperation between qualitative researchers and practitioners across all aspects of health promotion programme design, implementation, and evaluation. For researchers, this will better ensure that evidence is generated from the specific setting of practice, for practitioners, it means that their practice will reflect the best and most relevant evidence available, whilst the populations at risk have the opportunity to benefit most of all.

References

Ailinger, R.L. (2003). Contributions of qualitative research to evidence-based practice in nursing. *Revista Latino-Americana de Enfermagem* 11(3): 275–279.

Bishop, S. and Limmer, M. (2017). Performance, power and condom use: Reconceptualised masculinities amongst Western male sex tourists to Thailand. *Culture, Health & Sexuality* 20(3): 276–228.

Bowleg, L., Teti, M., Massie, J.S., Patel, A., Malebranche, D.J. and Tschann, J.M. (2011). 'What does it take to be a man? What is a real man?': Ideologies of masculinity and HIV sexual risk among black heterosexual men. *Culture, Health and Sexuality* 13(5): 545–559.

Bryman, A. (2008). *Social Research Methods*, 3rd ed. Oxford, UK: Oxford University Press.

Calabrese, S., Reisen, C., Zea, M., Poppen, P. and Bianchi, F. (2012). The pleasure principle: The effect of perceived pleasure loss associated with condoms on unprotected anal intercourse among immigrant Latino men who have sex with men. *AIDS Patient Care and STDs* 26(7): 430–435.

Colson, P. and Raoult, D. (2016). Fighting viruses with antibiotics: An overlooked path. *International Journal of Antimicrobial Agents* 48(4): 349–352.

Cooper, A., García, M., Petrovas, C., Yamamoto, T., Koup, R.A. and Nabel, G.J. (2013). HIV-1 causes CD4 cell death through DNA-dependent protein kinase during viral integration. *Nature* 498(7454): 376–379.

Crawford, C. (2006). Cultural, economic and legal factors underlying trafficking in Thailand and their impact on women and girls from Burma. *Cardozo Journal of Law Gender* 12(3): 821–854.

Decker, M., McCauley, H., Phuengsamran, D., Janyam, S. and Silverman, J. (2011). Sex trafficking, sexual risk, sexually transmitted infection and reproductive health among female sex workers in Thailand. *Journal of Epidemiology and Community Health* 65(4): 334–339.

Delpech, V. (2013). The HIV epidemic: Global and UK trends. *Medicine* 41: 417–419.

Dhalla, S. and Poole, G. (2011). Motivators of enrolment in HIV vaccine trials: A review of HIV vaccine preparedness studies. *AIDS Care* 23(11): 1430–1447.

Dove, D.C., Rosengard, C., Morrow, K. and Stein, M.D. (2006). Understanding reasons for condom non-use among adolescents based on sexual frequency: A qualitative analysis. *Journal of Adolescent Health* 38(2): 124.

Dowson, L., Kober, C., Perry, N., Fisher, M. and Richardson, D. (2012). Why some MSM present late for HIV testing: A qualitative analysis. *AIDS Care* 24(2): 204–209.

Evans, C., Turner, K., Suggs, L.S., Occa, A., Juma, A. and Blake, H. (2016). Developing a mHealth intervention to promote uptake of HIV testing among African communities in the conditions a qualitative study. *BMC Public Health* 16: 656.

Fairchild, A.L. and Bayer, R. (2011). HIV surveillance, public health, and clinical medicine – Will the walls come tumbling down? *New England Journal of Medicine* 365(8): 685–687.

Faugier, J. and Sargeant, M. (1997). Sampling hard to reach populations. *Journal of Advanced Nursing* 26: 790–797.

Garrick, D. (2005). Excuses, excuses: Rationalisations of Western sex tourists in Thailand. *Current Issues in Tourism* 8: 497–509.

Geter, A. and Crosby, R. (2014). Condom refusal and young black men: The influence of pleasure, sexual partners, and friends. *Journal of Urban Health* 91(3): 541–546.

Goldenberg, T., Finneran, C., Andes, K.L. and Stephenson, R. (2015). 'Sometimes people let love conquer them': How love, intimacy, and trust in relationships between men who have sex with men influence perceptions of sexual risk and sexual decision-making. *Culture, Health and Sexuality* 17(5): 607–622.

Greene, G.J., Andrews, R., Kuper, L. and Mustanski, B. (2014). Intimacy, monogamy, and condom problems drive unprotected sex among young men in serious relationships with other men: A mixed methods dyadic study. *Archives of Sexual Behavior* 43(1): 73–87.

Hammersley, M. (1992). *What's Wrong with Ethnography? Methodological Explorations.* London, UK: Routledge.

Hobbs, J., Na, P.P. and Chandler, R.C. (2011). Advertising Phuket's nightlife on the Internet: A case study of double binds and hegemonic masculinity in sex tourism. *Sojourn* 26: 80–104.

Kaye, W. and Field, B. (1997). *Stopping AIDS: AIDS/HIV Education and the Mass Media in Europe.* London, UK: Longman.

Khalesi, Z.B., Simbar, M., Azin, S.A. and Zayeri, F. (2016). Public sexual health promotion interventions and strategies: A qualitative study. *Electron Physician* 8(6): 2489–2496.

Khruakham, S. and Lawton, B. (2012). Assessing the impact of the 1996 Thai prostitution law: A study of police arrest data. *Asian Journal of Criminology* 7(1): 23–36.

Kippax, S. and Race, K. (2003). Sustaining safe practice: Twenty years on. *Social Science & Medicine* 57(1): 1–12.

Limmer, M. (2014). The pressure to perform: Understanding the impact of masculinities and social exclusion on young men's sexual risk taking. *International Journal of Men's Health* 13(3): 184–202.

Manieri, M., Svensson, H. and Stafstrom, M. (2013). Sex tourist risk behaviour – An on-site survey among Swedish men buying sex in Thailand. *Scandinavian Journal of Public Health* 41: 392–397.

Mercer, C.H., Fenton, K.A., Wellings, K., Copas, A.J., Erens, B. and Johnson, A.M. (2007). Sex partner acquisition while overseas: Results from a British national probability survey. *Sexually Transmitted Infections* 83: 517–522.

Monteiro, F., Canavarro, M.C. and Pereira, M. (2016) Factors associated with quality of life in middle-aged and older patients living with HIV. *AIDS Care* 28(Suppl 1): 92–98.

Murray, L., Moreno, L., Rosario, S., Ellen, J., Sweat, M. and Kerrigan, D. (2007). The role of relationship intimacy in consistent condom use among female sex workers and their regular paying partners in the Dominican Republic. *AIDS and Behavior* 11(3): 463–470.

Mykhalovskiy, E. (2015). The public health implications of HIV criminalization: Past, current, and future research directions. *Critical Public Health* 25(4): 373–385.

Okal, J., Chersich, M., Tsui, S., Sutherland, E., Temmerman, M. and Luchters, S. (2011). Sexual and physical violence against female sex workers in Kenya: A qualitative enquiry. *AIDS Care* 23(5): 612–618.

Peterson, J.A., Reisinger, H.S., Schwartz, R.P., Mitchell, S.G., Kelly, S.M., Brown, B.S. and Agar, M.H. (2008). Targeted sampling in drug abuse research: A review and case study. *Field Methods* 20: 155–170.

Peterson, Z.D., Janssen, E. and Heiman, J.R. (2010). The association between sexual aggression and HIV risk behavior in heterosexual men. *Journal of Interpersonal Violence* 25(3): 538–556.

Popay, J. and Williams, G. (1998). Qualitative research and evidence-based healthcare. *Journal of the Royal Society of Medicine* 91(Suppl 35): 32–37.

Public Health England. (2017). *Towards Elimination of HIV Transmission, AIDS and HIV-Related Deaths in the UK.* London, UK: Public Health England.

Regan, R. and Morisky, D.E. (2013). Perceptions about HIV and condoms and consistent condom use among male clients of commercial sex workers in the Philippines. *Health Education & Behavior* 40(2): 216–222.

Regushevskaya, E. and Tuormaa, T. (2014). How do prostitution customers value health and position health in their discussions? Qualitative analysis of online forums. *Scandinavian Journal of Public Health* 42(7): 603–610.

Reuters. (2018). Thailand plans for even more tourists as numbers top 35 million [online]. Available at http://www.reuters.com/article/thailand-tourism/update-1-thailand-plans-for-even-more-tourists-as-numbers-top-35-million-idUSL3N1PB1XU (Accessed 7 May 2018).

Rhodes, T. (2000). The multiple roles of qualitative research in understanding and responding to illicit drug use. In Greenwood, G. and Robertson, K. (Eds.), *Understanding and Responding to Drug Use: The Role of Qualitative Research.* Luxembourg: Office for Official Publications of the European Communities, pp. 21–36.

Rice, B., Gilbart, V.l., Lawrence, J., Smith, R., Kall, M. and Delpech, V. (2012). Safe travels? HIV transmission among Britons travelling abroad. *HIV Medicine* 13: 315–317.

Roberts, H. (1997). Qualitative research methods in interventions in injury. *Archives of disease in childhood* 76(6): 487–489.

Rosen, R.K., Kuo, C., Gobin, R.L., Peabody, M., Wechsberg, W., Zlotnick, C. and Johnson, J.E. (2018). How qualitative methods contribute to intervention adaptation: An HIV risk reduction example. *Qualitative Psychology* 5(1): 2–15.

Singh, J.P. and Hart, S.A. (2007). Sex workers and cultural policy: Mapping the issues and actors in Thailand. *Review of Policy Research* 2: 155–173.

Syvertsen, J.L., Bazzi, A.R., Martinez, G., Rangel, M.G., Ulibarri, M.D., Fergus, K.B., Amaro, H. and Strathdee, S.A. (2015). Love, trust, and HIV risk among female sex workers and their intimate male partners. *American Journal of Public Health* 105: 1667–1674.

Taithe, B. (2001). Morality is not a curable disease: Probing the history of venereal diseases, morality and prostitution. *Social History of Medicine* 14(2): 337–350.

Tansey, J. and O'Riordan, T. (1999). Cultural theory and risk: A review. *Health, Risk & Society* 1(1): 71–90.

Thompson, M., Ellis, R. and Wildavsky, A. (1990). *Cultural Theory*. Boulder, CO: Westview Press.

Treerutkuarkul, A. (2010). Thailand's new condom crusade. *Bulletin of the World Health Organization* 88(6): 404–405.

Urada, L.A., Morisky, D.E., Pimentel-Simbulan, N., Silverman, J.G. and Strathdee, S.A. (2012). Condom negotiations among female sex workers in the Philippines: Environmental influences. *PloS one* 7(3): 1–9.

Wariki, W.M., Ota, E., Mori, R., Koyanagi, A., Hori, N. and Shibuya K. (2012). Behavioral interventions to reduce the transmission of HIV infection among sex workers and their clients in low- and middle-income countries. *Cochrane Database of Systematic Reviews* 12: CD006045.

Webel, A.R., Longenecker, C.T., Gripshover, B., Hanson, J.E., Schmotzer, B.J. and Salata, R.A. (2014). Age, stress, and isolation in older adults living with HIV. *AIDS Care* 26(5): 523–531.

Williams, W.L. (2002). Endangered relations: Negotiating sex and AIDS in Thailand. *American Ethnologist* 29: 1016–1017.

WHO. (2016). Sexually transmitted infections (STIs) [online]. Available at http://www.who.int/en/news-room/fact-sheets/detail/sexually-transmitted-infections-(stis) (Accessed 7 May 2018).

5

The Phenomenological Experience of Family Caregiving following Traumatic Brain Injury

Charles Edmund Degeneffe

CONTENTS

Introduction

A brain injury refers to damage to the brain occurring after birth and is not the result of congenital, degenerative, hereditary, or birth trauma aetiologies. Clinicians and researchers characterise brain injuries with the term 'acquired brain injury' (ABI), which includes both traumatic and non-traumatic forms of brain injury. A traumatic brain injury (TBI) refers to injuries caused by an external force to the head, such as gun-shot wounds or improvised explosive devices, whilst non-traumatic forms of injury can be due to non-traumatic causes such as strokes and drug overdoses (Brain Injury Association of America, 2018a). TBI is a pervasive disability throughout the world, resulting for many in life-long disability, employment restrictions, and reliance on caregivers to manage daily living needs.

Several national ABI advocacy organisations document the high numbers of citizens incurring ABI through reviews of available data sources in their respective countries. In the United Kingdom, Headway (2018) noted there were 348,934 ABI-related hospital admissions in 2013–2014, a 10% increase from 2005 to 2006. Brain Injury Australia (2016) highlighted the fact that three out of the four of the over 700,000 Australian citizens with ABI-related activity limitations and participation restrictions are under the age of 65 years. Brain Injury Canada (n.d.) indicated 160,000 Canadians experience ABI annually, with over a million living with life-long impairments associated with ABI. In the United States, the Brain Injury Association of America (2018b) reported over 3.5 million persons incur ABI each year, with 1 in 60 of those injured each year living with a TBI-related functional impairment.

On a long-term basis, many persons with TBI are able to recover sufficiently to be able to work, live independently, and re-engage with many of their pre-injury activities.

However, those with more severe levels of TBI-related disability need assistance from caregivers to meet daily support needs. Because of limited funding and insufficient services in the United States and other parts of the world, this responsibility often falls to family caregivers (Degeneffe & Lee, 2015). TBI can result in a variety of physical, psychological, and cognitive changes that can result in life-long and at times pervasive support needs. Family caregiving can range from limited support to around the clock responsibilities, attending to all of the injured family member's needs. In recognition of the magnitude of this responsibility, the consequences of family caregiving have received considerable and growing attention by TBI professionals and researchers over the past 20 to 30 years primarily through quantitatively-based research.

Quantitative studies primarily focus on the negative aspects of caregiving. Several examples are presented. In an early investigation, Allen, Linn, Gutierrez, and Willer (1994) examined burdens experienced by 60 spouse and 71 parent caregivers of persons with TBI. Using the Questionnaire on Resources and Stress-Short Form, both groups reported high levels of caregiver burden. Kreutzer and associates (2009) examined depression, anxiety, and somatic complaints amongst 273 family caregivers of persons with TBI supported by six Traumatic Brain Injury Model System Center programs in the United States. As measured with the Brief Symptom Inventory-18, approximately one in five caregivers met the criteria for clinically significant distress in each of these three domains. Norup and associates (2015) examined needs endorsed by family caregivers in Mexico, Colombia, Spain, Denmark, and Norway. Using the Family Needs Questionnaire, the greatest number of needs across the collective sample related to health information about TBI, whilst the greatest area of unmet needs related to emotional support.

Additionally, quantitative research advances professional understanding of common caregiver needs (Schaaf et al., 2013). It provides researchers the means to test (e.g., Chronister & Chan, 2006) the applicability of caregiving theories and models to ABI and develop instruments that best capture the ABI caregiver experience (e.g., Degeneffe, Chan, Dunlap, Man, & Sung, 2011). In summary, quantitative research provides valuable insights into the quality of life consequences of providing care and support to persons with TBI. It increases professional recognition of the vital role that families hold for the long-term care of their injured family members, providing motivation for the development of policy and programs to alleviate caregiver distress.

Whilst the contributions of quantitative methods are clear, this form of research is limited in understanding the subjectively experienced worlds of family caregivers. In TBI and other rehabilitation populations, qualitative research offers scholars and clinicians the tools to understand caregiving through a lens not possible in quantitative research. Qualitative research advances contextual understanding (Tate, 2006) informed by factors such as race/ethnicity, gender, social class, and country of origin. It offers researchers a means for better understanding reactions to the implementation of policies, interventions, and programs (Chwalisz, Shah, & Hand, 2008). Qualitative research presents a means for understanding human behaviour in naturalistic settings beyond the artificial parameters established in quantitative studies (Hagner, 2010). Qualitative research gives study participants voice to shape public and professional understanding based on life experiences and needs (Koch, Niesz, & McCarthy, 2014). Qualitative studies present a nuanced perspective that the disability experience reflects a broad range of potentially negative *as well as* positive experiences.

In counselling and rehabilitation contexts, clinicians and researchers increasingly recognise these positive aspects of qualitative methodologies as a systematic and scientifically grounded approach to research. Also, qualitative research is recognised for its utility in addressing the complex and idiosyncratic worlds of persons with disabilities and other client populations (Koch et al., 2014). Whilst the use of qualitative research continues to expand, its presence pales in comparison to the use of quantitative studies. Berríos and Lucca (2006) analysed all articles published in *Counseling and Values*, the *Journal of Counseling and Development*, *Professional School Counseling*, and *The Counseling Psychologist* between 1997 and 2002. Only 98 of the 593 research-based articles published during this period were qualitative. Hanley-Maxwell, Al Hano, and Skivington (2007) found that over a 30-year period, only 23 studies published in *Rehabilitation Counseling Bulletin* employed qualitative methods. Searching for qualitative research via the PsycINFO and MEDLINE databases with the search terms 'qualitative' and 'rehabilitation', Chwalisz and associates (2008) located only 151 studies using qualitative and 22 studies using mixed methods approaches.

Because of its limited use as a research approach, many clinicians and researchers do not appreciate the value of qualitative research to understand the disability experience. This lack of understanding extends to research addressing family caregiving and adjustment following TBI. The purpose of this chapter is to review and evaluate the extant use of qualitative methods in TBI family research. By doing so, readers will gain an enhanced understanding of the unique and subjectively lived experiences of family caregivers of persons with TBI. In the text that follows, three categories of qualitative studies will be reviewed by identifying common issues and unique perspectives. A review of data collection strategies, research sites, analytic strategies, and participants is provided. The chapter concludes by offering recommendations for policy, clinical intervention, and future research.

Qualitative Research and Family Caregiving Following TBI

The review of qualitative research started with the goal of identifying all published research in peer-reviewed journals *only* from the perspective of the family caregiver. In TBI and ABI family caregiver research, there are several qualitative studies offering shared perspectives from the family caregiver along with the injured family member (e.g., Willer, Allen, Liss, & Miriam, 1991) and/or professionals (Gan, Gargaro, Brandys, Gerber, & Boschen, 2010). Also, articles were limited to caregivers of persons with TBI, to not include other forms of ABI such as strokes. Because impairments can differ (e.g., Zhang et al., 2016) between those with TBI compared to persons with other forms of ABI, the focus on caregiving was limited to TBI.

By focusing specifically on the family caregiver, the following review offers a phenomenological perspective specific to the experience of caregiving and adjustment following TBI. Phenomenology refers to research that focuses on participant subjective experiences and meaning (Patten, 2012) of events unique in nature (Creswell, 2007). In the context of this chapter, providing care and support to an individual with TBI is offered as a lived experience unlike any other form of caregiving.

The search for articles was guided by the use of multiple databases, within journal searches, reviews of article reference sections, and the author's knowledge of available research. Databases included Communication Sciences and Disorders, EBSCO, PsycINFO, SAGE, Web of Science, ERIC, PubMed, Education Full Text, Academic Search Premier, and Social Services Abstracts. Multiple search terms were used that related broadly to ABI, TBI, qualitative research, chronic disability, families, and family caregiving.

Tables 5.1 through 5.3 present a summary view of all identified studies, including information on the study focus, participants, methodology, key findings, and authors.

TABLE 5.1

Caregiver Quality of Life and Personal Development

Study Focus	Participants	Methods	Key Findings	Authors
Caregiver reactions in the initial recovery period following TBI	12 female family caregivers of persons with TBI in Western Cape, South Africa	Semi-structured interviews/ thematic analysis	From the very beginning, family caregivers need support, education, and training.	Broodryk and Pretorius (2015)
Military-related caregiver health-related quality of life	45 caregivers of military-service members or veterans with TBI in Maryland, Michigan Tennessee, and Washington, United States	Focus groups/ frequency analysis	The most common concern was caregiver social health.	Carlozzi et al. (2016)
Caregiver health-related quality of life	55 caregivers in Michigan, New Jersey, and Texas, United States	Focus groups/ deductive and inductive analytic approach	The most common concern was caregiver social health.	Carlozzi et al. (2015)
Family system changes	277 adult siblings of persons with TBI, with 80.5% from the Midwest part of the United States	Open-ended survey question/constant comparative method of textual analysis	TBI can both compromise and strengthen family systems	Degeneffe, Gagne, and Tucker (2013)
Perceptions of quality of life for family member with TBI	279 adult siblings of persons with TBI, with 80% from the Midwest part of the United States	Open-ended survey question/ grounded theory	Siblings express deeply felt and well-informed views of the quality of life for their injured brothers and sister.	Degeneffe and Lee (2010)
Sibling life changes	272 adult siblings of persons with TBI from 23 U.S. states and one outside the United States	Open-ended survey question/ grounded theory	TBI can result in profound positive and negative life changes.	Degeneffe and Olney (2010)
Sibling experiences of living with a brother or sister with TBI	Eight adolescent or young adult siblings of persons with TBI in Ontario, Canada	McCracken's long-interview method/data analysis guided by family system theory	The siblings' lives are forever changed.	Gill and Wells (2000)
Caregiving experiences of family caregivers	15 primary caregivers of persons with TBI in Japan	Semi-structured interviews/ Berelson method of content analysis	Caregiving includes both positive and negative dimensions	Ishikawa et al. (2011)

(Continued)

TABLE 5.1 (*Continued*)

Caregiver Quality of Life and Personal Development

Study Focus	Participants	Methods	Key Findings	Authors
Caregiver quality of life	52 caregivers in Michigan, New Jersey, and Texas, United States	Focus groups/ thematic content analysis and matrix analysis injured family member.	Quality of life is determined by role demands and changes with	Kratz et al. (2017)
Family member meaning of living with someone with TBI	11 close relatives of persons with moderate of severe TBI in Sweden	Qualitative research interviews/ phenomenological hermeneutic interpretation	Family members are challenged by own emotional reactions while also showing compassion for the injured family member.	Jumisko, Lexell, and Soderberg (2007)
Transition from the hospital to the community	10 family caregivers of persons with TBI discharged from 7 to 12 months after community reentry	Semi-structure interviews/ framework approach	Caregivers wished to move past the injury.	Nalder et al. (2012)
The maternal experience of parenting a young adult child with TBI	Seven mothers of young adults with TBI, injured from 8 months to 20 years	Conducted three neutral open-ended questions/ phenomenological data analysis methods	Each mother's experience was unique.	Wongvatunyu and Porter (2008)
Caregiver perceptions of change in themselves and the injured family member	Nine family caregivers from three families of persons with TBI	Three unstructured narrative interviews/Life Thread Model	Caregivers are agents of making change for themselves and their injured family members	Whiffin, Ellis-Hill, Bailey, Jarrett, and Hutchinson (2017)

Participant geographical information is provided when specifically identified by authors. Methods include the studies' primary data collection and analytic strategy. A total of 22 studies were found, published from 1993 to 2017, with most studies (n = 18; 81.8%) published since 2007. A majority of the studies (n = 13; 59.1%) employed individual interviews, whilst other data collection approaches included open-ended survey responses (n = 5; 22.7%) and focus groups (n = 4; 18.2%). Authors differed on the extent to which they identified analytic strategies, but most described some form of thematic, content, grounded theory, phenomenological, and/or constant comparative analysis. Specific countries participants were drawn from included Australia, Canada, Japan, New Zealand, South Africa, Sweden, the United Kingdom, and the United States. Most articles were published in nursing (n = 5; 22.7%) and brain injury (n = 5; 22.7%) journals.

In the introductory section of each article, authors described phenomenologically guided motivations to provide readers an understanding of the family caregiving experience not

TABLE 5.2

Family Role Specific Experiences

Study Focus	Participants	Methods	Key Findings	Authors
Parent's experience following TBI	Parents from 20 families with the person with TBI living with at least one parent	Semi-structured interviews/ grounded theory	Parents cope with TBI through a three-phrase process of providing care, fostering independence, and seeking stability	Carson (1993)
Sibling future concerns	280 adult siblings of persons with TBI from 24 U.S. states and one outside the United States	Open-ended survey question/grounded theory	The two most common concerns were the future recovery their injured siblings would obtain and their roles as future caregivers	Degeneffe and Olney (2008)
Marital relationship stability	Five male and five female spouses of persons with TBI	Two gender-specific focus groups/ constructivist approach to grounded theory	Post-TBI marital relationships can pull closer together or apart	Hammond et al. (2011)
Spouse/partner decision-making	Four spouses/partners of persons with severe TBI in the Eastern states of Australia	Two in-depth interviews with each participant/ constructivist approach to grounded theory	Decision-making is largely directed by the non-injured spouse	Knox et al. (2015)

previously examined or poorly understood. Authors described how qualitative methods gave families a voice not previously heard and took readers into the inner-world experiences of caregiving. Consistent across many articles was the need to justify the use of qualitative methods instead of traditional quantitative methods. For example, Kratz, Brickell, Lange, and Carlozzi (2017) argued:

> Qualitative methodology is well-suited to examine the complex lived experiences and perspectives of caregivers of individuals with TBI. In contrast to a quantitative approach where the investigator determines what is important to study (e.g., anxiety, depression), a qualitative approach allows the caregivers to describe and define what is important in their lives.

The collective set of articles described in Tables 5.1 through 5.3 provide a greater understanding of the *how* and *why* of family caregiving beyond the *what* (i.e., outcomes) focused on in most quantitative research. Studies were categorised by key findings into one of three areas including: (a) caregiver quality of life and personal development, (b) family role specific experiences, and (c) opinions on professional services. The following section describes and summarises each section of research.

TABLE 5.3

Opinions on Professional Services

Study Focus	Participants	Methods	Key Findings	Authors
Perceptions of the quality of professional services	267 adult siblings of persons with TBI from 23 U.S. states and one outside the United States	Open-ended survey question/constant comparison of textual analysis	Professional and service-system support is largely inadequate	Degeneffe and Bursnall (2015)
Perspectives on the service system	Eight primary family caregivers of persons with TBI in Canada	Semi-structured interviews/content analysis using NUD*IST	Caregivers did not want to give up this role but needed more support.	Smith and Smith (2000)
Responding to challenging behaviors	Six female relatives of persons with TBI in Melbourne, Australia	Interviews guided by three open-ended questions/thematic analysis	Family members had a broader understanding of challenging behaviors than professionals.	Tam et al. (2015)
Experiences of caregivers of young children who incurred TBI	21 caregivers of 15 children who incurred TBI before two years of age in Auckland, New Zealand	Semi-structured interviews/thematic analysis	Additional stress occurred because of lack of information, difficulty in accessing services, and inconsistent care.	Wharewera-Mika et al. (2016)
Mothers' experiences in helping young adults with TBI	Seven mothers of young adults with TBI in Missouri, United States	Three in-depth interviews with each mother/descriptive phenomenological method	The mothers continued their rehabilitation efforts with their children even with minimal support.	Wonngvatunyu and Porter (2005)

Caregiver Quality of Life and Personal Development

Consistent with the majority of quantitative articles that focus on negative outcomes such as stress, burden, and depression, most qualitative studies (n = 13; 59.1%) on family caregiving after TBI examine the underlying reasons for these responses. Authors examined these outcomes from multiple and interrelated perspectives, including caregiver quality of life, changed relationships, and personal development. Participants described caregiving and family response from a nuanced perspective that highlighted a range of negative to positive experiences. Authors provided results-guided recommendations on needed professional supports and interventions.

With regard to quality of life, researchers provided insights into caregiver burden, health, and perceptions of life satisfaction. A common thread across this area of research concerns how caregiving limits the ability to attend to positive health-related behaviours. For example, in two studies led by Carlozzi et al. (2015, 2016), family caregivers (parents, spouses/partners, children, siblings) in focus group discussions indicated their social health was most affected with regard to such areas as giving up careers, experiencing family disruption, and not performing pre-injury family roles, such as child or spouse. Through the development of a conceptual quality of life model developed by Carlozzi and her colleagues, both studies also described the quality of life implications of caregiving with regard to emotional, physical/medical, cognitive function, and feelings of loss outcomes.

Authors described how the relationship to the injured family member changed following TBI. Several studies shared how family caregivers engaged in a grieving process as they mourned the person they knew before TBI and learned new ways of understanding their injured family member. For example, Gill and Wells (2000) shared how a sibling could no longer socialise the same way with his brother with TBI:

> I'll say hello to him. Usually we have dinner together, but that's about it. I hung out with him a lot before his accident. We were close. It's just a disappointment. I'm a lot closer with his friends now. I should spend more time with him, but it's hard to hang out with someone who doesn't do the same things you do. (p. 51)

In talking about their injured family members, caregivers conveyed deep emotions such as guilt, anger, and sadness. For example, an adult sibling in a study by Degeneffe and Lee (2010) commented on her brother's limitations to live a happy and productive life:

> He wants so badly to get a job, to meet someone and have a family, and to get his driver's license. He will never be able to get his driver's license because of his behaviour and his physical disabilities. I don't know if he will ever find a job that works out, also because of his behaviour. Who knows, he may meet someone one day, but right now, he is so lonely. (p. 32)

Different than the focus of most quantitative studies, several studies described the positive dimensions of TBI. Caregivers discussed their ability to cope, draw on family and personal strengths, and achieve insights into personal values and goals. For example, Ishikawa, Suzuki, Okumiya, and Shimizu (2011) identified ways in which caregivers (parents and wives) were able to facilitate the involvement of family and friends to provide caregiving help. They also discussed how caregivers productively channelled energy into providing peer support and advancing public understanding of TBI. Also, Degeneffe and Olney (2010) described how adult siblings of persons with TBI experienced profound insights regarding spirituality and the development of new life goals and personal values.

Family Role Specific Experiences

Four studies focused on roles, experiences, and concerns specific to the family member type. These studies examined family caregiving processes and outcomes via perspectives particular to each family role. The inference of these studies is that TBI affects family members uniquely as a function of the nature of the relationship to the family member with TBI.

From a parent perspective, Carson (1993) guided interviews amongst parents from 20 families of persons with TBI (aged 17 to 35 years) with the question (p. 166), 'Tell me about your experiences since your child returned to the home setting'. Carson described how parents engaged in an intense process of providing care, reorganising their lives, fostering independence for their children with TBI, and coping with stresses and demands. Carson also discussed changes specific to the parental role, such as limited ability to attend to the needs of their other children and re-evaluating future plans. For example, in discussing retirement, one parent shared (p. 172), 'I think we're going to have a real different retirement than a lot of people do. We've really never talk about her not being with us'.

Two studies examined spousal/partner relationships following TBI. Both studies highlighted changed roles, communication patterns, and post-injury relationship quality. In a study of four spouses/partners of persons with TBI, Knox, Douglas, and Bigby (2015) focused on decisions the non-injured spouse/partner makes on behalf of the injured spouse/partner. Non-injured spouses/partners made almost all decisions for the family, and the ability to make decisions was enhanced by attending to the quality of the relationship, effective communication, and ability to see the injured person in a positive light. Through two gender-specific focus groups, Hammond, Davis, Whiteside, Philbrick, and Hirch (2011) examined relationship stability amongst 10 spouses of persons with TBI. Wives and husbands differently viewed caregiving responsibilities. Spouses described a variety of challenges with trust, communication, emotional attachment, changes with the injured spouse, and relationships becoming closer or pulling apart.

A fourth study examined future concerns amongst adult siblings of persons with TBI. Degeneffe and Olney (2008) asked (p. 240) a national sample of 280 adult siblings, 'What are your concerns regarding the future for your sibling with TBI?' Siblings shared impassioned concerns for the future health and welfare of their injured brothers and sisters. Specific to their role as siblings, participants also conveyed deep concerns about future caregiving responsibilities once parents were no longer able to serve in this role:

> While my parents are my sister's main caregivers, she will outlive them. As the only sibling, I will have to care for her. Will she be able to live on her own 2,000 miles aware from me? In addition to her, will there be other family members to take care of in later years? (p. 245)

Opinions on Professional Services

The third research area (five studies) addressed the quality and availability of long-term services following TBI. Studies ranged from 2000 to 2016 with participants living in Australia, Canada, New Zealand, and the United States. Participants included mothers, fathers, sisters, brothers, grandparents, and a spouse. Care recipients included those injured before the age of 2 years through adolescence and then adulthood. Despite these differences, the studies were consistent in noting the lack of long-term, community-based supports to meet the demands of caregiving. In some cases, families were pleased with professional services, however, more commonly participants felt professional services were unavailable, inconsistent, ineffective, and/or not respectful of family views and participation. Also, families were committed to providing long-term care, but at times felt they were on their own in doing so.

In one of the first studies focused on family caregiver views following TBI, Smith and Smith (2000) interviewed eight primary family caregivers of persons with TBI in Canada on their experiences navigating the service system. Care recipients resided in the community and had lived with TBI from 2 to 9 years. Participants complained of doctors who only conveyed negative information about their injured family member's deficits and prognosis. Participants experienced great difficulty navigating the service system and felt unprepared for the home return of family members with TBI in responding to their emotional problems. Participants lacked information about care decisions and often needed to advocate for the best interests of their family members with TBI with healthcare and rehabilitation services.

Since the publication of Smith and Smith's (2000) study, findings in the other four studies were in many ways consistent. Examples from the remaining studies are provided. In a study of seven mothers of young adults with TBI in the United States, Wongvatunyu and Porter (2005, p. 1068) shared how several participants felt doctors overly focused on the negative, 'Don't always listen to what the doctor tells you. They tell you the worst-case scenario'. In their study of 267 adult siblings of persons with TBI in the United States, Degeneffe and Bursnall (2015, p. 21) described struggles participants encountered in navigating the service system and shared that some siblings '...found the process difficult because of confusing, impersonal, and arbitrary approaches in service delivery'. Tam, McKay, Sloan, and Ponsford (2015, p. 7) addressed how six female caregivers (four mothers, one spouse, and one sister) responded to providing care to family members with TBI with challenging behaviours. Some participants addressed the lack of respite to give them a break from the demands of caregiving, 'More help with out of home respite, definitely, which we don't get. That would help a hundred times' (Mother). In their study of 21 caregivers (mothers, fathers, grandparents, and others) of children who incurred TBI before the age of two years in New Zealand, Wharewera-Mika, Cooper, Kool, Pereira, and Kelly (2016, p. 275) discussed how participants were not prepared for the home return of their injured child. One participated shared, 'We were overwhelmed with people for the first 6 months and then nothing (010)'.

Research and Policy Implications

The extant literature presenting family views on caregiving for a person with TBI yields important implications to guide future research and policy. Three areas of focus were found in the areas of: (a) caregiver quality of life and personal development, (b) family role specific experiences, and (c) opinions on professional services. In comparison to studies examining family caregiving following TBI from a quantitative perspective, only 22 studies utilised qualitative methods. To illustrate this disparity, of the 3142 research articles published in *Brain Injury* from 1987 (volume 1, issue 1) through 2018 (volume 32, issue 5), only three articles in the present review were published. Also, in the *Journal of Head Trauma Rehabilitation*, only one article in the present review was published amongst the 1,413 research articles published from 1986 (volume 1, issue 1) through 2018 (volume 32, issue 6). Clearly, researchers need to do more to capture family voices to understand their unique perspectives and experiences following TBI.

Whilst the available research provides clinicians, researchers, and the public important insights and information, there are many areas of the TBI family caregiver experience not yet addressed. With the exception of Japan (Ishikawa et al., 2011) and South Africa (Broodryk & Pretorius, 2015), most studies are based on the views on largely white participants from affluent countries like Australia and the United States. Missing are the perspectives of family caregivers from countries in Latin America, Asia, and Africa, incorporating racial and ethnic populations holding different views towards caregiving based on cultural norms, family structures, and economic status.

Qualitative research has not yet addressed the family experience in several areas of emerging professional and public interest. With the massive and worldwide prevalence of armed conflicts (Amnesty International, 2018), qualitative research is needed that gives voice to the civilian and military service member/veteran family caregiver experience following TBI caused by bombs, gunfire, and improvised explosive devices. To date, only one study in the present view (Carlozzi et al., 2016) focused on families of military service members or veterans with TBI. Also, with growing awareness of the connection between concussive and sub-concussive injuries with chronic traumatic encephalopathy (CTE) due to participation in sports like American football, rugby, and boxing (Solomon and Zuckerman, 2015), qualitative research is needed to generate insights into how families adjust and adapt over time to the progressive nature of CTE. Finally, falls are the second leading global cause of unintentional injury or death, with age being a primary risk factor for falls (World Health Organization, 2018). In the United States, from 2009 to 2010, persons over the 65 had the highest rate of TBI-related emergency department visits (Centers for Disease Control and Prevention, 2016). Qualitative research could, for example, examine how adult children adapt to meeting the needs of aging parents with TBI.

The articles in Table 5.3 found consensus across countries, family member types, and time since the onset of TBI regarding the lack of availability and quality of long-term TBI services and professionals. However, the potential of these studies to influence professional training, public policy, and service expenditures is little to none given the neglect of this area in qualitative TBI family caregiver research. Researchers need to use qualitative research to document the real costs of caregiving in an environment of insufficient services and poor professional preparation. Hearing the stories and real-life experiences of family caregivers can be more compelling to administrators, clinicians, policymakers, politicians, and the general public than simply relying on statistics and quantitative data.

Studies reviewed in Tables 5.1 through 5.3 were published in brain injury, nursing, social work, and rehabilitation journals. Qualitative research is needed beyond a human service focus to extend to academic disciplines better able to explore the economic, cultural, and policy implications of family caregiving following TBI, such as economics, anthropology, sociology, disability studies, and public health. An expanded scholarly focus holds promise for influencing the development of public policies and expenditures designed to reduce caregiver stress, develop targeted interventions, and maximise the quality of life for caregivers and their family members with TBI.

Conclusion

Following TBI, families provide a range of care and support. This role provides families a phenomenological experience unlike any other form of caregiving following disability or chronic illness. Most research on families of persons with TBI examines outcomes from a quantitative perspective. As reviewed in this chapter, qualitative research goes beyond the limitations of quantitative methods by giving readers an insider perspective on the experiences, needs, and negative and positive changes that emerge from this unique experience.

References

Allen, K., Linn, R. T., Gutierrez, H., & Willer, B. S. (1994). Family burden following traumatic brain injury. *Rehabilitation Psychology, 39*(1), 29–48.

Amnesty International. (2018). *Armed conflict.* Retrieved from https://www.amnesty.org/en/what-we-do/armed-conflict/ (Accessed 26 April 2018).

Berríos, R., & Lucca, N. (2006). Qualitative methodology in counselling research: Recent contributions and challenges for a new century. *Journal of Counseling & Development, 84*(2), 174–186.

Brain Injury Association of America. (2018a). *Brain injury overview.* Retrieved from https://www.biausa.org/brain-injury/about-brain-injury/basics/overview (Accessed 3 April 2018).

Brain Injury Association of America. (2018b). *Fact sheet.* Retrieved from https://www.biausa.org/public-affairs/public-awareness/campaigns/fa (Accessed 3 April 2018).

Brain Injury Australia. (2016). *About brain injury.* Retrieved from https://www.braininjuryaustralia.org.au/

Brain Injury Canada. (n.d.). *Brain injury info.* Retrieved from https://www.braininjurycanada.ca/acquired-brain-injury/ (Accessed 3 April 2018).

Broodryk, M., & Pretorius, C. (2015). Initial experiences of family caregivers of survivors of a traumatic brain injury. *African Journal of Disability, 4*(1), 1–7.

Carlozzi, N. E., Kratz, A. L., Sander, A., Chiaravalloti, N. D., Brickell, T., Lange, R., Tulsky, D. S. (2015). Health-related quality of life in caregivers of individuals with traumatic brain injury: Development of a conceptual model. *Archives of Physical Medicine and Rehabilitation, 96*(1), 105–113.

Carlozzi, N., Brickell, T., French, L., Sander, A., Kratz, A., Tulsky, D., Lange, R. (2016). Caring for our wounded warriors: A qualitative examination of health-related quality of life in caregivers of individuals with military-related traumatic brain injury. *Journal of Rehabilitation Research and Development, 53*(6), 669–680.

Carson, P. (1993). Investing in the comeback: Parent's experience following traumatic brain injury. *Journal of Neuroscience Nursing, 25*(3), 165–173.

Centers for Disease Control and Prevention [CDC]. (2016). *Rates of tBI-Related Emergency Department Visits by Age Group.* Retrieved from https://www.cdc.gov/traumaticbraininjury/data/rates_ed_byage.html (Accessed 26 April 2018).

Chronister, J., & Chan, F. (2006). A stress process model of caregiving for individuals with traumatic brain injury. *Rehabilitation Psychology, 51*(3):190–201.

Chwalisz, K., Shah, S.R., & Hand, K. M. (2008). Facilitating rigorous qualitative research in rehabilitation psychology. *Rehabilitation Psychology, 53*(3), 387–399.

Creswell, J. (2007). *Qualitative Inquiry & Research Design: Choosing Among Five Approaches* (2nd ed.). Thousand Oaks, CA: Sage.

Degeneffe, C. E., & Bursnall, S. (2015). Quality of professional services following traumatic brain injury: Adult sibling perspectives. *Social Work, 60*, 19–28.

Degeneffe, C. E., & Lee, G. (2015). Brain injury and the family. A guide for rehabilitation counselors. In M. Millington & I. Marini (Eds.), *Families in Rehabilitation Counseling: A Community-Based Rehabilitation Approach* (pp. 153–170). New York: Springer Publishing.

Degeneffe, C. E., & Olney, M. F. (2008). Future concerns of adult siblings of persons with traumatic brain injury. *Rehabilitation Counseling Bulletin, 51*(4), 240–250.

Degeneffe, C. E., & Olney, M. F. (2010). 'We are the forgotten victims': Perspectives of adult siblings of persons with traumatic brain injury. *Brain Injury, 24*(12), 1416–1427.

Degeneffe, C. E., Chan, F., Dunlap, L., Man, D., & Sung, C. (2011). Development and validation of the caregiver empowerment scale: A resource for working with family caregivers of persons with traumatic brain injury. *Rehabilitation Psychology, 56*(3), 243–250.

Degeneffe, C. E., Gagne, L. M., & Tucker, M. (2013). Family systems changes following traumatic brain injury: Adult sibling perspectives. *Journal of Applied Rehabilitation Counseling, 44*, 32–41.

Degeneffe, C.E., & Lee, G. (2010). Quality of life after traumatic brain injury: Perspectives of adult siblings. *Journal of Rehabilitation, 76*(4), 27–36.

Gan, C., Gargaro, J., Brandys, C., Gerber, G., & Boschen, K. (2010). Family caregivers' support needs after brain injury: A synthesis of perspectives from caregivers, programs, and researchers. *NeuroRehabilitation, 27*(1), 5–18.

Gill, D. J., & Wells, D. L. (2000). Forever different: Experiences of living with a sibling who has a traumatic brain injury. *Rehabilitation Nursing, 25*(2), 48–53.

Hagner, D. (2010). The role of naturalistic assessment in vocational rehabilitation. *Journal of Rehabilitation, 76*(1), 28–34.

Hammond, F. M., Davis, C. S., Whiteside, O. Y., Philbrick, P. A., & Hirsch, M. (2011). Marital adjustment and stability following traumatic brain injury: A pilot qualitative analysis of spouse perspectives. *Journal of Head Trauma Rehabilitation, 26*(1), 69–78.

Hanley-Maxwell, C., Al Hano, I., & Skivington, M. (2007). Qualitative research in rehabilitation counseling. *Rehabilitation Counseling Bulletin, 50*(2), 99–110.

Headway – The Brain Injury Association. (2018). *Statistics*. Retrieved from https://www.headway.org.uk/about-brain-injury/further-information/s (Accessed 3 April 2018).

Ishikawa, F., Suzuki, S., Okumiya, A., & Shimizu, Y. (2011). Writers' award winner experiences of family members acting as primary caregivers for patients with traumatic brain injury. *Rehabilitation Nursing: The Official Journal of the Association of Rehabilitation Nurses, 36*(2), 73–82.

Jumisko, E., Lexell, J., & Söderberg, S. (2007). Living with moderate or severe traumatic brain injury. *Journal of Family Nursing, 13*(3), 353–369.

Knox, L., Douglas, J., & Bigby, C. (2015). 'The biggest thing is trying to live for two people': Spousal experiences of supporting decision-making participation for partners with TBI. *Brain Injury, 29*(6), 745–757.

Koch, L., Niesz, T., & McCarthy, H. (2014). Understanding and reporting qualitative research. *Rehabilitation Counseling Bulletin, 57*(3), 131–143.

Kratz, A., Sander, A., Brickell, T., Lange, R., & Carlozzi, N. (2017). Traumatic brain injury caregivers: A qualitative analysis of spouse and parent perspectives on quality of life. *Neuropsychological Rehabilitation, 27*(1), 16–37.

Kreutzer, J.S., Rapport, L.J., Marwitz, J.H., Harrison-Felix, C., Hart, T., Glenn, M., & Hammond, F. (2009). Caregivers' well-being after traumatic brain injury: A multicenter prospective investigation. *Archives of Physical Medicine and Rehabilitation, 90*(6), 939–946.

Nalder, E., Fleming, J., Cornwell, P., & Foster, M. (2012). Linked lives: The experiences of family caregivers during the transition from hospital to home following traumatic brain injury. *Brain Impairment, 13*(1), 108–122.

Norup, A., Perrin, P., Cuberos-Urbano, G., Anke, A., Andelic, N., Doyle, S., Carlos Arango-Lasprilla, J. (2015). Family needs after brain injury: A cross cultural study. *NeuroRehabilitation, 36*(2), 203–214.

Patten, M. L. (2012). *Understanding research methods* (8th ed.). Glendale, CA: Pyrczak Publishing.

Schaaf, K. W., Kreutzer, J. S., Danish, S. J., Pickett, T. C., Rybarczyk, B. D., Nichols, M. G., & Wegener, S. (2013). Evaluating the needs of military and veterans' families in a polytrauma setting. *Rehabilitation Psychology, 58*(1), 106–110.

Smith, J. E., & Smith, D. L. (2000). No map, no guide: Family caregivers' perspectives on their journeys through the system. *Care Management Journals, 2*(1), 27.

Solomon, G. S., & Zuckerman, S. L. (2015). Chronic traumatic encephalopathy in professional sports: Retrospective and prospective views. *Brain Injury, 29*(2), 164–170.

Tam, S., McKay, A., Sloan, S., & Ponsford, J. (2015). The experience of challenging behaviours following severe TBI: A family perspective. *Brain Injury, 29*(7–8), 813–821.

Tate, D. (2006). The state of rehabilitation research: Art or science? *Archives of Physical Medicine and Rehabilitation, 87*(2), 160–166.

Wharewera-Mika, J., Cooper, E., Kool, B., Pereira, S., & Kelly, P. (2016). Caregivers' voices: The experiences of caregivers of children who sustained serious accidental and non-accidental head injury in early childhood. *Clinical Child Psychology and Psychiatry, 21*(2), 268–286.

Whiffin, C., Ellis-Hill, C., Bailey, C., Jarrett, N., & Hutchinson, P. (2017). We are not the same people we used to be: An exploration of family biographical narratives and identity change following traumatic brain injury. *Neuropsychological Rehabilitation*, 1–17. doi:10.1080/09602011.2017.1387577.

Willer, B., Allen, K., Liss, M., & Zicht, M. (1991). Problems and coping strategies of individuals with traumatic brain injury and their spouses. *Archives of Physical Medicine and Rehabilitation, 72*(7), 460–464.

Wongvatunyu, S., & Porter, E. (2005). Mothers' experience of helping young adults with traumatic brain injury. *Journal of Nursing Scholarship, 37*(1), 48–56.

Wongvatunyu, S., & Porter, E. (2008). Helping young adult children with traumatic brain injury: The life-world of mothers. *Qualitative Health Research, 18*(8), 1062–1074.

World Health Organization [WHO]. (2018). *Falls.* Retrieved from http://www.who.int/en/news-room/fact-sheets/detail/falls (Accessed 26 April 2018).

Zhang, H., Zhang, X.-N., Zhang, H.-L., Huang, L., Chi, Q.-Q., Zhang, X., & Yun, X.-P. (2016). Differences in cognitive profiles between traumatic brain injury and stroke: A comparison of the Montreal cognitive assessment and mini-mental state examination. *Chinese Journal of Traumatology, 19*(5), 271–274. doi:10.1016/j.cjtee.2015.03.007.

6

Using Interpretative Phenomenological Analysis to Study Patient and Family Members' Experiences of a Mechanical Ventilation Weaning Unit

Craig D. Murray, Jo Jury, Victoria Molyneaux, Jane Simpson and David J. Wilde

CONTENTS

Introduction

In this chapter, we set out a phenomenological approach to collecting and analysing qualitative data (that of interpretative phenomenological analysis, or IPA) and apply this in a study of patient and family members' experiences of a mechanical ventilation weaning unit. We then consider how the findings of this study may inform healthcare and rehabilitation for this patient group. Our description and application of IPA here serves an illustrative purpose for others interested in applying qualitative methods for similar purposes to other healthcare settings.

Interpretative Phenomenological Analysis

IPA was developed by Jonathan Smith (Smith, 2004, 2011; Smith & Osborn, 2008; Smith, Flowers, & Larkin, 2009; Smith, Jarman, & Osborn, 1999) with the vision to return the study of 'lived experience' to the centre ground of psychology research attention by cultivating a phenomenology-based methodology that was inherently psychological in nature. IPA treats language as disclosing participants' being-in-the-world and the meanings of this for them. It is an approach intended to explore how participants experience their world, and hence enable an insider's perspective of the topic under study.

IPA is principally phenomenological owing to the central importance it accords to the lived experience of a particular phenomenon as it is perceived and understood by the person concerned. The approach aims to capture the complexity inherent in individual experience and make transparent the person's sense making of that experience. Consequently, there is no attempt in the presentation of the findings to produce objective statements of 'truth' about a phenomenon. Instead, an interpretative account is produced, comprised of detailed expositions of participants' understandings and meanings, and drawing out the psychological entailments of these.

IPA acknowledges that achieving an understanding of another's lifeworld is a delicate and collaborative social enterprise between participant and researcher; as Smith et al. (1999) note, access to a participant's lifeworld, '...depends on and is complicated by the researcher's own conceptions... required in order to make sense of that other personal world through a process of interpretative activity' (pp. 218–219). Smith (2011) refers to this process of the researcher trying to make sense of the participant trying to make sense of their experience as a 'double hermeneutic'.

In order to foreground the distinctive nature of personal experience, IPA takes an idiographic approach to research (Smith, 2011) involving the painstaking, fine-grained analysis of individual cases and seeking to illuminate the meaning and sense-making of lived phenomena as divulged within personal narratives. Because of this, IPA studies may focus on single case studies, where the commitment to idiography is most evident in the detailed reporting of one person's experience. However, it is more common for IPA studies to involve a small number of participants, where concerns centre around '...the balance of convergence and divergence within the sample, not only presenting both shared themes but also [...] the particular way in which these themes play out for individuals' (Smith, 2011, p. 10).

As already discussed, IPA is primarily a phenomenological methodology with an acute emphasis on the psychological study of lived experience and how people make sense of their experiences. Nonetheless, it also has links with more mainstream psychology in that it recognises that inherent in the sense-making process there is a '...chain of connection between people's talk and their thinking and emotional state' (Smith & Osborn, 2008, p. 54). However, as one might expect when carrying out psychological research, this 'chain of connection' is not straightforward – people often find it difficult to say what they mean, finding it challenging to put into words complex feelings and thoughts. Accordingly, it is incumbent on the researcher to draw out and interpret what people are thinking and feeling from the data obtained. When engaging in this kind of interpretative activity, IPA acknowledges that it is impossible to 'get into the head' of another human being and know their thoughts directly. Instead, the IPA researcher tries to develop a critically formed viewpoint from which they can then try to understand what it is like to have a given experience.

Given the close attention to detail and the intense idiographic nature of the approach taken, IPA research necessitates the purposive recruitment of a small sample of people who share a common experience and possibly other characteristics as well. Consequently, IPA studies are typically conducted with small samples of 4–10 participants that form a homogenous sample. Homogeneity can occur on a variety of levels. At the most fundamental level, participants in an IPA study are homogenous because they share an experience of a similar phenomenon. Other levels of homogeneity can apply to a given sample, however, these parameters will vary according to the particular research question and topic area (Smith, 2004). The analysis itself will pay concerted attention to the thorough examination of each participant case in turn until a point is reached where '...some degree of closure or gestalt has been achieved' (Smith, 2004, p. 41) for each individual. Only then will the researcher consider a cross-case analysis with a view to teasing out the convergences and divergences available within the data.

In terms of output, the proof of the idiographic focus of the analysis should be evident in the writing up of the findings. A detailed, nuanced, and resonant account of the participants' lifeworlds and meaning-making of their experiences of a given phenomenon should be presented. Smith (2004) notes that a good quality IPA write-up should aim to strike a balance between addressing the common elements that participants as a sample experienced, whilst retaining the uniqueness of each participant in such experiences.

As IPA has grown in stature and popularity, a variety of methods have been used to collect the experientially rich data necessary to perform a suitable analysis: for example, data have been culled from naturally occurring data sources existing on the Internet such as web discussion/message forums (Mulveen & Hepworth, 2006); through email interviews (Murray & Rhodes, 2005); diaries (Boserman, 2009); and focus groups (Palmer, Larkin, de Visser, & Fadden, 2010). However, the most popular and utilised method of data collection in the vast majority of IPA studies remains the semi-structured interview.

Mechanical Ventilation and Weaning Unit

The study reported here used interpretative phenomenological analysis to examine experiences of a mechanical ventilation unit. Mechanical ventilation (MV) is used when a person is unable to breathe unaided, usually as a result of chronic illness such as heart failure (Ayalon, 2007). Machinery delivers air to a person's lungs, either invasively through a tracheostomy or non-invasively, for example, via a sealed mask. The experience of MV can be a short one, for most people removal of the ventilator causes little distress or difficulty and is a quick process (Boles et al., 2007). However, up to 10% of users can become physically or psychologically dependent on MV and therefore have to be weaned from the equipment (Wise et al., 2011).

Weaning can be difficult and complex (Henneman et al., 2002). Dependency can be seen for a number of reasons, including lung disease, cardiac impairment, or psychosocial and psychological factors (Arslanian-Engoren & Scott, 2003; Cook, Meade, & Perry, 2001; NHS Modernisation Agency, 2001; Wunderlich, Perry, Lavin, & Katz, 1999). Greater understanding of the emotions that people experience during MV and the weaning process has been derived from qualitative studies. In a systematic review of five qualitative studies (Jablonski, 1994; Jenny & Logan, 1996; Logan & Jenny, 1997; Mendel & Khan, 1980; Wunderlich et al., 1999), Cook et al. (2001) highlighted the need to consider the emotions of the person being weaned. They argued that the weaning process evoked feelings of frustration, hopelessness, and fear.

Due to the range of difficulties and complications seen in weaning, it is important to have a specialist multi-disciplinary team (MDT) around the person being weaned (Henneman et al., 2002; Hoffman, Tasota, Zullo, Scharfenberg, & Donahoe, 2005). Specialist units can be more financially viable than weaning on the ICU (e.g., Seneff, Wagner, Thompson, Honeycutt, & Silver, 2000). The study described in this chapter is set within a specialist weaning unit in the United Kingdom. The unit is made up of an MDT which includes respiratory physicians with a special interest in weaning, nurses, physiotherapists, occupational therapists, and psychologists.

Whereas previous research has highlighted the importance of psychological and psychosocial aspects of MV and weaning, there is an absence of research on experiences of a weaning unit taken from a psychological perspective. IPA, with its focus on lived experience, meaning-making, and psychology, provides an appropriate, rigorous methodological approach to study this topic. In addition, given the central role that family members play in patients' recovery – be it within the hospital whilst the inpatient is sedated (Dreyer & Nortvedt, 2008), during the transition from hospital to home (Mustfa et al., 2006), or caring for the person at home (Huang & Peng, 2010) – it is important to gain insight into their experiences also (Happ et al., 2007).

Given the above considerations, the study presented here aimed to gain a better understanding of the experience of former patients and their family members who became involved with a mechanical ventilation weaning unit. By interviewing discharged patients and their significant others, the study aimed to develop healthcare professionals' understanding of the lived experiences of these people as well as the psychological impact of being involved with the unit.

Study Setting

The specialist weaning unit that is the focus of the current research was set up in the United Kingdom and opened in early 2010. It was one of only two in the country at the time of opening and provides specialist weaning care within a hospital setting. The unit itself consists of four dedicated weaning beds within a ventilation ward. A MDT, which includes respiratory physicians with a special interest in weaning, nurses, physiotherapists, occupational therapists, and psychologists, staffs the unit.

This study aimed to gain a better understanding of the experience of former patients and their significant others who become involved with the mechanical ventilation weaning unit.

By interviewing people who had been discharged and their significant others, it aimed to develop healthcare professionals' understanding of the lived experiences of these people as well as the psychological impact of being involved with the unit. It was a timely piece of work because at the time of data collection, the weaning unit had just completed its second year of operation, and therefore the research aimed to guide developing practices and procedures. It was also intended to be of benefit to other units already in operation or looking to open up in the future. Additionally, the study could provide clinical implications for those who carry out weaning within an ICU or similar setting, as it might guide the support provided to people who spend time there.

Data Collection and Analysis

Sampling and Participants

This study was approved by a National Health Service Research Ethics Committee and the weaning unit's National Health Service Research and Development office. All participants gave informed consent to be interviewed and permission for their data to be used in this study. The Ventilation Business Manager identified 21 people who had undergone weaning at the unit, of which four were still inpatients. Of the 17 discharged patients, five had died, or judged close to death by the Ventilation Business Manager. This left 12 people who were invited to take part in this study. As part of this invitation, patients were asked to identify a family member or a friend who had spent time with them on the unit who might also wish to take part. All potential participants were asked to express their interest to the research team directly either by email, post, or telephone. As a result, seven people took part: three patients and their partners and an additional family member (mother) of a patient who did not take part (see Table 6.1). Thus, the sample size and composition comprised a small and relatively homogenous group, as appropriate for IPA.

TABLE 6.1

Participant Pseudonyms and Relationship to Other Participants

Participant Pseudonym	Status	Relationship to Another Participant
Alan	Former inpatient on weaning unit	Partner of Bernice
Bernice	Significant other (spouse)	Partner of Alan
Carol	Significant other (mother of Ian, former patient, who was not interviewed)	N/A
Dan	Former inpatient on weaning unit	Partner of Helen
Eddie	Significant other (spouse)	Partner of Fiona
Fiona	Former inpatient on weaning unit	Partner of Eddie
Helen	Significant other (spouse)	Partner of Dan

TABLE 6.2

Example Topics and Prompt Questions from Interview Schedules

Example Topics for Person Who Had Been Weaned	Example Topics for Significant Other
Expectations of the unit (What did you expect from staff?) Psychological impact of being on the unit (How did you feel when you moved there? Emotional support (Did you get any? Where did this come from?)	Experience of visiting the unit Experience of the weaning process (Were you there for any this process?) Psychological impact of having a loved one on the unit (Did this change at all?)

Interview Procedure

Semi-structured interviews were conducted and audio recorded in participants' homes, with interviews lasting between 33 minutes and 70 minutes each. The interview schedule was developed by the research team, including the MDT within the weaning unit, and was designed to let participants recount their experiences with as little direction as possible (see Table 6.2). Example questions included 'How did you feel when moved there (the weaning unit)?' and (in relation to discharge) 'How was planning this managed?'

Data Analysis

There are many guides available on how to conduct IPA, discussing different levels of analysis that may be attempted (Smith et al., 2009) and different ways of presenting IPA findings. IPA is an epistemological and methodological approach that can tolerate some variation in procedures and presentation (Smith & Osborn, 2008). For example, we focus our own description of analysis here on identifying themes within and across transcripts.

To begin with, transcripts were read a number of times to increase the researcher's level of familiarity with the data. Each transcript was read to identify themes from a psychological perspective. Notations were made on parts of the text of relevance to the central research focus (patients' and their family members' experiences of the mechanical ventilation weaning unit). This included summarising material, making connections between passages and statements, and providing preliminary interpretations. Following this, the fundamental substance of the text was recorded in the form of keywords and phrases that captured the essence of these emergent themes. These keywords served as early placing or interpretative reflections on what was thought to be present in the text. Analysing each transcript individually allowed the researchers to be open to new themes from each participant, rather than being driven by themes from previous transcripts. Once this process was completed for each transcript, a list of the emergent themes was collated so that connections across the transcripts could be examined. Patterns across participants were then explored, including commonalities and nuances within and between participants' data. Related themes were grouped together and the final theme titling modified to reflect the depth and breadth within and across accounts. This stage of analysis focused on producing a parsimonious and saturated account of the study data that resulted in a three-theme narrative structure: being different; the unit as both a community and a lonely place; and the transition from unit to home. Each of these themes is presented below and illustrated using data excerpts from the interviews conducted.

Findings

Being Different

The weaning unit gave participants the opportunity to feel special or different in some way. This unit is not a typical hospital ward and therefore does not operate in the same way that more traditional wards might have to, where people are typically admitted not based on choice, but based on physical need. Participants understood that the weaning unit actively selected people who might benefit from the service it offered and tried to make sense of this:

> They felt that I was a suitable candidate to go to the unit. They wanted to try the system on me and wean me off ventilation... They thought they could do something, there's no point in making someone who wasn't going to do any good. I must have been fighting the good fight and not giving up. (Alan)

Alan made sense of this decision as being about the personality of the individual, rather than being based on a medical decision. To be chosen meant that the individual was actively behaving in a particular way and this will cause them to have a good weaning outcome, something that would be wasted on a person who was not going to be able to make the most of the opportunity. Therefore, the responsibility for the success or failure of weaning is partly put onto the individual rather than the medics, although some of this responsibility does stay with the staff, who will be able to 'do something'. Alan recognised himself that he was 'fighting the good fight', therefore making him stand out from others who might not be putting as much effort into recovering. This sense of feeling unique was also discussed by Helen, who described how her husband, Dan, was seen as someone special to the weaning unit doctors:

> Cardiology had been, you know monitoring him closely, and they probably wanted him to go onto the cardio ward, but they weren't sure, are you with me, I think Dr. [name omitted] had sort of like decided that wasn't happening, and he was going his way. He wanted him as sort of like a, a prodigy. (Helen)

Dan was seen as being special, and this resulted in a battle between different specialities within the hospital, where Dan was wanted by both teams. However, although the doctors might make the decision that someone is suitable to go onto the unit, the decision remains a joint one, and people are given the option whether to accept or decline a place. In the following extract, Eddie is talking about his partner, a former patient on the unit:

> They offered us the option of going to the Unit. And Dr. [name omitted] came, we said, Fiona said yes, and Dr. [name omitted] came down to assess her, and was very glad to accept her as a patient, with the objective of weaning her off the tracheostomy. (Eddie)

This decision can be one that is made by both the person admitted to the unit and the significant other, however, is ultimately up to the individual who is to be admitted. Whilst there was a sense that this is a joint decision, it is actually the person admitted to the unit who is in control of saying yes or no. This was something that was conveyed by all participants except Carol – mother of a former patient – who showed that control is not always something that the person admitted to the unit or the significant other can keep:

> So he did stay there on that ward [another ward in hospital] and then he had, he had a respiratory arrest. Which then, he needed resuscitation really, which then forced the move down to the [weaning] unit. So although we were relieved that he was going, it wasn't quite as straightforward as that, you know. It was more difficult. But when he actually went down there, it was very clear that he needed to be somewhere other than a ward. (Carol)

These extracts show how the weaning unit was seen as somewhere different and, whether they have control over the decision or not, being moved to the unit can bring positive emotions and make a person feel special in some way.

The Unit as Both a Community and a Lonely Place

The unit was discussed as a special place throughout the interviews, and this was expressed most clearly by the idea of the unit being like a community. It was portrayed as different in this aspect to other hospital settings, despite being within a hospital setting:

> ... being in the hospital, little more of a community feeling than a big block of wards. Although having, because I wasn't in a ward, luckily that felt a little bit special too in a way... Didn't think of it being as a, a general ward. (Fiona)

By thinking of the unit as being unlike a general ward, the idea of feeling special was maintained, and removed from the hospital setting in which it was surrounded. This sense of community led Fiona to feel a bond with the other people on the unit, who were going through similar experiences:

> We all became, you know, not friends as such but we got to know each other, have a laugh about each other's' masks and stuff, and helped each other as we got stronger, to go to the loo and stuff. (Fiona)

This bond meant that emotional support could be offered, sometimes through the more practical care that staff would otherwise provide. There was a sense of the people on the unit getting better together, and this instilled a sense of group cohesion. However, Fiona made the clear distinction between this bond and friendship, these people are not close to her, but rather a temporary support structure that will give and take help where needed.

As continuing support was often needed, participants still felt part of the unit. Several participants spoke about revisiting the unit once they had been discharged, and two spoke about going back to give gifts of appreciation. Hence, the sense of community and support continued even after people left the unit:

> People were coming and visiting... who had been in... they'd just come visiting and say, I need a mask, or I need a whatever, or breathing was a bit out last night, and they'd either say to them I'll get you a mask or, let's have a, we'll keep you overnight and have a look you know. I just thought that was amazing. (Helen)

The unit was perceived as a calm, supportive, and 'good' place to be:

> I actually feel very comfortable going there cos you know there's such a good, such a good place. You feel good. (Eddie)

Conversely, there were times when this sense of community and support dissipated. The term 'lonely' was used a lot throughout the data set and encapsulated a time for those on the unit when significant others were not around:

> I realised it was lonely. And also in a small, in a room on your own like that. ... I found I couldn't concentrate. (Alan)

Alan's sense of isolation and loneliness was also recognised by his partner, Bernice:

> He was lonely... And when he was getting a lot of constant care, it was ok because there was somebody there, but when he was getting better, there wasn't anybody there, and he would have to ring for attention if he needed it you know, and he was lonely then. (Bernice)

The Transition from Unit to Home

Contrary to the experience of having a choice to move to the unit, leaving was something that was out of participants' control, and at times fraught with battles, leaving participants unsure about when they or their loved one could leave:

> Then they said, 'Well if everything's ok, you can go home Thursday'. ... And then I would think, oh great, Thursday. Thursday night, guaranteed, the physiotherapist would be on because I've not been able to get my breath. So another week, and then eventually, they said, I could go home...I got out of there. (Fiona)

Therefore, for some people on the unit, a discharge date could be given tentatively, however, as the person's physical status could vary, this might change, meaning that people had to wait to be re-assessed. Fiona described the delay as being due to her physical condition, as she was not able to get her breath, and it remained something outside of her control. Being out of control was something that other participants felt, none more so than Carol, who described having a difficult battle to get her son discharged from the unit.

> When somebody needs to come out to the community with a tracheostomy and, use of the ventilator and other pieces of equipment, it's a very long process. It's just a very difficult time so we just, we were just playing a kind of waiting game. (Carol)

Carol's son had not been weaned from his tracheostomy, and this along with other complicated health difficulties meant that discharge was not as simple as getting oxygen levels to an acceptable standard. For Carol, this was a battle she had to fight, and she found that they were waiting, not because of the unit, but because of other agencies that needed to be co-ordinated: 'I think the unit staff are, it, it's out of their hands' (Carol). Processes like this could be difficult for the significant other as they are keen to have their loved one back home, and therefore they can experience the same frustration as the person who has been admitted.

There was a sense of hope in recognising that people did find their way out of the weaning unit, and progress towards this could be seen by moving from a tracheostomy to non-invasive ventilation. Similarly to other participants, Eddie portrayed the discharge process as having delays and 'diversions', but these were minimised as the hope for an exit was placed as paramount importance. All participants spoke about the transition to getting home, and although adjusting to life after the unit was seen as difficult, only one participant described the difficult emotions he felt over leaving the unit:

> … there was a fear of coming home, you know because I'd been there and maybe, maybe because I was in a comfort zone, and you knew if anything went wrong they were there you know, and I was coming home here and I'd have to get up the stairs and, stuff like that you know. (Dan)

Dan became safe at the unit and did not need to think about the care he would receive. There was a fear that something would go wrong at home, although this was related to practical issues rather than worries about his breathing. This worry was not limited to people who had been admitted, and Carol, a significant other, was also worried about the practicalities of managing without staff:

> So we were then forced to be there, cos if we'd have brought him home, it would have been very tricky cos one of us would have been up all night with him. (Carol)

Here, Carol describes feeling as though she had no choice but to remain in the unit, and although she was fighting for her son to return home, she was aware of the difficulties this transition would bring. Carol had the distinction that her son had not been weaned, unlike all the other people who had been on the unit. This placed a pressure on her to continue the level of care that would have been available when on the unit.

Although difficulties with the transition from the unit to home were recounted, one participant summed up the feeling of eventually returning home after a long time away: 'I was glad to be home. Free to do what I wanted' (Fiona). There was a sense of relief and of breaking free from the routine that was placed upon people at the unit. The transition to home was a difficult one, but positive, as the person was back in their own surroundings where they could regain a sense of control over their life.

Healthcare Implications of the Study Findings

The aim of this chapter was to present a particular qualitative approach suited to understanding lived experience, meaning-making, and the psychological responses of patients (and their significant others) within a certain healthcare setting. We chose to illustrate this via a study of a mechanical ventilation weaning unit, using the method of IPA.

The aim of the study was to gain an understanding of the experiences of patients and family members who had spent time on a mechanical ventilation weaning unit, with a view to understanding psychological considerations. There are key implications for weaning units, such as that drawn on in this research.

'Being different' was an experience highlighting participants' feelings of being special in some way. The unit actively selects people for admission. This led to a feeling amongst people admitted that they were special and had something different about them which meant they would be a good candidate. The feeling of being different and special by participants could be used to shape how conversations are had prior to people being admitted to the hospital. It was important for participants that they were offered a service over which they had a choice whether to attend or not. Therefore, conversations with patients and family about moving to the unit should revolve around what makes them a suitable candidate and how they might be different to other people who would not be admitted to the unit.

The ability to be together during this difficult period was vital for patients and their significant others, and the environment of the unit afforded both opportunities for community, but also times of isolation and loneliness. Being visited helped to prevent patients from feeling low or depressed. When visitors left, people admitted to the unit relied on the sense of community that the unit offered. The study also echoes previous research which has identified the importance patients place on being able to rely on family members for support (e.g., Arslanian-Engoren & Scott, 2003). The current study extends this work to show how, by taking the importance of support on board and being flexible with visiting hours, people are made to feel special and display resilience to low mood, anxiety, and other psychological difficulties. Clearly, the features that supported community or added to feelings of isolation and loneliness should be maximised and minimised, respectively, as much as possible (e.g., flexible visiting, opportunities for patients to socialise, outpatient care that maintains the continuity of care).

Contrary to other research (e.g. Arslanian-Engoren & Scott, 2003; Cook et al., 2001; Wunderlich et al., 1999), no mention was made of psychological difficulties which impeded the weaning process. However, participants did indicate they experienced psychological difficulties at the time of transition from the unit to home. Both people who had been admitted to the unit and their family members felt this distress. The process of going home is a simple one, but for most it is long and difficult with considerable psychological barriers. Therefore, the provision of psychological support would be of particular use here in supporting both patients and family members in continuing their recovery at home, as this transition period evokes particular and difficult emotions.

Conclusion

Within this chapter, we have presented the qualitative approach of interpretative phenomenological analysis and applied it to the setting of a mechanical ventilation weaning unit. The study demonstrates how the application of qualitative research methods can be used to guide and develop practices and procedures in healthcare delivery settings. Although the present findings offer particular issues of consideration for specialist mechanical ventilation weaning units and ICUs, our description and application of IPA here serves an illustrative purpose for others interested in applying qualitative methods for similar purposes to other healthcare settings.

References

Arslanian-Engoren, C., & Scott, L. D. (2003). The lived experience of survivors of prolonged mechanical ventilation: A phenomenological study. *Heart & Lung: The Journal of Acute and Critical Care, 32*, 328–334.

Ayalon, L. (2007). The potential role of dependency in the weaning process: The case of a 57-year-old woman connected to a mechanical ventilator. *Clinical Case Studies, 6*(6), 459–467.

Boles, J. M., Bion, J., Connors, A., Herridge, M., Marsh, B., Melot, C., Pearl, R., Silverman, H., Stanchina, M., Vieillard-Baron, A., & Welte, T. (2007). Weaning from mechanical ventilation. *European Respiratory Journal, 29*(5), 1033–1056.

Boserman, C. (2009). Diaries from cannabis users: An interpretative phenomenological analysis. *Health, 13*(4), 429–448.

Cook, D. J., Meade, M. O., & Perry, A. G. (2001). Qualitative studies on the patient's experience of weaning from mechanical ventilation. *Chest, 120*(6 suppl), 469S–473S.

Dreyer, A., & Nortvedt, P. (2008). Sedation of ventilated patients in intensive care units: Relatives' experiences. *Journal of Advanced Nursing, 61*(5), 549–556.

Happ, M. B., Swigart, V. A., Tate, J. A., Arnold, R. M., Sereika, S. M., & Hoffman, L. A. (2007). Family presence and surveillance during weaning from prolonged mechanical ventilation. *Heart & Lung: The Journal of Acute and Critical Care, 36*(1), 47–57.

Henneman, E., Dracup, K., Ganz, T., Molayeme, O., & Cooper, C. B. (2002). Using a collaborative weaning plan to decrease duration of mechanical ventilation and length of stay in the intensive care unit for patients receiving long-term ventilation. *American Journal of Critical Care, 11*(2), 132–140.

Hoffman, L. A., Tasota, F. J., Zullo, T. G., Scharfenberg, C., & Donahoe, M. P. (2005). Outcomes of care managed by an acute care nurse practitioner/attending physician team in a subacute medical intensive care unit. *American Journal of Critical Care, 14*(2), 121–130.

Huang, T. T., & Peng, J. M. (2010). Role adaptation of family caregivers for ventilator-dependent patients: Transition from respiratory care ward to home. *Journal of Clinical Nursing, 19*(11–12), 1686–1694.

Jablonski, R. S. (1994). The experience of being mechanically ventilated. *Qualitative Health Research, 4*, 186–207.

Jenny, J., & Logan, J. (1996). Caring and comfort metaphors used by patients in critical care. *Journal of Nursing Scholarship, 28*(4), 349–352.

Logan, J., & Jenny, J. (1997). Qualitative analysis of patients' work during mechanical ventilation and weaning. *Heart & Lung: The Journal of Acute and Critical Care, 26*, 140–147.

Mendel, J. G., & Khan, F. A. (1980). Psychological aspects of weaning from mechanical ventilation. *Psychosomatics, 21*, 465–471.

Mulveen, R., & Hepworth, J. (2006). An interpretative phenomenological analysis of participation in a pro-anorexia internet site and its relationship with disordered eating. *Journal of Health Psychology, 11*(2), 283–296.

Murray, C., & Rhodes, K. (2005). The experience and meaning of adult acne. *British Journal of Health Psychology, 10*(2), 183–202.

Mustfa, N., Walsh, E., Bryant, V., Lyall, R. A., Addington-Hall, J., Goldstein, L. H., Donaldson, N., Polkey, M. I., Moxham, J., & Leigh, P. N. (2006). The effect of noninvasive ventilation on ALS patients and their caregivers. *Neurology, 66*(8), 1211–1217.

NHS Modernisation Agency. (2001). Critical care programme: Weaning and long term ventilation. Leicester, England: NHS Modernisation Agency. Retrieved from http://www.ics.ac.uk/intensive_care_professional/critical_care_programme_-_weaning_and_long_term_ventilation_

Palmer, M., Larkin, M., de Visser, R., & Fadden, G. (2010). Developing an interpretative phenomenological approach to focus group data. *Qualitative Research in Psychology, 7*(2), 99–121.

Seneff, M. G., Wagner, D., Thompson, D., Honeycutt, C., & Silver, M. R. (2000). The impact of long-term acute-care facilities on the outcome and cost of care for patients undergoing prolonged mechanical ventilation. *Critical Care Medicine, 28*(2), 342–350.

Smith, J. A. (2004). Reflecting on the development of interpretative phenomenological analysis and its contribution to qualitative research in psychology. *Qualitative Research in Psychology, 1*(1), 39–54.

Smith, J. A. (2011). Evaluating the contribution of interpretative phenomenological analysis. *Health Psychology Review, 5*(1), 9–27.

Smith, J. A., Flowers, P., & Larkin, M. (2009). *Interpretative phenomenological analysis: Theory, method and research*. London, UK: Sage.

Smith, J. A., & Osborne, M. (2008). Interpretative phenomenological analysis. In J. A. Smith (Ed.), *Qualitative Psychology: A Practical Guide to Research Methods* (2nd ed., pp. 53–79). London, UK: Sage.

Smith, J. A., Jarman, M., & Osborn, M. (1999). Doing interpretative phenomenological analysis. In M. Murray, & K. Chamberlain (Eds.), *Qualitative health psychology: Theories and methods* (pp. 218–240). London, UK: Sage.

Wise, M. P., Hart, N., Davidson, C., Fox, R., Allen, M., Elliott, M., … Campbell, J. (2011). Home mechanical ventilation. *British Medical Journal, 342*, d1687.

Wunderlich, R. J., Perry, A., Lavin, M. A., & Katz, B. (1999). Patients' perceptions of uncertainty and stress during weaning from mechanical ventilation/Educational STATPack. *Dimensions of Critical Care Nursing, 18*(1), 2.

7

Using Narrative Analysis to Study Coping and Adjusting to Cardiothoracic Transplant

Craig D. Murray, Catherine Elson, Zoey Malpus and Stephen Weatherhead

CONTENTS

Introduction

In this chapter, we set out a qualitative approach to collecting and analysing qualitative data (that of narrative analysis) and apply this in a study of coping and adjusting to cardiothoracic transplant. We then consider how the findings of this study may inform healthcare and rehabilitation for this patient group. Our description and application of narrative analysis here serves an illustrative purpose for others interested in applying qualitative methods for similar purposes to other healthcare settings.

Cardiothoracic Transplant and Psychological Challenges

The term 'cardiothoracic transplant' refers to the transplantation of the heart and/or lung organs and is the final treatment option for those experiencing organ failures (Hertz et al. 2002). In recent years, cardiomyopathy has become the most frequently cited reason for heart transplants (Stehlik et al. 2011). For lung transplant recipients, chronic obstructive pulmonary disease, cystic fibrosis, and emphysema are the most common reasons (Christie et al. 2012). Approximately 3500 lung transplants and 100 heart/lung transplants are carried out worldwide each year (Christie et al. 2012), in addition to 4000 heart transplants (Stehlik et al. 2011). The international median survival rate for heart transplant recipients is 10 years (Stehlik et al. 2011) and for lung transplant recipients it is 5 and 1/2 years (Christie et al. 2012).

The period of time that candidates spend on the transplant waiting list can be psychologically challenging (Stukas et al. 1999). It is characterised by uncertainty as candidates often experience worsening health and repeated hospital admissions until a suitable donor organ is found (DiMartini et al. 2008). Candidates may experience both hope for the possibility of a successful outcome and fear of the upcoming surgery and its potential failure (DiMartini et al. 2008). Thoughts of death are common during this stage and candidates often experience feelings of guilt and shame due to assuming a connection between their need for an organ and the death of donor (Sanner 2003).

During the immediate time period following transplantation, psychological difficulties, including depression, anxiety, and post-traumatic stress disorder are common (Dew & DiMartini 2005). Transplant recipients may feel a sense of disillusionment with the realisation that one diminished health state has been exchanged for another (Dudley et al. 2007). They face an extensive post-transplant medication regime, with accompanying side effects (Sadala & Stolf 2008). There is also the ever-present threat of acute and chronic graft rejection, in addition to complications associated with immunosuppression, such as diabetes and kidney failure (Dew & Dimartini 2005). Psychological difficulties may be further exacerbated by the psychosocial challenges encountered by transplant recipients. These include physical disability and body image difficulties (Engle 2001), sexual dysfunction (Rainer et al. 2010), and a lack of coping strategies and social support (Dew & DiMartini 2005).

It is clear from the above literature that undergoing a cardiothoracic transplant is a difficult and demanding process for recipients and their families. To date, the emphasis in quantitative research has largely been on post-transplant quality of life which focuses on a return to activities of daily living (Hyland 1998). The data for quality of life studies are generally gathered using questionnaires, leaving little room for exploration of the subjective experiences of the recipient (Joralemon & Fujinaga 1996). In contrast, there is limited qualitative evidence regarding coping, adjustment, and the support needs of transplant recipients, particularly in relation to receiving organs from a deceased donor (Rainer et al. 2010). Such research has the potential to increase the understanding of researchers and practitioners regarding the events and experiences in which transplant recipients require support.

Narrative Analysis

Whilst qualitative methods in general can illuminate the above issues, researchers have suggested that qualitative narrative research allows novel understandings to be gleaned about an individual's self-identity, perceptions of illness states, and healthcare needs (McMahon et al. 2012). A narrative perspective posits that people tell stories as a way of putting events in a temporal order and establishing meaning and coherence to their changing life circumstances (Murray 2008). As discussed by McMahon et al. (2012, p. 1124):

> Narrative researchers propose that people are meaning-generating beings who are continually constructing their identities from building blocks available to them in their common culture, above and beyond their individual experience… Narratives or stories are thought to be central in this process, providing the means by which people organise actions and events in their lives, bringing a sense of meaning, coherence and continuity to their wide ranging experiences… Therefore narrative approaches are concerned with accessing the meaning within personal narratives and in doing so learning about the life-world and personality of the narrator. … Furthermore, we are born into a storied world in which we are exposed to a whole host of stories which capture our imagination and impart shared wisdom in relation to acceptable behaviour, values and morality within our culture… As such, the stories that we tell are connected to and limited by wider stories, or dominant narratives which reveal culturally shared meanings and expectations.

In relation to healthcare and rehabilitation, narrative approaches view the onset of illness, especially chronic illness, as disrupting a person's everyday life, challenging 'taken for granted' assumptions and prompting a re-evaluation and re-formulation of the self (Bury 1982; Charmaz 1991; Frank 1995). Eliciting narratives of these experiences in research offers a way in which this meaning-making process can be observed, whilst also disclosing how the social context contributes to this (Murray 2008).

Narrative analysis is particularly well-suited for exploration of the trajectory cardiothoracic transplant recipients experience during the course of their illness and treatment. For example, Flynn et al. (2013) employed this approach in relation to heart and lung transplantation and intensive care unit delirium. Within a narrative approach, events and occurrences are taken to be experientially configured into a temporal whole, with a beginning, middle, and an end. A person's experience of the present reciprocally informs their understanding of both their past and their future. This theoretical and analytical interest of narrative approaches makes them particularly suited, from a suite of possible qualitative approaches, for the study of accounts of illness over an extended period. Therefore, the present study takes a narrative approach seeking to understand participants' experiences of coping and adjusting to cardiothoracic transplant. In addition, the study detail presented here provides a guiding example for applying narrative analysis to other healthcare and rehabilitation settings where the research objectives are similar in scope.

Data Collection and Analysis

Sampling and Participants

In order to explore coping and adjusting to cardiothoracic transplant, eight participants who had all undergone a heart (n = 6) or double lung transplant (n = 2) were recruited from two outpatient cardiothoracic transplant services in the United Kingdom. Participants' ages ranged from 32 to 65 and consisted of six men and two women. The length of time post-transplant ranged from 2 years to 20 years. Demographic information for participants is summarised in Table 7.1.

TABLE 7.1

Participant Demographic Details

Participant Number and Pseudonym	Gender	Age	Type of Transplant	Length of Time Since Transplant	Length of Time on Waiting List for Transplant
1. Sally	F	41	Heart	1 years 8 months	3 weeks
2. Simon	M	56	Double lung	24 months	3 weeks
3. Dan	M	62	Heart	10 years 11 months	3 months
4. John	M	46	Double lung	6 years	9 months
5. Gerard	M	65	Heart	20 years	1 week
6. Tim	M	54	Heart	6 years	1 day
7. Peter	M	51	Heart	3 years	7 months
8. Laura	F	32	Heart	2 years	3 weeks
Whole sample	**M = 6 F = 2**	***Range* = 32–65**	***Heart* = 6 *Double lung* = 2**	***Range* = 1 year 8 months–20 years**	***Range* = 1 day–9 months**

Recruitment and Interview Procedure

The National Research Ethics Service and the Research and Development departments of both National Health Service Trusts provided ethical approval. Participants were recruited by responding to posters displayed within the premises of the cardiothoracic services over a 4-week period (a sample pool n of approximately 66). Six participants chose to be interviewed at the transplant service and two chose to be interviewed in their home. As is common in narrative research, a minimal interview schedule was used and was designed to facilitate participants in recounting their story, in their own words. Each interview began with the question 'Can you tell me the story of your transplant, what it has meant to you and how it fits in with the rest of your life?' Whilst eliciting their story, additional prompt questions were asked as needed in order to encourage participants to elaborate.

The interviews lasted between 60 minutes and 90 minutes. They were audio recorded and transcribed verbatim. All personally identifiable information was removed, with pseudonyms used in place of real names. A summary story was subsequently provided to each participant so that they could provide any changes that they felt were needed. Three participants requested minor changes.

Analysis

Narrative analysis distinguishes itself from other approaches by its focus on 'particular actors, in particular social places, at particular social times' (Abbott 1992, p. 48). A number of key texts in the field of narrative analysis were drawn upon in order to inform the present analysis (Andrews et al. 2008; Crossley 2000; Riessman 1993, 2008). The first stage of the analysis process involved actively listening to the interview recordings and noting down initial reactions and assumptions (McCormick 2004). Interviews were subsequently transcribed verbatim and re-read several times in order to produce a summary story for each participant. These stories summarised key events and characters, in addition to noting significant thoughts and emotions associated with the different stages of the transplant experience. Once any changes suggested by participants had been incorporated into the summary stories, additional readings of each transcript were made. Initially, attention was focused on the content (Hoshmand 2005) and the structure of the narration (Riessman 2008). Each subsequent read of the transcript was concerned with a different aspect of the narrative, such as metaphors and imagery (Lieblich et al. 1998), tone (Crossley 2000), and character (which included significant others) (McCormick 2004). Finally, individual accounts were synthesised together through a process of comparison between stories, merging areas of commonality, and incorporation of elements of each participant's story that illuminated or extended that of other participants.

Findings

The narrative analysis of the interview transcripts is presented in the form of a composite story, incorporating the stories of all eight participants. This story is made up of five 'chapters', which reflect the way in which participants organised their stories of transplantation. Each chapter is presented in turn: 'A life changed, contracted or on hold'; 'Hoping for the best whilst preparing for the worst'; 'From person to patient'; 'Adapting expectations'; and 'The price of the gift'.

Chapter One: 'I Felt in Limbo': A Life Changed, Contracted, or on Hold

This chapter was the starting point for all of the narratives, and the listener was orientated to the period of time before the transplant when participants had begun to experience organ failure. For some, the decline into chronic illness had been gradual, whereas for others it had been very sudden. Nevertheless, as participants' health deteriorated they became increasingly incapacitated: 'I couldn't walk, I couldn't breathe, I couldn't do anything' (Peter), 'it ends up being really difficult to breathe and it gets harder' (Simon).

During this time, participants described searching for an answer to their physical ill-health. Medical professionals were discussed as authoritative characters and often experienced as dismissive of their symptoms: 'He looked at me and said you don't look like you're dying do you?' (Sally). Participants felt disempowered and there was a sense of having to fight to get the right diagnosis: 'I kept going to the doctors, they'd say there was nothing up with me and so I kept going back and it turned out I had cardiomyopathy' (Peter).

Participants described feeling shocked when they learned that transplant was an option: 'I'd never thought about it before, I knew I was getting weaker, but the thought of a transplant never crossed my mind' (Tim). Diagnosis brought with it the introduction of a biomedical narrative, in which physical symptoms were named and placed within a medical discourse. There was an experience of choice having been taken away: 'He asked me if I'd like a transplant and then told me that if I didn't have one I'd die' (Dan). For some, feelings of injustice were present: 'I was angry because I don't really drink and I don't smoke and I don't do drugs, I almost felt like, why didn't I just do the whole bloody lot' (Sally). This sense of unjustness could lead to a search for meaning regarding their organ failure: 'I went through a stage of thinking, why not him and why me?' (Gerard).

When describing their afflicted organ, participants used language reflecting their perceptions of the damage that had occurred to their bodies as a result of chronic illness: 'The right side of my heart was useless and just hanging there' (Laura); 'My heart had blown up, they think it was a virus and my heart had become scarred and wounded' (Gerard). The conversational pace that participants used when recounting this part of their story was fast and the language repetitive, reflecting the unrelenting nature of organ failure: 'I continued to get worse and worse and worse' (John); 'I was getting weaker and weaker' (Tim). The language used to describe the evaluation process highlighted the experienced intrusiveness, unnaturalness, and depersonalisation of the evaluation process: 'They were prodding and cutting' (Simon); 'They poked around inside you, checked all your other organs and bits were ok' (Peter).

Within each of the narratives, there was a feeling that life had shrunk and contracted around the individual: 'My life became going to work, getting home, and going to bed because I was so tired physically' (Sally); 'I was confined to the telly and the computer and sleep, that's all I would do' (John). Living with a chronic illness meant losing a sense of purpose in life and resulted in reluctant and distressing surrender of both social and occupational roles: 'I was absolutely devastated because it was the one thing I had left and I loved my job' (Sally); 'I missed the everyday things; going to work and being able to pop to the shops' (Tim). The predictable routine and consistency of everyday life had been disrupted and it was experienced as drastically altered from the way things once were: 'I went from being completely fit to a cardiac cripple' (Gerard). This language reflected the devastating loss of functioning and level of disability that had occurred.

These interruptions to daily life resulted in the future being narrowed, leading participants to become focused on the immediate 'here and now'. For participants, life was on hold: 'It was difficult because I couldn't plan anything with my life, I felt in limbo' (Laura). There was, then, a sense that life had been slowed down and become dominated by the monotonous routine of medication regimes and hospital appointments.

Chapter Two: 'Balancing Between Life and Death': Hoping for the Best whilst Preparing for the Worst

Once listed for transplant, anxiety became an increasingly prominent feature of participants' narratives: 'I thought at best I'd be disabled and I was worried, really worried' (Dan); 'I'd started looking it up on the Internet, and it was even more terrifying' (Laura). Central to these anxieties were thoughts of death: 'I really thought I was going to die' (Sally); 'I started to think that I might not survive' (Peter). Dan recalled wondering 'What it would feel like to die' and found it 'impossible to stay positive' when his life consisted of simply 'lying in bed'. However, other participants found that denying the seriousness of their illness was a protective strategy: 'I don't think I let the risks that I knew of come to the surface whilst I was going through it' (John).

The physical health of all of the participants had significantly deteriorated by this point and they had begun to experience a feeling of being trapped by their 'failing' bodies: 'It was like torture, sensory deprivation… a prisoner's regime' (Dan). There was a feeling that life was not being lived, but rather, it was being endured: 'I was so ill, I was existing in my bedroom, I was sleeping there, eating, drinking there' (Simon).

Participants described the paradoxical situation they found themselves in of hoping for the best outcome, whilst preparing for the worst: 'You're balancing between life and death, you could die or you could go on to have a revolutionary change of life for the best' (John); 'I wanted to live, I wanted to be well, but at the same time I wrote a will and thought about what my funeral would be like' (Dan). This period was experienced as desperately lonely as participants found loved ones reluctant to discuss the possibility of their death: 'I had nobody to talk to; nobody wanted to hear that I thought I was going to die' (Sally).

Within each of the narratives, receiving 'the call' that a suitable donor organ was available was highly significant. For some, it represented the possibility of 'brighter days ahead' (Peter), whilst others convinced themselves that it would be a 'false alarm' as a way to manage their anxiety: 'I kept saying, well it's not going to happen anyway' (Sally). The experience of shock numbed other feelings: 'I was like a zombie' (Simon); 'I think its panic and shock that takes over, you're not in the mood for emotion' (John). This numbness lasted into the final moments before going into theatre: 'When they told me it was going to happen and I had twenty minutes, it kicks in then' (Sally); 'All of a sudden, I was in theatre, totally terrified' (Simon). The language that participants used when narrating this part of their story exemplified how momentous it was to be finally going ahead with their transplant: 'I just couldn't believe it, it's such an odd thing, it feels sort of like you hear of the First World War, going over the top, sort of, here we go, let's do it. It's totally unreal' (Dan).

Chapter Three: 'Your Personality Is Taken Away from You': From Person to Patient

After the transplant operation, a heightened awareness of mortality resulted in participants developing a feeling of being dependent on having medical professionals around them: 'I didn't want to leave hospital, I got myself in a real state, thinking, this hurts and that hurts' (Sally); 'I got this feeling of institutionalisation' (Tim). This powerful prison metaphor conveyed the feeling of being trapped and the lack of control that is experienced during this stage of hospitalisation: 'I wanted to just scream and shout… to get away but you can't, you're stuck' (Laura).

During this time in hospital after the transplant, participants had to adapt to the role of a 'patient' who was dependent on others: 'Your personality is taken away from you, you go from being able to make all the decisions about your life to being treated as though you can't make any decisions for yourself, everything from your past is gone' (Dan). Inherent in Peter's narrative, and seemingly at the core of his self-identity, was his desire to care for others. However, in the immediate aftermath of the transplant he had been forced to abandon this part of himself: 'It was hard because I'd always had people relying on me and now I was relying on other people to do everything' (Peter). Laura highlighted her distress at being physically unable to fulfil her central role as a parent: 'I needed to be a mother to him and I wasn't able to… I felt like I was stopping him in some way from being a child'. Participants described a loss of independence and increased sense of fragility: 'I had to learn to do everything again, I couldn't walk, I couldn't brush my teeth' (John); 'I felt like an egg shell' (Simon).

Throughout the transplant process, the medical professionals were perceived as powerful figures who left participants feeling powerless: 'Some of the nurses are very directive as well, shout at you if you try to get out of bed or something, so you are in a very powerless position' (Dan). This perceived power imbalance was particularly marked when participants were talking about the transplant doctors: 'The consultants, you're in awe of them… I put them on a pedestal in a way, but I mean I'm just glad they kept me alive' (John). Participants also felt their emotional well-being was sometimes neglected: 'Sometimes you can feel like it's all about the figures and they haven't really asked about you, how you are… [but] their main aim is to keep you alive' (Simon).

Chapter Four: 'It's Not a Magic Cure': Adapting Expectations

Participants described the immense struggle of adapting to life as a transplant recipient. They found their confidence had been knocked and found it difficult to regain a sense of autonomy: 'When I first got home I felt really nervous, quite vulnerable' (Tim). This seemed to be especially apparent in those who had become ill quite suddenly: 'I always used to be quite confident, but I think it was because I was suddenly for no apparent reason really ill, it was a big shock when I was in the realms of what might happen next' (Dan).

Participants lost faith in their own health and normal physical functions, becoming sensitive to physical symptoms which could be indicative of rejection: 'So every time I pick up a bug, every time, I think, is this it?' (Laura). This increased vigilance was rooted in fear of returning to the life lived just before the transplant: 'I couldn't stand for my lungs to start packing up, rejecting, I can't imagine myself being back there, not being able to breathe and being on morphine, I'm not doing that so I try not to dwell on it' (Simon).

For some, it was difficult to adjust to being at home: 'Psychologically I suppose it was a shock. I relate it to the First World War, the extreme conditions of being at war and then the veterans come home and it is hard to get used to at first' (Dan). This combat metaphor characterised participants' experiences both before the transplant and during their recovery: 'You feel like you're losing [the] battle' (Peter). It reflected 'the fight' that transplant recipients faced, both for their life and for the survival of their identity: 'I've known what it is to be on the edge of losing something… like my life' (Laura).

There was a feeling that friends and family did not fully appreciate the implications of being a transplant recipient. The invisibility of the struggles of daily living post-transplant left some with a feeling of anger and frustration: 'People think that once you've had the transplant, that's it, you're totally fine, back to normal' (Sally). Some found it a comfort to go back to the transplant unit because they felt safe and understood: 'If they'd have asked me to come in every week then I would've done quite happily, it was like getting this reassurance that everything was ok' (Simon).

A successful transplant carried with it the implication of finality, of the end of a life of chronic illness and the beginning of a new life. However, participants found that they were still 'patients', with regular hospital appointments to attend and a lifetime of immune suppressing medication: 'So suddenly I've got this whole load of problems, all of that to take on board, blood clots, all of that, it seems that as soon as you've sorted something, something else goes wrong' (Peter). Indeed, within each of the narratives there was an acknowledgement that expectations had to be adapted to fit with the post-transplant reality: 'I thought, all of a sudden you're going to spring back into life and everything would be fine but, it's not and you've just got to learn to accept that you're never going to get back what you had' (Peter).

Alongside the struggle with their physical recovery, all participants experienced some psychological difficulties post-transplant, for which there was a feeling of being unprepared for: 'They were brilliant with the medical side; rejection, preparing you for surgery, but nobody ever addressed the psychological side, what was going to happen to you' (Gerard).

Participants who had to give up their work as a result of their ill-health struggled to assimilate their post-transplant selves to their pre-transplant selves:

> Some days I don't want to get out of bed, I wonder what my life is about because I think beforehand I had such a sense of purpose… I had sport, a big circle of friends and then suddenly it's like, bang. (Sally)

Chapter Five: 'It's a Heavy Load on My Shoulders': The Price of 'The Gift'

As recovery post-transplant progressed, this composite story reflected participants' thoughts about the organ donor and the donor's family. When difficulties in recovery were experienced a sense of obligation to their organ donor motivated participants to persevere: 'You've got to get yourself straight, someone has died and you've got their lungs and it's happened for a reason' (John); 'I think that's what makes you take your medication because your trying to look after yourself to make the most of your life, so that person didn't die for nothing' (Sally).

The donor became a central character in each of the narratives and there was a sense that the two lives had become inextricably linked: 'It sounds daft, but last year I played quite a lot of golf, I was getting out, I enjoyed myself. So sometimes I thought, "I wonder if he enjoyed golf?" You know, he was out there with me' (Simon); 'I think about my donor every day, in terms of what his life was like, what his family was like, what did he like doing, the circumstances of how he passed away' (John).

Feelings of guilt regarding the death of the donor were present across the narratives, with participants equating their life with the donor's death:

> I still feel very guilty that someone had to die for me to live and I think that's at the back of your head... somebody else will have died so you can have it... (Sally)

Simon had been a smoker and he described his unresolved feelings of guilt with regards to his chronic illness being 'self-induced': 'There was a lot of guilt, like there were more deserving cases and I don't know what I did with that actually, I never dealt with that so it's probably still floating around somewhere'. Peter also had difficulty accepting that he was deserving of the donor organ because he did not perceive himself as 'ill enough': 'I don't know, I just felt "why me?" I didn't deserve it. Somebody else should have had it'.

Participants expressed strong feelings of gratitude towards the donor. When thoughts turned to expressing this thanks to the donor's family, some struggled to put the enormity of their gratefulness into words: 'I'm incredibly grateful... and there may come a day when I know what to say and I will write, but at the moment, I don't' (Simon). Peter, on the other hand, had wanted to write a thank you letter, but 'the co-ordinator wouldn't let me because I was in and out of hospital all the time, she didn't think it would be helpful for them to know I wasn't well'. Laura had written a letter to her donor's family and when she did not get a response from them she began to worry: 'maybe they have regrets... and that troubles me when I think of it like that'. Participants also spoke of a sense of societal pressure and expectation to do 'extraordinary things, like a marathon or a bungee jump' (Laura), and by not doing such things they felt they were 'not making the most of things' (Simon).

As this composite story concludes, the focus of the narratives turns to the future. For participants, thoughts of the future were closely linked to thoughts of death. For Laura, having a transplant had given her a feeling of living on 'borrowed time' and she felt the 'future is inevitable'. Some found these thoughts threatening and difficult to reconcile: 'From death never being on your mind to it occupying quite a lot of your thoughts, dying is now the thing that scares me the most' (Sally). Expectations and assumptions for the future had been disrupted by the implications of being a transplant recipient. For Sally, the life limiting nature of her condition had left her feeling alienated from other people because she knew they did not understand her reality:

> When I think about the future, I think about me not in it... it's something that's always there, it torments me... I would say the mental side is harder than the physical side... telling everyone you're absolutely fine when actually, you just want to curl up and cry...

Peter struggled to come to terms with the reality of his physical capabilities following his transplant: 'They've told me that my health will never be what it was, they reckon I'll need a mobility chair from now on... hopefully I'll prove them wrong one day, you've just got to cling onto it'. Laura described feeling changed as a result of her experiences and as such, struggled to relate to others in the same way: 'It's like I'm looking in on a glass ball, like I'm on the outside of a goldfish bowl and I'm looking in at everyone else'. Although Laura had experienced a considerable amount of psychological distress throughout her transplant journey, she also described some positive psychological change: 'I've had an experience that most people never have in a lifetime... I do think back to the person I used to be, but I don't wish to be that person'. The experience had left her 'stronger as a person' and able to 'see things in a different perspective' and 'appreciate even the simplest of things'.

Discussion

This study explored the narratives of cardiothoracic transplant recipients through individual stories of the transplant journey. Here, the findings are considered in relation to how they might be addressed in service delivery.

The story threads through the initial stage of being diagnosed with a chronic illness, to the transplant, and subsequent recovery. Participants' struggle to locate a cause and assign meaning to their symptoms was accompanied by diagnosis and a biomedical focus being introduced to their narrative. The assessment process potential recipients undergo in order to determine their suitability for transplant (e.g., to identify possible risk factors such as pre-existing mental health difficulties; Dew et al. 2002) presents an opportunity at which these issues could be addressed. It is common practice for candidates to be asked to complete cardiac or pulmonary rehabilitation to optimise physical function. This study suggests that it is also an opportune time to complete psychological interventions to improve mood and resilience prior to transplant. Certainly the value of improving physical fitness to reduce the length of post-transplant rehabilitation is well understood. This could also be enhanced by emphasising the importance of building coping strategies and managing expectations as part of a holistic rehabilitation plan.

Medical professionals were experienced as authoritative and powerful characters. Attention could be given here to making the assessment process more participative in order to empower patients and involve them in shared decision making. Perhaps involving patients in this training programme would allow them to voice their shared experience and increase understanding amongst medical professionals.

As participants' trajectory through their transplant experience progressed, they found themselves balanced between life and death as they waited and hoped for a donor organ to become available. Candidates and their families, as well as the health professionals working with them, are often focused on continuing healthcare and the hope of a suitable donor organ, so conversations about end of life issues may be neglected (Wright et al. 2007). Whilst care teams will take great care to remind patients that donors were not dying so that they would live, participants often experienced feelings of guilt and shame due to assuming a connection between their need for an organ with the death of a potential donor (Sanner 2003). During this time, participants felt unable to share their fears and anxieties with those around them, such as family and friends, and felt unprepared and uninformed. These experiences indicate the possible utility of an experienced transplant group who could provide a much-needed source of social support and informational needs. A recent critical review has also highlighted the role of social support in meeting the emotional needs of transplant patients (Conway et al. 2013). This can be facilitated by pre-transplant support groups, post-transplant patient led forums, and formal support systems where recipient volunteers can offer support and advice to pre-transplant candidates. Given the complex infection risks, the teams might consider how else to provide such support, for example, via online discussion groups or through a booklet written by patients for patients.

Participants described a sense of disappointment upon the realisation that their transplant had not offered *a magic cure* and that ongoing health problems persisted. Participants discovered that they were in fact still 'patients' (Crowley-Matoka 2005). Expectations had to be adapted to fit with the post-transplant reality, and they fought to regain their sense of purpose in life. In some circumstances, this was a protective factor because avoidance and denial are common strategies used to prevent individuals from feeling overwhelmed or shocked by the prospect of a transplant (Mai 1986). However, for others, it was a crushing disappointment not to be restored to their pre-deterioration self. Some recipients were able to find a new meaning and purpose to their post- transplant lives, either by focusing upon time with their family, or by caring for others. Transplant buddy networks are one way recipients could be encouraged to repay the 'gift of life' and manage feelings of guilt.

For all participants, there was a sense that they felt unprepared for the psychological impact and the realities of life following transplant surgery. Whilst such expectations could be partly addressed in the ways indicated above (e.g., addressing informational needs in the evaluative process or through contact with experienced transplant patients), some recipients may also benefit from psychological interventions, such as acceptance and commitment therapy (Hayes et al. 2006). Acceptance and commitment therapy is premised on the idea that, sometimes, helpful change can only take place when some aspects of the problem are accepted as they are. Participants are thus encouraged to embrace an active willingness to engage in meaningful activities in life despite experiences, thoughts, and other related feelings that might otherwise hinder that engagement. Other third wave contextual approaches may be equally useful, compassion focused therapy (Gilbert 2010) is particularly effective for recipients who have a strong sense of guilt and shame regarding their donor and the shame that their donor died to donate their organ so that they may live longer.

When the participants in this study were given the opportunity to share their experiences of their transplant they were keen to do so and gave detailed and insightful narratives of their journey. The benefit of storytelling has been recognised in testimonial psychotherapy (Lustig et al. 2004), which was developed for adults who have experienced trauma over a sustained period and consists of the individual telling their story to a clinician who subsequently creates a written document of the narrative at the end of therapy. This process also enables the person to recognise the strength and resources they have employed (Lustig et al. 2004). A similar model has been employed in the dignity therapy model developed by Chochinov et al. (2005), a narrative approach to end of life care that encourages people to share and make sense of their life story, resolving tensions, and providing a legacy to pass on after their death.

Conclusion

Within this chapter, we have presented the qualitative approach of narrative analysis and applied it to coping and adjusting to cardiothoracic transplant. The journey of cardiothoracic transplantation is an ongoing process that is a lifetime challenge. The composite story presented illustrates the challenges that transplant recipients encounter. It is clear that it is 'normal' to be distressed at each stage of the transplant process. By investing in time and resources to improving psychological care, the quality of the transplant experience may be improved, and so too recipients' psychological health. If recipients can be encouraged and supported to find purpose and meaning in their post-transplant life, then they will achieve better adjustment and well-being. Although the present findings offer particular issues of consideration for cardiothoracic transplant services, our description and application of narrative analysis here serves an illustrative purpose for others interested in applying narrative analysis for similar purposes to other healthcare settings.

References

Abbott, A. (1992) 'What do cases do?' Some notes on activity in sociological analysis. In Ragin, C.C. & Becker, H.S. (Eds.). *What Is a Case? Exploring the Foundations of Social Inquiry*. Cambridge, UK: University Press, pp. 53–82.

Andrews, M., Squire, C., & Tamboukou, M. (2008) *Doing Narrative Research*. Los Angeles, CA: Sage.

Bury, M. (1982) Chronic illness as biographical disruption. *Sociology of Health and Illness*, 4, 167–182.

Charmaz, K. (1991) *Good Days, Bad Days: The Self in Chronic Illness and Time*. New Brunswick, NJ: Rutgers University Press.

Chochinov, H.M., Hack, T., Hassard, T., Kristjanson, L.J., McClement, S., & Harlos, M. (2005). Dignity therapy: A novel psychotherapeutic intervention for patients near the end of life. *Journal of Clinical Oncology*, 23(24), 5520–5525.

Christie, J.D., Edwards, L.D., Kucheryavaya, A.Y., Benden, C., Dipchand, A.I., Dobbels, F. et al. (2012). The registry of the international society for heart and lung transplantation: Twenty-ninth adult lung and heart-lung transplant report – 2012. *The Journal of Heart and Lung Transplantation*, 31(10), 1074–1085.

Conway, A., Schadewaldt, V., Clark, R., Ski, C., Thompson, D.R., & Doering, L. (2013) The psychological experiences of adult heart transplant recipients: A systematic review and meta-summary of qualitative findings. *Heart & Lung: The Journal of Acute and Critical Care*, 42(6), 449–455.

Crossley, M.L. (2000) *Introducing Narrative Psychology: Self, Trauma and the Construction of Meaning*. Buckingham, UK: Open University Press.

Crowley-Matoka, M. (2005) Desperately seeking 'normal': The promise and perils of living with kidney transplantation. *Social Science & Medicine*, 61(4), 821–831.

Dew, M.A., & DiMartini, A.F. (2005) Psychological disorders and distress after adult cardiothoracic transplantation. *Journal of Cardiovascular Nursing*, 20(5), 51–66.

Dew, M.A., Manzetti, J., Goycoolea, J. R., Lee, A., Zomak, R., Vensak, J.L., & Kormos, R.L. (2002) Psychosocial aspects of transplantation. In Smith, S. & Ohler, L. (Eds.). *Organ Transplantation: Concepts, Issues, Practice and Outcomes*. New York: MedicaLogic/Medscape.

DiMartini, A., Crone, C., Fireman, M., & Dew, M.A. (2008) Psychiatric aspects of organ transplantation in critical care. *Critical Care Clinics*, 24, 949–981.

Dudley, T., Chaplin, D., Clifford C., & Mutimer, D.J. (2007) Quality of life after liver transplantation for hepatitis C infection. *Quality of Life Research*, 16, 1299–1308.

Engle, D. (2001) Psychosocial aspects of the organ transplant experience: What has been established and what we need for the future. *Journal of Clinical Psychology*, 57, 521–549.

Flynn, K., Daiches, A., Malpus, Z., Sanchez, M., & Yonan, N. (2013) 'A post-transplant person': Narratives of heart or lung transplantation and intensive care unit delirium. *Health*, 18, 352–368.

Frank, A.F. (1995) *The Wounded Story Teller: Body, Illness and Ethics*. Chicago, IL: University of Chicago Press.

Gilbert, P. (2010) *Compassion Focused Therapy: Distinctive Features*. London, UK: Routledge.

Hayes, S.C., Luoma, J.B., Bond, F.W., Masuda, A., & Lillis, J. (2006) Acceptance and commitment therapy: Model, processes and outcomes. *Behaviour Research and Therapy*, 44(1), 1–25.

Hertz, M.I., Taylor, D.W., Trulock, E.P., Boucek, M.M., Mohacsi, P.J., Edwards, L.B., & Keck, B.M. (2002) The registry of the international society for heart and lung transplantation: Nineteenth official report. *The Journal of Heart and Lung Transplantation*, 21, 950–970.

Hoshmand, L. (2005) Narratology, cultural psychology, and counselling research. *Journal of Counselling Psychology*, 52(2), 178–186.

Hyland, M.E. (1998) The problem of quality of life in medicine. *The Journal of the American Medical Association*, 279(6), 30.

Joralemon, D., & Fujinaga, M.K. (1996) Studying the quality of life after organ transplantation: Research problems and solutions. *Social Science & Medicine*, 44(9), 1259–1269.

Lieblich, A., Tuval-Mashiach, R., & Zilber, T. (1998) *Narrative Research: Reading, Analysis, and Interpretation*. Thousand Oaks, CA: Sage Publications.

Lustig, S.L., Weine, S.M., Saxe, G.N., & Beardslee, W.R. (2004) Testimonial psychotherapy for adolescent refugees: A case series. *Transcultural Psychiatry*, 41, 31–45.

Mai, F.M. (1986) Graft and donor denial in heart transplant recipients. *The American Journal of Psychiatry*, 143(9), 1159–1161.

McCormick, C. (2004) Storying stories: A narrative approach to in-depth interview conversations. *International Journal of Social Research Methodology*, 7, 219–236.

McMahon, L., Murray, C., & Simpson, J. (2012) The potential benefits of applying a narrative analytic approach in understanding the experience of fibromyalgia: A review. *Disability and Rehabilitation*, 34, 1121–1130.

Murray, M. (2008) Narrative psychology. In Smith, J.A. (Ed.). *Qualitative Psychology: A Practical Guide to Research Methods*. London, UK: Sage, pp. 111–132.

Rainer, J.P., Thompson, C.H., & Lambros, H. (2010) Psychological and psychosocial aspects of the solid organ transplant experience–A practice review. *Psychotherapy: Theory, Research, Practice, Training*, 47, 403–412.

Riessman, C. (1993) *Narrative Analysis*. London, UK: Sage Publications.

Riessman, C. (2008) *Narrative Methods for the Human Sciences*. Thousand Oaks, CA: Sage Publications.

Sadala, M.L.A., & Stolf, N.A.G. (2008) Heart transplantation experiences: A phenomenological approach. *Journal of Clinical Nursing*, 17, 217–225.

Sanner, M.A. (2003) Transplant recipients' conceptions of three key phenomena in transplantation: The organ donation, the organ donor, and the organ transplant. *Clinical Transplantation*, 17, 391–400.

Stehlik, J., Edwards, L.B., Kucheryavaya, A.Y., Benden, C., Christie, J.D., Dipchand, A.I. et al. (2011). The Registry of the International Society for Heart and Lung Transplantation: Twenty-ninth adult heart transplant report – 2012. *The Journal of Heart and Lung Transplantation*, 31(10), 1053–1064.

Stukas, A.A., Dew, M.A., Switzer, G.E., Dimartini, A., Lormos, R.L., & Griffith, B.P. (1999) PTSD in heart transplantation and their primary family caregivers. *Psychosomatics*, 40, 21.

Wright, L., Pape, D., Ross, K., Campbell, M., & Bowman, K. (2007) Approaching end-of-life care in organ transplantation: the impact of transplant patients' death and dying. *Progress in Transplantation*, 17(1), 57–62.

8

Qualitative Research and Osteoarthritis of the Knee

Nicholas F. Taylor, Samantha Bunzli, Jason A. Wallis and Nora Shields

CONTENTS

Brief Outline and Introduction

Knee osteoarthritis is one of the most common chronic diseases (Pereira et al. 2011). In 2015, 1 in 11 Australians (2.1 million) were estimated to have osteoarthritis (Australian Institute of Health and Welfare 2015) with direct costs to the health system of over $2 billion (Ackerman et al. 2016). Knee osteoarthritis, in particular, impacts the health system with over 60,000 total knee replacements performed in Australia in 2016 (Australian Orthopaedic Association National Joint Replacement Registry 2017). Lower limb osteoarthritis is also a major contributor to the burden of disease globally, ranked 11th out of 291 diseases according to years lived with disability (Cross et al. 2014), and is responsible for reduced health-related quality of life (Abbott et al. 2017, Salaffi et al. 2005, Wilson and Abbott 2018).

The main symptom associated with knee osteoarthritis is pain, with or without stiffness and swelling around the joint. It is recommended that osteoarthritis is diagnosed clinically without investigations if a person is over 45 years and has activity-related joint pain and either no morning joint-related stiffness or morning stiffness that lasts no longer than 30 minutes (National Institute for Health and Care Excellence 2014). People with knee osteoarthritis often have difficulty with mobility and other everyday activities (Creamer et al. 2000), which in turn can affect participation in work and leisure activities. As pain has a central role in the experience of people living with knee osteoarthritis, qualitative enquiry is particularly relevant. The experience and construct of pain associated with knee osteoarthritis may be better explored with qualitative analysis than quantitative analysis.

Clinical care standards emphasise the importance of embedding patient-centred care principles in the management of patients with knee osteoarthritis (Australian Commission on Safety and Quality in Health Care 2017). Patient-centred care for patients with knee osteoarthritis encourages patient participation in decision-making and communication with patients about their management options. Qualitative analysis with its focus on exploring the views and perceptions of participants is consistent with this principle of patient-centred care.

Qualitative analysis can also play an important complementary role to quantitative methods in knee osteoarthritis research. In evaluating the effects of interventions using quantitative methods, researchers are limited to a relatively small number of outcome measures. Indeed, reporting guidelines for randomised controlled trials recommend the choice of a single primary quantitative outcome (Schulz et al. 2010). Whilst such recommendations increase rigour and reduce bias, it does mean that potentially important outcomes from an intervention may not be identified. Qualitative analysis as part of a mixed-methods design (Creswell 2014), often using an inductive rather than a deductive approach, can address this limitation of quantitative research. Similarly, qualitative methods can be useful as part of a process evaluation of an intervention, providing insights into the reasons why an intervention was acceptable, adhered to, or why it did or didn't work (Moore et al. 2015).

This chapter will systematically review the literature on qualitative analysis of management of knee osteoarthritis. The review will include patient, caregiver, and clinician perceptions on management. The aims of this chapter are: (1) to investigate the scope of qualitative knee osteoarthritis research and (2) to explore how a qualitative approach can provide insights into the management of knee osteoarthritis.

Methods

The review was reported consistent with the Enhancing Transparency in Reporting the Synthesis of Qualitative Research (Tong et al. 2012).

Identification and Selection of Studies

Five electronic data bases (CINAHL, EMBASE, MEDLINE, PsycINFO, SPORTDiscus) were searched from inception until April 2018. The search strategy comprised two key concepts: knee osteoarthritis and qualitative research. For each concept, key words and Medical Subject Headings (MeSH) terms were combined using the 'OR' operator, and the results were combined using the 'AND' operator. An example of the search in one database can be viewed in Table 8.1. The search results were downloaded into bibliographic software. Reference lists of selected articles were manually searched for additional relevant articles.

Two reviewers independently reviewed the titles and abstracts yielded according to the inclusion criteria (Table 8.2). If eligibility was uncertain based on title and abstract, a full text version of the study was obtained. Studies reporting the perceptions of people with knee osteoarthritis, their carers, or their clinicians were included. Studies of perceptions on management and attitudes to living with knee osteoarthritis were included. Studies that explored perceptions to perioperative management to the intervention of total knee replacement were excluded. However, studies exploring attitudes about the decision to proceed to total knee replacement were included.

TABLE 8.1

Search Strategy in Medline

Search
1. knee osteoarthritis mp or Osteoarthritis, Knee/
2. knee/
3. knee arthroplasty.mp or Arthroplasty, Replacement, Knee/
4. Knee joint/
5. (knee adj3 osteoarthritis).mp
6. qualitative research.mp or Qualitative Research/
7. qualitative analysis.mp
8. qualitative evaluation.mp
9. qualitative study.mp
10. 1 or 2 or 3 or 4 or 5
11. 6 or 7 or 8 or 9
12. 10 and 11

/ denotes MeSH term; mp denotes keyword.

TABLE 8.2

Inclusion Criteria

	Inclusion Criteria	Exclusion Criteria
Design and report	Qualitative studies • Full text article published in peer-reviewed journal • Systematic review of qualitative research	• Questionnaires/surveys • Non-English language • Single case studies
Participants	Knee osteoarthritis • Perceptions of participants with knee osteoarthritis, their carers or their clinicians • May include other conditions providing perceptions about knee osteoarthritis are reported separately	• Participants not identified as having knee osteoarthritis (e.g. knee pain)
Interventions	No interventions required • May include perceptions about interventions for the management of knee osteoarthritis	• Perceptions of peri-operative management of knee replacement

Data Extraction and Analysis

Data were extracted from each study regarding participant age, sex, disease severity, body mass index, and current management, where available. Data were also extracted on qualitative design including sample size, data collection (individual interview or focus group), and qualitative framework informing the analysis.

Data analysis had two stages. The first stage involved coding studies to identify the area of knee osteoarthritis qualitative research. Then, the codes were organised into themes of enquiry. This process was completed independently by two reviewers. Reviewers read and re-read text to develop codes to describe the type of qualitative enquiry of each study. Codes were recorded with notes of definitions provided. A third reviewer was consulted if consensus was not reached.

The second stage of analysis involved a brief descriptive synthesis of each major theme identified, thereby providing an overview of the breadth of qualitative research of knee osteoarthritis. For each theme of enquiry, included studies were analysed by assigning codes to the themes and subthemes reported in each study. Patterns of codes between studies were then identified as themes. The descriptive synthesis was consistent with a content analysis approach, with the number of studies supporting an identified theme noted. Case studies of individual studies from two themes were highlighted.

Results

The search strategy yielded 680 articles. After title and abstract screening, 71 articles remained for full text review, with good agreement between the reviewers (Kappa = 0.654, 95% CI 0.552–0.757). Fifteen articles were excluded after full text review resulting in a final library of 56 articles (Figure 8.1).

The most common reasons for exclusion were that articles were abstracts, and the results of knee osteoarthritis were not reported separately from arthritis at other sites. The 56 articles reported the results of 49 qualitative studies and included 3 systematic reviews.

Three themes of enquiry were identified: the experience of living with knee osteoarthritis (12 articles from 9 studies); management of knee osteoarthritis (28 studies and 1 systematic review); and waiting for and deciding whether to have a total knee replacement (13 articles from 12 studies and 2 systematic reviews). The theme 'management of knee osteoarthritis' included the subthemes of: overall management; specific interventions; and physical activity and exercise.

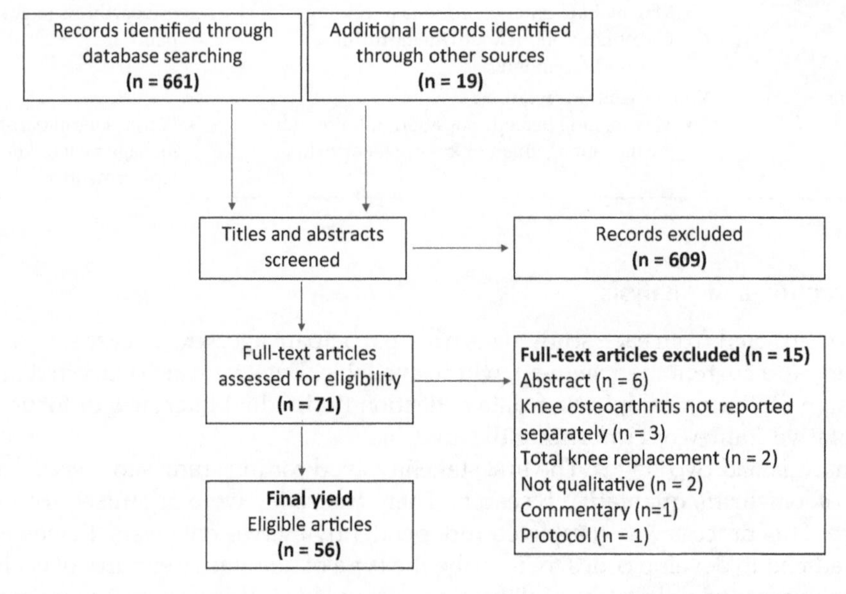

FIGURE 8.1
Yield of studies.

Methodological Approach of Included Studies

The methodological frameworks among the studies included the Lazarus stress model, constructive grounded theory, descriptive and interpretive phenomenology, framework analysis and meta-ethnography. Data were most often collected via semi-structured interviews, focus groups, or a combination of both, with structured field interviews and patient diaries also included. Three studies systematically reviewed the literature. Participant sampling was either convenience, purposive, or theoretical sampling. Data were analysed in various ways including content analysis, thematic analysis, grounded theory, constant comparative methods, or the van Kaam method of phenomenological data analysis.

The Experience of Living with Knee Osteoarthritis

Twelve articles reporting data from nine studies described the experience of living with knee osteoarthritis of 170 people (114 women; mean age 61 years, age range 25–87) and 28 carers of people with osteoarthritis (13 women; mean age 48 years) (Table 8.3). These studies were completed in Asia (n = 4), North America (n = 3), and Europe (n = 2) and most were recently published (six studies of nine studies published since 2013). Participants were diagnosed with knee osteoarthritis by a physician, rheumatologist, or orthopaedic surgeon between 1 year and 10 years prior. Participants' comorbidities as described in five studies included diabetes, depression/anxiety, polyarthritis, hypertension, heart disease, haemophilia, silicosis, vascular problems, cancer, gout, and multiple knee surgeries. Most people were symptomatic at the time of the study: participants in four studies self-assessed their pain as mild to severe, and participants in three studies reported functional limitations, including difficulties with squatting and limitations in activities of daily living and sport and recreation, and reduced quality of life. Five studies provided details on participant employment status, all participants in three studies were retired, and the majority of participants in two studies were employed at the time of the study.

The studies explored the experience of living with knee osteoarthritis from the perspectives of the participants themselves (n = 7) and their caregivers (n = 1). One study focused specifically on quality of life in people with knee osteoarthritis. The main themes reported were: (1) perceived causes of knee osteoarthritis and prognosis; (2) pain experience and management; (3) functional impact of knee osteoarthritis; (4) social impact of knee osteoarthritis; (5) emotional impact of knee osteoarthritis; (6) interactions with health professionals; and (7) adjusting to knee osteoarthritis.

The perceived causes of knee osteoarthritis discussed in five studies (Chan and Chan 2011, Hsu et al. 2015, Kao and Tsai 2012, 2014, MacKay et al. 2016, Pouli et al. 2014) included internal factors such as being overweight, family history of osteoarthritis, ageing, working in occupations requiring extensive kneeling or lifting, past sporting activities, and menopause, and external factors such as trauma and the weather. Participants perceived knee osteoarthritis as preventable or partially attributable to actions or incidents that were modifiable (e.g. pushing too far or knee injury) had they changed their behaviour earlier in life. Caregivers of people with knee osteoarthritis attributed the cause of their relative's knee osteoarthritis to ageing, working too hard, or to unknown causes (Hsu et al. 2015). The prognosis of knee osteoarthritis was discussed by participants in two studies (Clarke et al. 2014, MacKay et al. 2016). Participants believed their symptoms would get worse over time, as knee osteoarthritis was 'a progressive

TABLE 8.3

Characteristics of Included Studies of Experiences of Living with Knee Osteoarthritis

Study	Country	Population	Demographics (N, Age, Sex, BMI)	Method: Framework/ Analysis	Sampling	Data Collection	Research Questions
Carmona-Teres et al. (2017)	Spain	Knee osteoarthritis • Symptomatic	N = 10 Mean age 70 yrs, 70% women	Content thematic analysis based on Lazarus stress model categories	Theoretical	Individual interviews • Semi-structured	Understand current practice from perspective of people with knee osteoarthritis Understand experiences of people with osteoarthritis
Chan and Chan (2011)	Hong Kong	Knee osteoarthritis • Mild to very severe	N = 20 Mean age 57 yrs, 65% women	Grounded theory	Convenience	Individual interviews • Semi-structured	Evaluate influence of different pain patterns on quality of life Investigate coping strategies
Clarke et al. (2014) Pouli et al. (2014)	UK	Knee osteoarthritis • Symptomatic	N = 24 Mean age 62 yrs, 71% women	Descriptive thematic analysis	Purposive	Individual interviews • Semi-structured	Explore participant's experience of living with knee osteoarthritis and their beliefs about knee osteoarthritis and its treatment
Hsu et al. (2015)	Taiwan	Caregivers of people with knee osteoarthritis	N = 28 Mean age 48 yrs, 46% women	Descriptive content analysis	Convenience	Individual interviews • Semi-structured	Explore primary caregivers perceptions of their older relatives' knee osteoarthritis pain and management

(Continued)

TABLE 8.3 (*Continued*)

Characteristics of Included Studies of Experiences of Living with Knee Osteoarthritis

Study	Country	Population	Demographics (N, Age, Sex, BMI)	Method: Framework/ Analysis	Sampling	Data Collection	Research Questions
Keysor et al. (1998)	USA	Knee osteoarthritis • Presence of functional limitations	N = 4 Age range 25–43 yrs, 75% women	van Kaam method of phenomenological data analysis	Purposive	Individual interviews • Semi structured (each participant interviewed twice)	Understand the experience of living with osteoarthritis as young and middle-aged adults
Kao and Tsai (2012, 2014)	Taiwan	Knee osteoarthritis • Symptomatic	N = 17 Mean age 50 yrs, 82% women Mean BMI 28.6	Constant comparison	Purposive	Individual interviews • Semi structured	Understand the living and illness experiences of middle-aged adults with early knee osteoarthritis
MacKay et al. (2014b, 2016)	Canada	Knee osteoarthritis • Moderately symptomatic	N = 51 Median age 49 yrs, 61% women	Constructivist grounded Theory/constant comparative method	Purposive	Focus groups Individual interviews • Semi-structured	Explore the meaning and perceived consequences of knee symptoms
Maly and Krupa (2007)	Canada	Knee osteoarthritis	N = 3 Age range 62–87 yrs, 67% women	Descriptive phenomenology	Convenience	Individual interviews • Semi structured	Understand the experience of living with knee osteoarthritis in older adults
Xie et al. (2006)	Singapore	Knee osteoarthritis • Symptomatic	N = 41 Mean age 64 yrs, 66% women	Grounded theory/ Content analysis	Purposive	Focus groups	Determine health-related quality of life domains affected by knee osteoarthritis Identify ethnic variations in the importance of these domains

degenerative disease' and could not be 'cured'. However, participants in one study (MacKay et al. 2016) also felt they could halt or slow the progression of their symptoms through diet and exercise.

Pain experience and management emerged as a theme in all nine studies. Pain was described by participants as the predominant 'omnipresent' feature of knee osteoarthritis. Pain was perceived to interrupt daily activities such as walking, to make people less confident in their bodies, and to slow people down. Participants in one study described two distinct patterns of pain: 'mechanical' pain described as 'sharp' pain related to discrete movements or activities and 'inflammatory' pain described as a 'burning' pain which was more unpredictable and associated with the weather or prolonged activity (Chan and Chan 2011). Pain was perceived as insurmountable when there was no foreseeable end to it and made some participants feel 'old'. Participants reported managing their pain with medication, but that this was not always a satisfactory strategy due to feelings of dependence, undesirable side effects, and only partial relief from symptoms. Other pain management strategies described were activity-related (including exercise, avoidance of certain activities, pacing, and 'physiotherapy'), psychological-related (having a positive life philosophy, humour, continuing to engage in pleasurable activities), passive treatment modalities (ice, heat, massage, Chinese traditional medicine), and weight loss.

Participants in all studies reported functional limitations due to their knee osteoarthritis, particularly mobility restrictions. Participants predominantly reported limitations in movements involving weight-bearing such as standing, stair climbing, squatting, kneeling, bending; limitations in self-care activities such as dressing, toileting, sleeping, cooking; or limitations in leisure pursuits such as walking, gardening, sport, and other forms of exercise. Living with knee osteoarthritis was reported by participants to reduce their physical activity, and to become sedentary. Participants described that the impact on physical activities was associated with the severity of their knee osteoarthritis. The combined impact of pain and functional limitations was an inability for some participants to participate in paid employment, a reduction in work hours affecting household income, or other impacts on work such as requiring modifications, tiring easily, or being less efficient. For others, living with knee osteoarthritis meant a loss of independence.

Participants in five studies felt knee osteoarthritis had a substantial social impact (Chan and Chan 2011, Keysor et al. 1998, MacKay et al. 2014b, Maly and Krupa 2007, Xie et al. 2006). It reduced their ability to stay socially connected because of reduced participation in leisure activities and because of difficulties with taking public transport. For some participants, the inability to take part in socially based physical activity, such as walking with friends or playing sport was the most difficult aspect of this condition. Participants described social isolation marked by doing fewer activities outside of home. Participants felt mobility limitations made them conspicuous to others that they had poor health which facilitated social isolation. Living with knee osteoarthritis reduced their enjoyment of activities, particular when travelling. Others described a change in their social relationships conveying that they related more to older individuals with health problems. Participants also described the repercussions of knee osteoarthritis on family life, including a need to stop looking after their grandchildren or difficulties playing with their children.

Eight studies reported data on the emotional impact of osteoarthritis (Carmona-Teres et al. 2017, Chan and Chan 2011, Hsu et al. 2015, Keysor et al. 1998, MacKay et al. 2014b, 2016, Maly and Krupa 2007, Pouli et al. 2014, Xie et al. 2006). Living with knee osteoarthritis was described as having a negative impact on mood, resulting in feelings of anxiety, irritability, emotional distress, depression, and fear for the future. Some participants expressed that their mobility limitations in particular devalued their sense of self-worth because mobility was integral to their identity and having knee osteoarthritis made them feel like 'a partial person', or 'less valuable'. Other participants talked of a reduced sense of control or of being 'lost' after being 'told' to eliminate athletic activities and change their lifestyles. Other participants reported grieving for activities they could no longer take part in, or their vision of ageing. Participants in one study (Chan and Chan 2011) felt the unpredictability and uncertainty of living with knee osteoarthritis caused the most stress.

Four studies explored the interactions of people with knee osteoarthritis with health professionals (Carmona-Teres et al. 2017, Clarke et al. 2014, Kao and Tsai 2012, Keysor et al. 1998). Participants described the impact of their diagnosis as a positive step towards successful management, although for people with low expectations of treatment, the impact of diagnosis resulted in limited contact with health professionals. Participants who had positive interactions with health professionals described being listened to, being offered hope for the future, and being provided with recommendations for managing knee osteoarthritis including weight loss and exercise. Participants who had negative experiences interacting with health professionals described their dissatisfaction with receiving limited information about treatment options available including behavioural management, a sense of not being listened to, not being given sufficient attention, or not understanding the information provided to them. For example, in one study (MacKay et al. 2016) participants recounted how their symptoms were viewed by health professionals as something that could not be changed, which they 'just had to live with' or were dismissed as an inevitable part of ageing.

Eight studies (Carmona-Teres et al. 2017, Chan and Chan 2011, Clarke et al. 2014, Hsu et al. 2015, Kao and Tsai 2014, Keysor et al. 1998, MacKay et al. 2014b, Maly and Krupa 2007) reported participants' descriptions of adjusting to having knee osteoarthritis in terms of role changes or modifications, ownership of their health management, awareness of their condition, and development of coping strategies. Participants described taking measures to alleviate symptoms and protect their knee joint including lifestyle adjustments by keeping active and controlling their weight, adapting their work, modifying activities or postures to manage everyday routines (e.g. climbing stair less frequently, not carrying heavy things, planning ahead), and seeking out health-related information.

These findings provide important insights into the unique psychosocial factors that characterise the experience of knee osteoarthritis. Some of these factors, for example, emotional distress and the unpredictability of pain, have also been identified among people with other chronic musculoskeletal conditions such as low back pain (Bunzli et al. 2013). Other factors, for example, the perception that knee osteoarthritis is an inevitable part of ageing and the perceived absence of a cure, appear to be more unique to the experience of living with knee osteoarthritis. By helping clinicians to better understand the lived experience of knee osteoarthritis, these findings can optimise the patient-clinician interaction, and may suggest potentially modifiable psychosocial targets for intervention.

Overall Management

Ten studies explored the perceptions of 392 participants with knee osteoarthritis and 62 health professionals (including 22 general practitioners, 14 orthopaedic surgeons and residents, and 8 physiotherapists) about management of knee osteoarthritis (Table 8.4).

TABLE 8.4

Characteristics of Included Studies of Overall Management

Study	Country	Population	Demographics (N, Age, Sex, BMI)	Intervention	Method: Framework/ Analysis	Sampling	Data Collection	Research Questions
Alami et al. (2011)	France	Knee osteoarthritis Health professionals	N = 81 71% women, N = 29: 11 general practitioners, 4 surgeons, 6 rheumatologists, 8 alternative therapists	No intervention	Descriptive • Inductive	Purposive	Individual interviews • Semi-structured	Explore views of patients and health professionals about management of knee osteoarthritis
Egerton et al. (2017)	Australia	Health professionals	N = 11 general practitioners	Telephone service to support self-management • Not yet received	Descriptive • Inductive	Purposive	Individual interviews • Semi-structured	Explore general practitioners expectations to use a telephone service for patients with knee osteoarthritis
Elwyn et al. (2018)	UK	Health professionals	N = 6 Physiotherapists	A patient decision support tool • Completed	Descriptive • Inductive	Convenience	Individual interviews • Semi-structured	Explore reactions of health professional to using a patient decision support tool
Kinsey et al. (2017)	UK	Knee osteoarthritis	N = 72 Man age 66 yrs 60% women	A patient decision support tool • Completed	Descriptive • Thematic analysis	Purposive	Individual interviews • Semi-structured	Explore patients experiences of using a decision support tool
Li et al. (2013)	Canada	Health professionals	N = 10 Orthopaedic surgeons and residents	Load absorbing implant • Not yet received	Descriptive	Purposive	Individual interviews Focus group	Perceptions on management of knee osteoarthritis and opinion on implants

(*Continued*)

TABLE 8.4 (*Continued*)

Characteristics of Included Studies of Overall Management

Study	Country	Population	Demographics (N, Age, Sex, BMI)	Intervention	Method: Framework/ Analysis	Sampling	Data Collection	Research Questions
MacKay et al. (2014a)	Canada	Knee osteoarthritis • Moderate	N = 41 Mean age 51 yrs, 63% women	No intervention	Constructivist grounded theory • Constant comparison	Purposive	Focus groups	Explore how people with knee osteoarthritis manage their symptoms
Morden et al. (2011)	UK	Knee osteoarthritis • Moderate to severe	N = 22 Age range 50–75+ yrs, 59% women	Self-management • Unstructured	Descriptive • Constant comparison	Purposive	Individual interviews • Semi-structured Diaries	Explore self-management of knee osteoarthritis
Prasanna et al. (2013)	Canada	Knee osteoarthritis Health professionals	N = 5 Age >50 yrs 60% women N = 6: Allied health	No intervention	Content analysis	Convenience	Focus groups	Explore reasons for delay in management
Spitaels et al. (2017)	Belgium	Knee osteoarthritis	N = 11 Mean age 66 yrs 64% women	No intervention	Content analysis	Convenience	Individual interviews • Semi-structured	Explore patient perceptions of guideline recommendations
Tallon et al. (2000)	UK	Knee osteoarthritis • Mild to moderate	N = 7	No intervention	Content analysis	Convenience	Focus group	Explore perception of treatment preferences

The majority of participants with knee osteoarthritis were women over 50 years. Five studies did not include an intervention, but sought participants' views on aspects of overall knee management (Alami et al. 2011, MacKay et al. 2014a, Prasanna et al. 2013, Spitaels et al. 2017, Tallon et al. 2000). Two studies explored experiences of participants and health professionals in using a decision support tool (Elwyn et al. 2018, Kinsey et al. 2017), 1 study explored the experiences of participants classified as providing self-management for their condition (Morden et al. 2011), and two studies sought health professionals' views on proposed interventions of a telephone service to support behavioural change (Egerton et al. 2017) and a load absorbing implant for the knee (Li et al. 2013).

There were two main themes. One theme was about the perceptions of participants with knee osteoarthritis and health professionals about interventions and management. The other theme was about what participants and health professionals thought about each other.

Both participants with knee osteoarthritis and health professionals agreed controlling symptoms, especially pain, and improving function were important treatment goals (four studies). There was concerns expressed in three studies (MacKay et al. 2014a, Morden et al. 2011, Tallon et al. 2000) about the over reliance on drugs to control pain. Participants with knee osteoarthritis in three studies expressed the view that 'active management', 'carrying on regardless', and making 'adaptations to get on with life' were important in managing their condition. However, in contrast, participants in two studies with very small sample sizes (Prasanna et al. 2013, Spitaels et al. 2017) expressed views that differed with guideline recommendations: 'insisting on the need for imaging', 'having a fear that physiotherapy may aggravate their condition', and 'perceiving surgery as the only option'.

Participants with knee osteoarthritis and health professionals each had negative perceptions of the other group. Participants with knee osteoarthritis perceived health professionals communicated poorly (two studies), thought they were not seen as a priority by health professionals, and that treatment was of little use in helping their condition (two studies). Health professionals viewed that patients with knee osteoarthritis could have unrealistic expectations (one study) and that it was difficult to explain treatment options (one study). Health professionals in one study expressed the view of a need for a decision aid to address the issue of communication (Alami et al. 2011). Experiences with a decision aid tool were explored in two studies. Both participants with knee osteoarthritis (Kinsey et al. 2017) and physiotherapists (Elwyn et al. 2018) expressed the view that the decision aid tool aided communication and added value to management.

Specific Management

Nine studies explored the experiences of 293 participants receiving or delivering specific interventions or management for knee osteoarthritis (Table 8.5). The interventions were varied. Six interventions were behavioural, including self-management, weight loss management (two studies), a form of cognitive behavioural therapy, health promotion, and the use of wearable technology. Three interventions could be considered passive involving a therapy being administered to a participant with knee osteoarthritis, including massage, prolotherapy (injections), and moxibustion (application of burnt mugwort to the skin). All studies explored the experiences of participants with knee osteoarthritis, except one which explored the experiences of physiotherapists delivering a cognitive behavioural therapy addressing pain coping skills for their patients with

TABLE 8.5

Characteristics of Included Studies of Specific Interventions

Study	Country	Population	Demographics (N, Age, Sex, BMI)	Intervention	Method: Framework/ Analysis	Sampling	Data Collection	Research Questions
Ali et al. (2017)	USA	Knee osteoarthritis • Relatively independent	N = 18 Mean age 65 yrs, 78% women, Mean BMI 33	Massage • 8 weeks • Weekly or biweekly • Completed	Descriptive Content analysis	Purposive • Participation in trial	Individual interviews • Semi-structured	Explore effects of massage
Belsi et al. (2016)	UK	Knee osteoarthritis • Receiving rehabilitation	N = 21 Age range 45–65 yrs, 90% women	Wearable technology • Not yet received	Framework analysis	Convenience	Focus groups	Explore expected impact of wearable technology
Isla Peria et al. (2016)	Spain	Knee osteoarthritis	N = 10 Mean age 67 yrs, 80% women, Mean BMI 41	Health education weight loss program • Completed	Phenomenology Thematic content analysis	Purposive	Focus group	Explore meaning of obesity and factors associated with weight loss or gain
Nielsen et al. (2014)	Australia	Physiotherapists • Providing therapy for patients with knee osteoarthritis	N = 8 90% women	Cognitive behaviour therapy • Pain coping skills therapy • 10 weekly sessions • Completed	Framework analysis	Purposive	Individual interviews • Semi structured	Explore therapists' experience with pain coping skills therapy
Ong et al. (2011)	UK	Knee osteoarthritis • Moderate to severe	N = 22 Age range 50–75+ yrs, 59% women	Self-management • Ongoing	Constant comparison	Purposive	Individual interviews • in-depth Diaries	Explore the meaning and enactment of self-management in everyday life

(*Continued*)

TABLE 8.5 ***(Continued)***

Characteristics of Included Studies of Specific Interventions

Study	Country	Population	Demographics (N, Age, Sex, BMI)	Intervention	Method: Framework/ Analysis	Sampling	Data Collection	Research Questions
Rabago et al. (2016)	USA	Knee osteoarthritis	N = 22 Mean age 57 yrs, 22% women	Prolotherapy • Hypertonic dextrose injections • 3–5 injections over 17 weeks • Completed	Descriptive	Purposive • Participation in trial	Individual interviews • Semi-structured	Explore experiences of participants who received prolotherapy
Toye et al. (2017)	UK	Knee osteoarthritis • Listed for total knee replacement	N = 6 Age range 59–76 yrs, 100% men, BMI range 31–38	Weight loss management • Unstructured	Constructivist grounded theory	Convenience	Individual interviews • Flexible guide	Experience of weight loss or gain
Son et al. (2013)	Korea	Knee osteoarthritis • Mild	N = 16 Age range 40–69 yrs 69% women	Moxibustion • Application of burnt dried mugwort to skin • 12 weeks, –x3 per week • Completed	Content analysis	Convenience • Participation in trial	Individual interviews	Explore experience of moxibustion
Victor et al. (2004)	UK	Knee osteoarthritis	N = 170 Mean age 63 yrs, 73% women	Health promotion • Nurse led 4 × 1 hr groups • Ongoing	Content analysis	Convenience • Participation in trial	Individual interviews Group discussion Diaries	Explore meaning of osteoarthritis for those receiving health promotion

knee osteoarthritis (Nielsen et al. 2014). Participants with knee osteoarthritis were typically older, with increased body mass index (where this was reported), with a greater proportion of women, with the exception of a study that explored the experiences of men to weight loss management (Toye et al. 2017). The severity of knee osteoarthritis was not well described; two studies included participants with moderate to severe knee osteoarthritis (Ong et al. 2011, Toye et al. 2017), and one study described participants as having mild osteoarthritis (Son et al. 2013).

Themes were reported about the effect of the intervention, about practical issues related to the implementation of the intervention, and about the personal experience of living with knee osteoarthritis. There were very few common themes reported across the nine studies.

The three studies reporting therapies administered to participants with knee osteoarthritis reported very positive results (Ali et al. 2017, Rabago et al. 2016, Son et al. 2013). Reported improvements included quality of life (two studies), relaxation/comfort (two studies), function (two studies), and reduced pain (one study). The four studies reporting the perceived effects of behavioural interventions reported neutral or negative findings. Self-management was regarded by participants as 'hard work' (Ong et al. 2011). Participants acknowledging the difficulty of losing weight expressed the view of 'what's the point?' (Toye et al. 2017). Less than half of participants enrolled in a health promotion program were satisfied with their management (Victor et al. 2004).

Four studies reported themes about implementation. Despite their positive experience, participants who had received a massage intervention were concerned that ongoing access to the intervention would be difficult due to cost (Ali et al. 2017). Participants interviewed about the prospect of using wearable technology to help their condition were concerned with practical issues about access and use of the technology (Belsi et al. 2016). Training or pre-treatment counselling was valued by physiotherapists delivering a form of cognitive behaviour therapy (Nielsen et al. 2014) and by participants with knee osteoarthritis.

The third broad theme concerned participants' experience of living with knee osteoarthritis whilst receiving their intervention. These personal experiences included: the experience of living with pain and the adjustments required to complete daily tasks (Ong et al. 2011). It also included the experience of living with obesity including negative societal labelling, plus attitudes and knowledge about obesity for men such as not thinking that they had to lose weight to be healthy (Toye et al. 2017). One study identified limited knowledge about osteoarthritis (Victor et al. 2004).

The synthesis of data from the nine studies exploring specific interventions suggests participants were more ambivalent about the benefits they received from behavioural interventions than from therapies where they were the passive recipients. These results were surprising, given theory suggests behavioural change should be important to address the lifestyle factors that contribute to and exacerbate knee osteoarthritis, and that some of the passive interventions studied are not recommended in clinical guidelines (McAlindon et al. 2014, National Institute for Health and Care Excellence 2014). Participants may have more faith in interventions to fix or to ease their symptoms rather than undertake the 'hard work', motivation, and commitment required to change behaviour. The negative attitudes and lack of knowledge demonstrated by participants in some studies reinforce the importance of basing behaviour change approaches on established theoretical frameworks, acknowledging stages of change, and utilising methods to address ambivalence.

Exercise Interventions

Six studies explored the perceptions of 95 participants (54% women) with knee osteoarthritis and 22 health professionals (18 physiotherapists) about their experiences after participation in, or delivery of, exercise interventions (Table 8.6). Five studies included physiotherapist-delivered exercise programs of between 8 weeks and 26 weeks duration as part of the intervention arm of randomised controlled trials (Campbell et al. 2001, Hinman et al. 2016, 2017, Lawford et al. 2018b, Wallis et al. 2017a). In one study, participants took part in an exercise program although no specific details were provided (Thorstensson et al. 2006). Various exercise delivery methods were used including face to face home exercise programs (two studies), telephone-delivered exercise (one study), Skype Internet technology to enable physiotherapists to prescribe and supervise exercise programs (one study), and a community-based walking program with supervised and unsupervised walking sessions (one study). One systematic review summarised findings from primary qualitative articles exploring people's opinions and experiences with exercise programs (Hurley et al. 2018). Two additional studies explored the perceptions of 49 participants (67% women) with knee osteoarthritis about exercise and physical activity who were not involved in an intervention (Gay et al. 2018, Hendry et al. 2006). One study explored the experiences of eight physiotherapists trained to deliver a behavioural intervention for people with knee osteoarthritis (Lawford et al. 2018a).

Participants with knee osteoarthritis in these studies were typically older, with a greater proportion of women and with an average body mass index of at least 30 (where this was reported). The severity of knee osteoarthritis based on either radiological or clinical findings was described as mild to severe.

Three main themes were reported. These were: (1) the effects and experiences from participation in, or delivery of exercise and behavioural interventions for patients with knee osteoarthritis; (2) the experiences related to implementing and compliance with exercise and behavioural interventions; and (3) people's attitudes and beliefs about exercise and physical activity who were not involved in an intervention.

Five studies described important positive effects of exercise and behavioural interventions delivered by physiotherapists and telephone coaches (Hinman et al. 2016, 2017, Lawford et al. 2018b, Thorstensson et al. 2006, Wallis et al. 2017a). Participants with knee osteoarthritis commented on the benefits of exercise such as ability to walk further, improved knee strength, sense of well-being and increased participation in meaningful activities. Physiotherapists' commonly noticed improvements in strength and functional outcomes.

Five studies reported on the theme 'experiences related to implementing and compliance with exercise and behavioural interventions' (Campbell et al. 2001, Hinman et al. 2016, 2017, Lawford et al. 2018b, Wallis et al. 2017a). Whilst the studies involved a range of intervention settings (face-face, phone, Internet, and community), most participants with knee osteoarthritis in the included studies valued support, information, supervision, and structure of exercise programs delivered by physiotherapists and telephone coaches that helped with motivation and incorporating prescribed exercise into weekly routines. Factors which enhanced compliance with exercises prescribed in the interventions included the ability to exercise at home, positive exercise beliefs, experience of positive outcomes, and support from clinicians and coaches. Comorbidities, age, the weather (for an outdoor exercise program), and negative beliefs about osteoarthritis reduced compliance. Some participants reported dissatisfaction with the intervention if the exercises were boring, if they had to travel long distances to perform interventions, and if the exercises were not supervised.

TABLE 8.6

Characteristics of Included Studies of Exercise Interventions

Study	Country	Population	Demographics (N, age, sex, BMI)	Intervention	Method: Framework/ Analysis	Sampling	Data Collection	Research Questions
Campbell et al. (2001)	UK	Knee osteoarthritis	N = 20 Age range 40–70+ yrs, 70% women	Physiotherapy • Face to face delivered home exercise program to strengthen VMO, patella taping, advice, and information leaflets • 9 × 30 min sessions over 8 weeks	Inductive	Convenience • Participation in RCT	Individual interviews • In-depth	To understand reasons for compliance or non-compliance with home exercise program for people with knee osteoarthritis
Gay et al. (2018)	France	Knee osteoarthritis • Mild to moderate symptoms	N = 20 (interviews) Mean age 67 yrs 60% women N = 7 (focus groups) Mean age 69 yrs 86% women	No intervention	Content analysis	Convenience • Recruited from Spa Therapy	Individual interviews • Semi-structured Focus groups	Explore the motivators for, and barriers to, regular physical activity in people with knee osteoarthritis
Hendry et al. (2006)	UK	Knee osteoarthritis • Mild to severe symptoms	N = 22 Age range 52–86 yrs 73% women	No intervention	Conceptual Framework	Convenience • Recruited from General Practice	Individual interviews Focus Groups (N = 6)	Explore the views of primary care patients with knee osteoarthritis towards exercise, and explore factors that determine acceptability and motivation to exercise, and barriers that limit its use

(*Continued*)

TABLE 8.6 (*Continued*)

Characteristics of Included Studies of Exercise Interventions

Study	Country	Population	Demographics (N, age, sex, BMI)	Intervention	Method: Framework/ Analysis	Sampling	Data Collection	Research Questions
Hinman et al. (2016)	Australia	Knee osteoarthritis • Mild to moderate symptoms Physiotherapists • Mean 19 years' experience Telephone coaches • Two had prior experience • 3 health disciplines	N = 6 Mean age 62 yrs, 50% women N = 10 50% women Mean age 43 yrs N = 4 100% women Mean age 42 yrs	Physiotherapy • Face to face delivered home exercise program including 4–6 exercises performed 3 x week • Advice to increase physical activity, and information booklet about exercise, physical activity, and behaviour change • 5 × 30 min sessions over 26 weeks Telephone coaching • 6–12 calls over 26 weeks • Mean duration 28 mins • HealthChange Australia model	Symbolic interactionism Grounded theory	Convenience • Participation in RCT	Individual interviews • Semi structured	Explore perceptions of participants, physiotherapists and telephone coaches engaged in an integrated program of physiotherapy and telephone coaching for people with knee osteoarthritis
Hinman et al. (2017)	Australia	Knee osteoarthritis • Mild to moderate symptoms Physiotherapists • Mean 15 years' experience	N = 12 50% women Mean age 62 yrs N = 8 50% women Mean age 39 yrs	Physiotherapy • Skype delivered home exercise program including 5–6 exercises performed 3 x week, • 7 Internet-based Skype-delivered sessions over 12 weeks	Donabedian framework Thematic and constant comparative analysis	Convenience • Participation in RCT	Individual interviews • Semi structured	Explore the experiences of people with knee osteoarthritis and physiotherapists with using Skype for exercise management of knee osteoarthritis

(*Continued*)

TABLE 8.6 (*Continued*)

Characteristics of Included Studies of Exercise Interventions

Study	Country	Population	Demographics (N, age, sex, BMI)	Intervention	Method: Framework/ Analysis	Sampling	Data Collection	Research Questions
Hurley et al. (2018)	–	Knee (and hip) osteoarthritis	N = 12 studies	Exercise-based rehabilitation programs including land-based or aquatic-based exercise	Systematic review of the literature	–	–	To people's opinions and experiences of exercise-based programs (e.g. their views, understanding, experiences and beliefs about the utility of exercise in the management of chronic pain/OA).
Lawford et al. (2018a)	Australia	Knee osteoarthritis • Mild to moderate symptoms	N = 20 Mean age 59 yrs 65% women Mean BMI 30	Physiotherapy • Telephone delivered home exercise program including 5–6 exercises performed 3 x week, over 26 weeks • Advice to increase physical activity, and information booklet about exercise, physical activity, and behaviour change, access to videos demonstrating the exercises	Donabedian framework Interpretivist paradigm Thematic analysis	Convenience • Participation in RCT	Individual interviews • Semi-structured	Explore participants perceptions of telephone delivered exercise therapy and behavioural change strategies

(*Continued*)

TABLE 8.6 (*Continued*)

Characteristics of Included Studies of Exercise Interventions

Study	Country	Population	Demographics (N, age, sex, BMI)	Intervention	Method: Framework/ Analysis	Sampling	Data Collection	Research Questions
				Telephone coaching • 5–10 calls over 26 weeks by physiotherapist using HealthChange Australia model • Calls duration 20–40 mins				
Lawford et al. (2018b)	Australia	Physiotherapists • Mean 14 years' experience	N = 8 Mean age 35 yrs 50% women	No intervention Physiotherapists completed HealthChange training to deliver person centred care	Constructivist paradigm Thematic analysis	Convenience • Participation in RCT	Individual interviews • Semi-structured	Explore the experiences and impacts from a behavioural management training course for physiotherapists
Thorstensson et al. (2006)	Sweden	Knee osteoarthritis • Moderate to severe radiographically (at least Grade 3 Kellgren Lawrence score)	N = 16 Age range 39–64 yrs 38% women, Mean BMI 30	Exercise program	Phenomenographic analysis	Convenience • Participation in trial	Individual interviews • Semi-structured	Describe how middle-aged patients conceive exercise as a treatment for knee osteoarthritis
Wallis et al. (2017a)	Australia	Knee osteoarthritis • Severe radiographically	N = 21 43% women Mean age 67 yrs Mean BMI 34	Physiotherapy • Walking program, moderate intensity • 70 minutes per week, in minimum of 10-minute sessions • One walking session per week supervised by physiotherapist	Phenomenological	Convenience • Participation in RCT	Individual interviews • Semi structured	Explore the perceptions of people with severe knee osteoarthritis and increased cardiovascular risk about participating in a walking program

Health professionals and coaches delivering the study interventions also reported mostly positive experiences. Physiotherapists perceived participation in the trials as an opportunity for professional development, to acquire new skills through training and practice in a supervised environment, and valued working together in multidisciplinary models of care (Hinman et al. 2016). Physiotherapists prescribing exercise interventions remotely via Skype technology in one study perceived this could enhance their clinical practice by improving access for patients living in remote areas (Hinman et al. 2017). However, telephone coaches highlighted difficulties with gaining rapport with participants when communicating via telephone without visual contact (Hinman et al. 2016). Some physiotherapists in the included studies felt that the structured trial protocol meant they could not use their clinical reasoning to deliver the study intervention, conflicting with their usual practice. Others saw this as a positive, removing the temptation to 'get bogged down with hands on stuff' that was perceived to be less effective treatments for people with knee osteoarthritis.

Two studies reported on the theme attitudes and beliefs about exercise and physical activity from people with knee osteoarthritis who did not participate in an intervention (Gay et al. 2018, Hendry et al. 2006). Commonly positive attitudes were related to perceived benefits in function and general well-being. Despite the benefits, common misconceptions about the cause of knee osteoarthritis were reported, with some participants believing physical activity caused osteoarthritis and pain. Pain was a common barrier to exercise as well as age, fear avoidance, low self-efficacy, anxiety, physical capacity, and illness. Participants with knee osteoarthritis reported dissatisfaction when health professional advice was conflicting or vague about exercise and physical activity. For example, participants being told to 'look after their knees' may imply that rest rather than exercise is beneficial (Hendry et al. 2006).

People with knee osteoarthritis often have low levels of physical activity and high risks of mortality from cardiovascular disease (Nüesch et al. 2011, Wallis et al. 2013). To address this, a recent randomised controlled trial showed 70 minutes/week of moderate intensity physical activity delivered via a walking program for 12 weeks for patients with severe knee osteoarthritis lead to cardiovascular benefits without increasing pain (Wallis et al. 2017b). The effectiveness of exercise interventions, including walking programs, is dependent on adherence, which is strongly influenced by people's thoughts, perceptions, attitudes, and beliefs about the risks and benefits of participation. A qualitative study alongside this trial explored 21 participants' subjective perspectives about the 12-week program (Wallis et al. 2017a). Semi-structured interviews were audiotaped, transcribed verbatim, member-checked, coded, and themes developed using thematic analysis. The main theme identified was the participants' overriding concern with their knee, including pain, knee damage (unrelated to the walking program), and the view that knee replacement surgery was required. As one participant said: 'It's not going to fix my knees because you can't. There's only one way and that's the operation', and another: 'I've got a knee that's absolutely shot, and buggered'.

Three subthemes were also identified: (1) the perception of functional, cardiovascular, and psychosocial benefits with the walking program; (2) that supervision, monitoring, and commitment were important enablers: 'Without it (pedometer) I probably wouldn't have done the 10-min walk every day…so it's been motivating'; and (3) external factors such as the weather, ill-health, and the environment were key barriers: 'If it's stormy out, I won't go walking, if it's hot or 30 odd degrees I probably won't go for a walk either.' The three subthemes are consistent with results from the five qualitative studies described above (Campbell et al. 2001, Hinman et al. 2016, 2017, Lawford et al. 2018b,

Thorstensson et al. 2006) and a previous systematic review (Hurley et al. 2018) that explored the perceptions of people with knee osteoarthritis following participation in exercise or behavioural interventions.

The dominant theme from Wallis et al. (2017a) regarding patients overriding concern about their knee joint, did not emerge from any other qualitative study that involved participation in exercise and behavioural interventions for people with knee osteoarthritis. There are a number of unique aspects from Wallis et al. (2017a) that may explain this: (1) participants had severe knee osteoarthritis diagnosed radiologically and had been referred for surgical opinion with an orthopaedic surgeon. Therefore, it is possible participants may have gained this negative perception about their knee from messages received about the x-rays, compared with the other qualitative trials that mainly involved participants with mild to moderate osteoarthritis; (2) the trial did not include formal education or behavioural management to challenge negative beliefs about their knee; and (3) the walking program was not a joint-specific program and was focused on increasing physical activity via walking, rather than focusing on addressing the patients knee impairments.

Together, these findings provide important insights into the thoughts, perceptions, attitudes, and beliefs about the risks and benefits of exercise among people with knee osteoarthritis and help us understand why people may or may not engage in exercise. It highlights the importance of exercise interventions tailored to individual's preferences, with appropriate levels of support and supervision. It also highlights the importance of providing information and advice about the safety and value of physical activity and exercise, and to address negative health beliefs. Whilst this theme of enquiry described the perceptions of health professionals involved in delivering exercise interventions as part of a clinical trial, there is a lack of understanding about the attitudes and beliefs towards exercise among health professionals who are not part of a clinical trial. Given evidence that health professionals have a substantial influence on the beliefs and attitudes of their patients presenting with musculoskeletal pain (Darlow et al. 2012), this is a worthy subject for future qualitative investigation.

Total Knee Replacement Decision Making

Thirteen articles (12 studies) explored the experiences of 340 participants considering or waitlisted for total knee replacement surgery (Table 8.7). Two systematic reviews summarised findings from 12 primary qualitative articles exploring patient decision making for total knee replacement (Barlow et al. 2015, O'Neill et al. 2007). Six primary studies included in the two reviews were also included in this review. The remaining six studies were excluded due to their focus on peri-operative or post-operative experiences of total knee replacement or because they included patients undergoing total hip replacement.

Among the 13 primary studies, seven countries were represented: Australia (n = 1), Canada (n = 1), Kuwait (n = 1), United Kingdom (n = 3), United States (n = 5), Sweden (n = 1), and Taiwan (n = 1). From details of participant ethnicity provided, 126 participants were African American, 9 were Hispanic, 39 were Kuwaiti women, and 26 were Taiwanese.

Three studies involved participants scheduled for total knee replacement surgery (Hall et al. 2008, Johnson et al. 2016, Nyvang et al. 2016) and four involved participants waitlisted for surgery (Al-Taiar et al. 2013, Man et al. 2017, Toye et al. 2006, Woolhead et al. 2002). One study involved participants actively considering total knee replacement surgery

TABLE 8.7

Characteristics of Included Studies of Total Knee Replacement Decision-Making

Study	Country	Population	Demographics (N, Age, Sex)	Method: Framework/ Analysis	Sampling	Data Collection	Research Questions
Al-Taiar et al. (2013)	Kuwait	Severe knee osteoarthritis Kuwaiti women waitlisted for total knee replacement	N = 39 Mean age 62 yrs 100% women	Thematic analysis	Convenience sample from waiting list in one public orthopaedic hospital	Focus groups	Explore the pain experience and mobility limitation as well as the patient' s decision making process to undertake total knee replacement among women with knee pain in the waiting list for surgery.
Barlow et al. (2015)	–	Qualitative studies examining patients' decision making for total knee replacement	N = 7 studies	Summary of literature with no attempt at synthesis	Systematic review of literature to January 2015	–	Systematically examine the qualitative literature surrounding patients' decision making in knee arthroplasty.
Bunzli et al. (2017)	Australia	Orthopaedic surgeons performing TKR	N = 20	An implementation approach involving deductive and inductive analysis	All orthopaedic surgeons performing TKR at one tertiary hospital	Individual interviews • Semi-structured	Explore the barriers and facilitators to total knee replacement decision aid uptake among orthopaedic surgeons.
Chang et al. (2004)	US	Severe knee osteoarthritis 20 White and 17 African Americans actively considering total knee replacement	N = 37 Mean age 60 yrs 68% women	Content analysis	Consecutive patients actively considering TKR from one orthopaedic surgeon's office	Focus groups	Examine differences in patients' concerns regarding total knee replacement by race/ethnicity and gender.
Figaro et al. (2004)	US	Knee osteoarthritis Not actively seeking total knee replacement	N = 94 Mean age 71 yrs African American	Content analysis Constant comparative methods	Purposive sampling to recruit from a church and seniors centre proportionately.	Structured field interviews	Explore older urban Blacks with knee osteoarthritis to determine their preferences and expectations of total knee replacement

(Continued)

TABLE 8.7 (*Continued*)

Characteristics of Included Studies of Total Knee Replacement Decision-Making

Study	Country	Population	Demographics (N, Age, Sex)	Method: Framework/ Analysis	Sampling	Data Collection	Research Questions
					Network, convenience and snowball sampling to extend the sample		
Hall et al. (2008)	Canada	Unilateral knee osteoarthritis Scheduled for total knee replacement	N = 15 Mean age 67 yrs 40% women	Grounded theory	Purposive sampling of preoperative patients at one orthopaedic hospital	Individual interviews • Semi-structured	Explore views of total knee replacement and the role of physiotherapy
Johnson et al. (2016)	UK	Knee osteoarthritis Scheduled for total knee replacement	N = 10 Age range 61–78 yrs 40% women	Interpretive Phenomenological Analysis	Purposive sampling for age and sex from preoperative patients at a large hospital	Individual interviews • Semi-structured	Explore how the process of undergoing and recovering from total knee replacement alters patients' experiences and use of their support networks.
Kroll et al. (2007) Suarez-Almazor et al. (2010)	US	Knee osteoarthritis Not actively seeking total knee replacement	N = 37 Mean age 64 yrs 62% women 15 African American, 9 Hispanic, and 13 Caucasian	Grounded theory	Purposively sampled attending primary care clinics at the same outpatient institution	Focus groups	Explore the experiences, knowledge, beliefs, and attitudes of African American, Hispanic, and Caucasian patients regarding their knee arthritis and total knee replacement, in order to understand how differing perceptions may influence decision-making about total knee replacement.

(*Continued*)

TABLE 8.7 (*Continued*)

Characteristics of Included Studies of Total Knee Replacement Decision-Making

Study	Country	Population	Demographics (N, Age, Sex)	Method: Framework/ Analysis	Sampling	Data Collection	Research Questions
Man et al. (2017)	US	Knee osteoarthritis Waitlisted for total knee replacement	N = 8 Age range 46–80 yrs 50% women	Thematic analysis	Secondary analysis of 8 purposively sampled transcripts from a primary study exploring why people with OA do or do not re-engage in pre-operative occupations following hip or knee replacement	Individual interviews • Semi-structured	Explore the meaning and importance of occupational changes experienced by individuals during the pre- total knee replacement period
Nyvang et al. (2016)	Sweden	Knee osteoarthritis Scheduled for total knee replacement	N = 12 Mean age 66 yrs 58% women	Thematic analysis	Purposive sampling for sex and age from patients scheduled for surgery at one hospital	Individual interviews • Semi-structured	Explore patients' experiences of living with knee osteoarthritis when scheduled for total knee replacement and further their expectations for future life after surgery.
O'Neill et al. (2007)	–	Qualitative studies examining the experience of total knee replacement	N = 10 studies	Meta-ethnography	Systematic review of literature to March 2006	–	Explore the factors that influence the decision-making process of TKR surgery by synthesising the available evidence from qualitative research

(*Continued*)

TABLE 8.7 (*Continued*)

Characteristics of Included Studies of Total Knee Replacement Decision-Making

Study	Country	Population	Demographics (N, Age, Sex)	Method: Framework/ Analysis	Sampling	Data Collection	Research Questions
Toye et al. (2006)	UK	Knee osteoarthritis Waitlisted for total knee replacement	N = 18 Age range 54–77 yrs 33% women	Interpretive Phenomenological Analysis	Purposive sampling of patients listed for TKR at one orthopaedic hospital with below average scores on the WOMAC	Individual interviews • Semi-structured	Explore patients' personal meanings of knee osteoarthritis and total knee replacement
Wen-Ling et al. (2017)	Taiwan	Older people with knee osteoarthritis Recommended a total knee replacement by surgeon, but are indecisive	N = 26 Mean age 74 yrs 77% women	Thematic analysis	Convenience sampling from two medical centres and one regional hospital	Individual interviews • Semi-structured	Explore factors related to the indecision of older adults with knee osteoarthritis about receiving physician-recommended total knee replacement and their needs during the decision-making process.
Woolhead et al. (2002)	UK	Knee osteoarthritis except for 1 person with rheumatoid arthritis and systemic lupus erythematosus. Waitlisted for total knee replacement	N = 25 Mean age 65 yrs 58% women	Constant comparison	Purposive sampling for sex and age from patients wait listed for surgery with 3 orthopaedic surgeons	Individual interviews • Semi-structured	Explore patients' views on who should have priority for total knee replacement

(Chang et al. 2004) and one involved participants who had been recommended a knee replacement, but were indecisive about whether or not to have it (Wen-Ling et al. 2017). Two studies (three articles) involved participants with knee osteoarthritis that were not actively considering total knee replacement surgery (Figaro et al. 2004, Kroll et al. 2007, Suarez-Almazor et al. 2010). One study involved orthopaedic surgeons that perform total knee replacement (Bunzli et al. 2017).

The majority of studies aimed to understand decision making processes for total knee replacement to address unmet needs in light of evidence of regional variation and inequities in uptake of total knee replacement. Common themes reported included: (1) arriving at the tipping point at which participants would seriously consider total knee replacement; (2) sources of information about total knee replacement and the information needs of people considering surgery; and (3) barriers to uptake of total knee replacement.

The theme 'tipping point' was reported in eight studies (Al-Taiar et al. 2013, Hall et al. 2008, Johnson et al. 2016, Man et al. 2017, Nyvang et al. 2016, Suarez-Almazor et al. 2010, Toye et al. 2006, Wen-Ling et al. 2017). Participants described the occupational, functional, social, and emotional impact of knee osteoarthritis. They believed knee osteoarthritis was a progressive disease that would get worse over time. Many had experienced a worsening trajectory, feeling less able to cope with pain and the impact of pain as time progressed. Coping strategies and non-operative interventions became continually less effective as participants arrived at the 'tipping point', the point at which they felt that their best option was a total knee replacement.

Eight studies reported themes related to sources of information about total knee replacement (Al-Taiar et al. 2013, Chang et al. 2004, Hall et al. 2008, Johnson et al. 2016, Nyvang et al. 2016, Suarez-Almazor et al. 2010, Toye et al. 2006, Wen-Ling et al. 2017). Participants turned to general practitioners and surgeons for information about total knee replacement, however, the information participants sought varied according to sex and race. The study by Chang et al. (2004) found white men had questions that typically aligned with the information provided by surgeons such as what intraoperative techniques were involved. White women had questions about the preoperative and post-operative phases such as functional recovery and limitations. African American women had more practical questions about support needs after surgery. Across many studies there was a perceived lack of information from doctors about likely surgical outcomes. Participants' outcome expectations were influenced by the positive and negative experiences of others in their social network. Among those waitlisted for surgery, there was an expectation surgery would 'cure' the disease process with subsequent improvements ranging from a significant improvement in pain and function to a return to their 'normal', pre-knee osteoarthritis lives.

Seven studies (eight articles) reported themes related to the barriers of uptake of total knee replacement (Al-Taiar et al. 2013, Chang et al. 2004, Figaro et al. 2004, Kroll et al. 2007, Nyvang et al. 2016, Suarez-Almazor et al. 2010, Wen-Ling et al. 2017, Woolhead et al. 2002). The decision to undergo a knee replacement was frequently described as a social one, involving not only the surgeon and participant, but also the participant's family. In the study by Al-Taiar et al. (2013) of Kuwaiti women, approval had to be sought from family members to undergo knee replacement surgery. In other studies, conflict between family members about the need or readiness for surgery and their availability to provide care post-operatively was a barrier to uptake. One study in the United Kingdom focused on system barriers to uptake such as waiting lists in public hospitals (Woolhead et al. 2002). Studies conducted in the United States highlighted participant concerns about the cost of total knee replacement. Fear related to the anaesthetic was identified in several studies. In one study, participants indecisive about surgery felt they were too old and worried that their significant comorbidities placed them at increased risk of adverse effects (Wen-Ling et al. 2017). Uncertainty about the surgical outcome was reported in several studies, with some participants stating a preference to continue in their current state, summed up powerfully by the comment: 'I know what I have, I don't know what I am going to get'. Studies involving minority groups identified a number of barriers to uptake including fear of surgery, scepticism about the longevity of the prosthetic device, and a distrust of clinicians and the medical system.

Consistent with previous reviews (Barlow et al. 2015, O'Neill et al. 2007), these findings provide valuable insight into the social processes that influence patient candidacy, expectations for and uptake of total knee replacement processes that may be targeted to better meet the needs of people with knee osteoarthritis, and improve equity in total knee replacement. Social processes also influence surgeon decision making for total knee replacement, and one study explored these processes by interviewing orthopaedic surgeons about their decision-making processes and biases, and their beliefs and attitudes towards decision aids for total knee replacement.

Decision aids have been shown to reduce variations in clinical judgements and promote shared decision making by helping patients understand their likely outcomes from surgery (Knops et al. 2013, Sacks et al. 2016). Implementing decision aids into routine orthopaedic practice may be one way to improve equity in total knee replacement, but only if surgeons are ready, willing, and able to use them.

Bunzli et al. (2017) adopted an implementation approach, using a validated theoretical framework to systematically explore the barriers and facilitators to uptake of a decision aid through interview questions structured on the framework. The theoretical framework, describing 14 mediators of clinician behaviour change, has been used in the health literature to design studies that are better able to facilitate behaviour change and provide a basis for better understanding the processes underpinning behaviour change (Michie et al. 2005).

The authors interviewed 20 orthopaedic surgeons performing total knee replacement at one large tertiary hospital. They used deductive coding techniques to classify interview responses into the 14 mediator domains and inductive techniques to identify beliefs underlying common responses in each domain. The results described key beliefs likely to influence surgeons' uptake of a decision aid. These were: the belief that the surgeons' own patient outcomes from total knee replacement were better than those reported in the literature (Knowledge domain) and an acknowledgement that objective feedback on patient outcomes was lacking (Behavioural regulation domain). Surgeons expressed difficulty assessing patient-related factors known to influence outcomes from knee replacement (Capability domain). They relied on their 'gut-feelings' about the patient (Skills domain) and perceived surgery to be an art and a science (Professional identity domain). Most believed decision aids could enhance communication and patient informed consent (Consequences domain), but expressed concerns about mandatory cut-offs that would exclude some patients from surgery, particularly as they perceived a lack of effective non-operative alternatives (Environmental context domain).

The findings suggest multifaceted strategies may be needed to promote uptake of a decision aid among orthopaedic surgeons. For example, audit/feedback methods may be needed to address current decision-making biases such as overconfidence about patient outcomes, enhancing readiness to uptake. Policy changes and/or incentives may enhance willingness of surgeons to uptake. Ensuring there are avenues surgeons can access to provide effective non-operative treatments for disabling knee osteoarthritis may also enhance uptake by ensuring that surgeons have the resources they need to carry out decisions.

Qualitative research involving orthopaedic surgeons is rare. Surgeons are time-poor and may be reluctant to participate in interview studies in which they may perceive their beliefs and practices are being challenged. However, the surgeons' perspective is an important pavestone that together with the perspectives of the patient, caregivers, primary care practitioners, advocacy groups, and policy makers, can help lay the path to improved equity for total knee replacement and better meet the needs of people with knee osteoarthritis.

Discussion

This systematic review has demonstrated the breadth of qualitative research on knee osteoarthritis, a total of 56 articles reporting the results of 49 qualitative studies. Participants reported on the experience of living with knee osteoarthritis, their experiences of interventions to manage their condition, and the decision-making process of deciding whether to proceed with total knee replacement surgery.

Collectively, the qualitative studies in this review demonstrate the important role that patient views and attitudes play in effective management of their condition and in choosing management options. Application of interventions considered to be appropriate in clinical practice guidelines such as exercise, self-management, and weight management (Australian Commission on Safety and Quality in Health Care 2017, McAlindon et al. 2014, National Institute for Health and Care Excellence 2014) was not always perceived positively by people with knee osteoarthritis. A crucial factor in the success of these evidence-based interventions appeared to be when patient factors and attention to behavioural change techniques were taken into account. Also, personal and social factors play an important role in the decision about whether to proceed to total knee replacement.

Exercise interventions that combine behavioural change interventions such as health coaching and a strong commitment and connection with supervising clinicians were viewed favourably by people with knee osteoarthritis. In contrast, when supportive elements appeared to be given little emphasis, people appeared more likely to perceive the intervention negatively. In these cases, patients with knee osteoarthritis also had negative perceptions of their clinicians. It seems that when evidence-based interventions work, an important factor may be how each intervention is implemented.

The emotional and psychosocial impact of knee osteoarthritis emerged as a key factor in the lived experience of people with knee osteoarthritis. The anxiety, depression, and feeling of hopelessness that emerged as a theme in our review have received little attention in clinical practice guidelines. For example, the Osteoarthritis Research Society International (OARSI) guidelines (McAlindon et al. 2014) make no mention of interventions to address the psychological impact of knee osteoarthritis. The recent Australian Osteoarthritis of the Knee Clinical Care Standard (Australian Commission on Safety and Quality in Health Care 2017) and NICE guidelines (National Institute for Health and Care Excellence 2014) acknowledge the importance of patient-centred care. They include specific recommendations for a psychosocial evaluation to identify unique factors that may affect a person's quality of life and participation in usual activities (Australian Commission on Safety and Quality in Health Care 2017). However, no mention is made of interventions to address the emotional impact of knee osteoarthritis.

Education is recommended in clinical practice guidelines (Australian Commission on Safety and Quality in Health Care 2017, National Institute for Health and Care

Excellence 2014). Education can address patient misconceptions about osteoarthritis, such as the effect of exercise (Gay et al. 2018, Hendry et al. 2006) and can help patients participate in decisions about their management. Qualitative analysis adds to clinical practice guidelines by providing insights into how patient education may be conducted. The use of decision aid tools has been viewed favourably by patients and clinicians (Elwyn et al. 2018, Kinsey et al. 2017). A key benefit of such tools may be in the way that they facilitate communication between patient and clinician to optimise education. However, recent qualitative analysis suggests that orthopaedic surgeons remain sceptical about the benefit of tools to assist the decision to proceed to total knee replacement (Bunzli et al. 2017). These findings suggest multifaceted strategies may be needed to promote uptake of a decision aid among orthopaedic surgeons, including taking into account the perceptions of patients.

A limitation of this review was that the methodological quality of the included studies such as credibility, transferability, dependability, and confirmability (Guba 1981) was not assessed. However, the aim was to explore the breadth of qualitative research in the area not to rate the rigour and trustworthiness of individual studies. Strengths of the review include the comprehensive search strategy and the thematic analysis approach.

In conclusion, the breadth of this review has highlighted the value of taking patient attitudes and experiences into account when planning and implementing management options for people with knee osteoarthritis.

References

Australian Commission on Safety and Quality in Health Care. 2017. *Osteoarthritis of the Knee Clinical Care Standard* [Online]. Available from: https://www.safetyandquality.gov.au/publications/osteoarthritis-of-the-knee-clinical-care-standard/.

Australian Institute of Health and Welfare. 2015. *AIHW Analysis of Australian Bureau of Statistics: National Health Survey (NHS) 2014–15* [Online]. Available from: https://www.aihw.gov.au/reports/arthritis-other-musculoskeletal-conditions/osteoarthritis/data.

Australian Orthopaedic Association National Joint Replacement Registry. 2017. *Hip, Knee and Shoulder Arthroplasty. Annual Report. Adelaide* [Online]. Available from: https://aoanjrr.sahmri.com.

Abbott, J. H., Usiskin, I. M., Wilson, R., Hansen, P. & Losina, E. 2017. The quality-of-life burden of knee osteoarthritis in New Zealand adults: A model-based evaluation. *PLoS ONE*, 12, e0185676.

Ackerman, I. N., Bohensky, M. A., Pratt, C., Gorelik, A. & Liew, D. 2016. Counting the cost. Part 1: Healthcare costs. The current and future burden of arthritis. Available from: http://www.arthritisaustralia.com.au/index.php/reports/counting-the-cost.html.

Al-Taiar, A., Al-Sabah, R., Elsalawy, E., Shehab, D. & Al-Mahmoud, S. 2013. Attitudes to knee osteoarthritis and total knee replacement in Arab women: A qualitative study. *BMC Research Notes*, 6, 406.

Alami, S., Boutron, I., Desjeux, D., Hirschhorn, M., Meric, G., Rannou, F. & Poiraudeau, S. 2011. Patients' and practitioners' views of knee osteoarthritis and its management: A qualitative interview study. *PLoS ONE*, 6 (5).

Ali, A., Rosenberger, L., Weiss, T. R., Milak, C. & Perlman, A. I. 2017. Massage therapy and quality of life in osteoarthritis of the knee: A qualitative study. *Pain Medicine*, 18, 1168–1175.

Barlow, T., Griffin, D., Barlow, D. & Realpe, A. 2015. Patients' decision making in total knee arthroplasty. *Bone Joint Research*, 4, 163–169.

Belsi, A., Papi, E. & McGregor, A. H. 2016. Impact of wearable technology on psychosocial factors of osteoarthritis management: A qualitative study. *BMJ Open*, 6, e010064.

Bunzli, S., Nelson, E., Scott, A., French, S., Choong, P. & Dowsey, M. 2017. Barriers and facilitators to orthopaedic surgeons' uptake of decision aids for total knee arthroplasty: A qualitative study. *BMJ Open*, 7, e018614.

Bunzli, S., Watkins, R., Smith, A., Schutze, R. & O'Sullivan, P. 2013. Lives on hold. A qualitative synthesis exploring the experience of chronic low back pain. *Clinical Journal of Pain*, 29, 907–916.

Campbell, R., Evans, M., Tucker, M., Quilty, B., Dieppe, P. & Donovan, J. L. 2001. Why don't patients do their exercises? Understanding non-compliance with physiotherapy in patients with osteoarthritis of the knee. *Journal of Epidemiology & Community Health*, 55, 132–138.

Carmona-Teres, V., Moix-Queralto, J., Pujol-Ribera, E., Lumillo-Gutierrez, I., Mas, X., Batlle-Gualda, E., Gobbo-Montoya, M., Jodar-Fernandez, L. & Berenguera, A. 2017. Understanding knee osteoarthritis from the patients' perspective: A qualitative study. *BMC Musculoskeletal Disorders*, 18, 225.

Chan, K. K. W. & Chan, L. W. Y. 2011. A qualitative study on patients with knee osteoarthritis to evaluate the influence of different pain patterns on patients' quality of life and to find out patients' interpretation and coping strategies for the disease. *Rheumatology Reports*, 3, 9–15.

Chang, H. J., Mehta, P. S., Rosenberg, A. & Scrimshaw, S. C. 2004. Concerns of patients actively contemplating total knee replacement: Differences by race and gender. *Arthritis Rheum*, 51, 117–123.

Clarke, S. P., Moreton, B. J., Das Nair, R., Walsh, D. A. & Lincoln, N. B. 2014. Personal experience of osteoarthritis and pain questionnaires: Mapping items to themes. *Disability & Rehabilitation*, 36, 163–169.

Creamer, P., Lethbridge-Cejku, M. & Hochberg, M. C. 2000. Factors associated with functional impairment in symptomatic knee osteoarthritis. *Rheumatology (Oxford)*, 39, 490–496.

Creswell, J. W. 2014. *Research Design: Qualitative, Quantitative, and Mixed Methods Approaches*. Thousand Oaks, CA: Sage Publications.

Cross, M., Smith, E., Hoy, D., Nolte, S., Ackerman, I., Fransen, M., Bridgett, B. et al. 2014. The global burden of hip and knee osteoarthritis: Estimates from the Global Burden of Disease 2010 study. *Annals of the Rheumatic Diseases*, 73, 1323–1330.

Darlow, B., Fullen, B. M., Dean, S., Hurley, D. A., Baxter, G. D. & Dowell, A. 2012. The association between health care professional attitudes and beliefs and the attitudes and beliefs, clinical management, and outcomes of patients with low back pain: A systematic review. *European Journal of Pain*, 16, 3–17.

Egerton, T., Nelligan, R., Setchell, J., Atkins, L. & Bennell, K. L. 2017. General practitioners' perspectives on a proposed new model of service delivery for primary care management of knee osteoarthritis: A qualitative study. *BMC Family Practice*, 18, 85.

Elwyn, G., Rasmussen, J., Kinsey, K., Firth, J., Marrin, K., Edwards, A. & Wood, F. 2018. On a learning curve for shared decision making: Interviews with clinicians using the knee osteoarthritis Option Grid. *Journal of Evaluation in Clinical Practice*, 24, 56–64.

Figaro, M. K., Allegrante, J. P. & Russo, P. W. 2004. Preferences for arthritis care among urban African Americans: 'I don't want to be cut'. *Health Psychology*, 23, 324–329.

Gay, C., Eschalier, B., Levyckyj, C., Bonnin, A. & Coudeyre, E. 2018. Motivators for and barriers to physical activity in people with knee osteoarthritis: A qualitative study. *Joint Bone Spine*, 85, 481–486.

Guba, E. G. 1981. Criteria for assessing the trustworthiness of naturalistic inquiries. *Educational Resources Infonnation Center Annual Review Paper*, 29, 75–91.

Hall, M., Migay, A., Persad, T., Smith, J., Yoshida, K., Kennedy, D. & Pagura, S. 2008. Individuals' experience of living with osteoarthritis of the knee and perceptions of total knee arthroplasty. *Physiotherapy Theory & Practice*, 24, 167–181.

Hendry, M., Williams, N. H., Markland, D., Wilkinson, C. & Maddison, P. 2006. Why should we exercise when our knees hurt? A qualitative study of primary care patients with osteoarthritis of the knee. *Family Practice*, 23, 558–567.

Hinman, R. S., Delany, C. M., Campbell, P. K., Gale, J. & Bennell, K. L. 2016. Physical therapists, telephone coaches, and patients with knee osteoarthritis: Qualitative study about working together to promote exercise adherence. *Physical Therapy*, 96, 479–493.

Hinman, R. S., Nelligan, R. K., Bennell, K. L. & Delany, C. 2017. "Sounds a bit crazy, but it was almost more personal:" A qualitative study of patient and clinician experiences of physical therapist-prescribed exercise for knee osteoarthritis via Skype. *Arthritis Care & Research*, 69, 1834–1844.

Hsu, K. Y., Tsai, Y. F., Lin, Y. P. & Liu, H. T. 2015. Primary family caregivers' observations and perceptions of their older relatives' knee osteoarthritis pain and pain management: A qualitative study. *Journal of Advanced Nursing*, 71, 2119–2128.

Hurley, M., Dickson, K., Hallett, R., Grant, R., Hauari, H., Walsh, N., Stansfield, C. & Oliver, S. 2018. Exercise interventions and patient beliefs for people with hip, knee or hip and knee osteoarthritis: A mixed methods review. *Cochrane Database of Systematic Reviews*, 4, CD010842.

Isla Pera, P., Ferrer, M. C. O., Juarez, M. N., Juarez, E. N., Soler, L. M., Matheu, C. L., Cuadra, A. R., Perez, M. H. & Marre, D. 2016. Obseity, knee osteoarthritis, and polypathology: factors favoring weight loss in older people. *Patient Preference and Adherence*, 10, 957–965.

Johnson, E. C., Horwood, J. & Gooberman-Hill, R. 2016. Trajectories of need: Understanding patients' use of support during the journey through knee replacement. *Disability & Rehabilitation*, 38, 2550–2563.

Kao, M. H. & Tsai, Y. F. 2012. Living experiences of middle-aged adults with early knee osteoarthritis in prediagnostic phase. *Disability & Rehabilitation*, 34, 1827–1834.

Kao, M. H. & Tsai, Y. F. 2014. Illness experiences in middle-aged adults with early-stage knee osteoarthritis: Findings from a qualitative study. *Journal of Advanced Nursing*, 70, 1564–1572.

Keysor, J. J., Sparling, J. W. & Riegger-Krugh, C. 1998. The experience of knee arthritis in athletic young and middle-aged adults: An heuristic study. *Arthritis Care & Research*, 11, 261–270.

Kinsey, K., Firth, J., Elwyn, G., Edwards, A., Brain, K., Marrin, K., Nye, A. & Wood, F. 2017. Patients' views on the use of an Option Grid for knee osteoarthritis in physiotherapy clinical encounters: An interview study. *Health Expectations*, 20, 1302–1310.

Knops, A. M., Legemate, D. A., Goossens, A., Bossuyt, P. M. & Ubbink, D. T. 2013. Decision aids for patients facing a surgical treatment decision: A systematic review and meta-analysis. *Annals of Surgery*, 257, 860–866.

Kroll, T. L., Richardson, M., Sharf, B. F. & Suarez-Almazor, M. E. 2007. "Keep on truckin'"or "It's got you in this little vacuum": Race-based perceptions in decision-making for total knee arthroplasty. *Journal of Rheumatology*, 34, 1069–1075.

Lawford, B. J., Delany, C., Bennell, K. L., Bills, C., Gale, J. & Hinman, R. S. 2018a. Training physical therapists in person-centered practice for people with osteoarthritis: A qualitative case study. *Arthritis Care and Research*, 70, 558–570.

Lawford, B. J., Delany, C., Bennell, K. L. & Hinman, R. S. 2018b. "I was really sceptical … But it worked really well": A qualitative study of patient perceptions of telephone-delivered exercise therapy by physiotherapists for people with knee osteoarthritis. *Osteoarthritis & Cartilage*, 26, 741–750.

Li, C. S., Pathy, R., Adili, A., Avram, V., Barasi, M. A., Mundi, R., Niroopan, G. & Bhandari, M. 2013. Is the treatment gap in knee osteoarthritis real? A qualitative study of surgeons' perceptions. *Journal of Long-Term Effects of Medical Implants*, 23, 223–240.

Mackay, C., Badley, E. M., Jaglal, S. B., Sale, J. & Davis, A. M. 2014a. "We're all looking for solutions": A qualitative study of the management of knee symptoms. *Arthritis Care & Research*, 66, 1033–1040.

Mackay, C., Jaglal, S. B., Sale, J., Badley, E. M. & Davis, A. M. 2014b. A qualitative study of the consequences of knee symptoms: 'It's like you're an athlete and you go to a couch potato'. *BMJ Open*, 4, e006006.

Mackay, C., Sale, J., Badley, E. M., Jaglal, S. B. & Davis, A. M. 2016. Qualitative study exploring the meaning of knee symptoms to adults ages 35-65 years. *Arthritis Care & Research*, 68, 341–347.

Maly, M. R. & Krupa, T. 2007. Personal experience of living with knee osteoarthritis among older adults. *Disability & Rehabilitation*, 29, 1423–1433.

Man, A., Davis, A., Webster, F. & Polatajko, H. 2017. Awaiting knee joint replacement surgery: An occupational perspective on the experience of osteoarthritis. *Journal of Occupational Science*, 24, 216–224.

McAlindon, T. E., Bannuru, R. R., Sullivan, M. C., Arden, N. K., Berenbaum, F., Bierma-Zeinstra, S. M., Hawker, G. A. et al. 2014. OARSI guidelines for the non-surgical management of knee osteoarthritis. *Osteoarthritis and Cartilage*, 22, 363–388.

Michie, S., Johnston, M., Abraham, C., Lawton, R., Parker, D. & Walker, A. 2005. Making psychological theory useful for implementing evidence based practice: A consensus approach. *Qualitative and Safety in Health Care*, 14, 26–33.

Moore, G. F., Audrey, S., Barker, M., Bond, L., Bonell, C., Hardeman, W., Moore, L. et al. 2015. Process evaluation of complex interventions: Medical Research Council guidance. *British Medical Journal*, 350.

Morden, A., Jinks, C. & Ong, B. N. 2011. Lay models of self-management: How do people manage knee osteoarthritis in context? *Chronic Illness*, 7, 185–200.

National Institute for Health and Care Excellence. 2014. *Osteoarthritis: Care and Management. UK* [Online]. Available from: https://nice.org.uk/guidance/cg177.

Nielsen, M., Keefe, F. J., Bennell, K. & Jull, G. A. 2014. Physical therapist-delivered cognitive-behavioral therapy: A qualitative study of physical therapists' perceptions and experiences. *Physical Therapy*, 94, 197–209.

Nüesch, E., Dieppe, P., Reichenbach, S., Williams, S., Iff, S. & Jüni, P. 2011. All cause and disease specific mortality in patients with knee or hip osteoarthritis: Population based cohort study. *British Medical Journal*, 342, d1165.

Nyvang, J., Hedstrom, M. & Gleissman, S. A. 2016. It's not just a knee, but a whole life: A qualitative descriptive study on patients' experiences of living with knee osteoarthritis and their expectations for knee arthroplasty. *International Journal of Qualitative Studies on Health and Well-being*, 11, 30193.

O'Neill, T., Jinks, C. & Ong, B. N. 2007. Decision-making regarding total knee replacement surgery: A qualitative meta-synthesis. *BMC Health Services Research*, 7, 52.

Ong, B. N., Jinks, C. & Morden, A. 2011. The hard work of self-management: Living with chronic knee pain. *International Journal of Qualitative Studies on Health and Well-being*, 6, 1–10.

Pereira, D., Peleteiro, B., Araujo, J., Brancoxa, J., Santoska, R. A. & Ramosyza, E. 2011. The effect of osteoarthritis definition on prevalence and incidence estimates: A systematic review. *Osteoarthritis and Cartilage*, 19, 1270–1285.

Pouli, N., Das Nair, R., Lincoln, N. B. & Walsh, D. 2014. The experience of living with knee osteoarthritis: Exploring illness and treatment beliefs through thematic analysis. *Disability & Rehabilitation*, 36, 600–607.

Prasanna, S. S., Korner-Bitensky, N. & Ahmed, S. 2013. Why do people delay accessing health care for knee osteoarthritis? Exploring beliefs of health professionals and lay people. *Physiotherapy Canada*, 65, 56–63.

Rabago, D., Van Leuven, L., Benes, L., Fortney, L., Slattengren, A., Grettie, J. & Mundt, M. 2016. Qualitative assessment of patients receiving prolotherapy for knee osteoarthritis in a multimethod study. *Journal of Alternative and Complementary Medicine*, 22, 983–989.

Sacks, G. D., Dawes, A. J., Ettner, S. L., Brook, R. H., Fox, C. R., Russell, M. M., Ko, C. Y. & Maggard-Gibbons, M. 2016. Impact of a risk calculator on risk perception and surgical decision making: A randomized trial. *Annals of Surgery*, 264, 889–895.

Salaffi, F., Carotti, M. & Grassi, W. 2005. Health-related quality of life in patients with hip or knee osteoarthritis: Comparison of generic and disease-specific instruments. *Clinical Rheumatology*, 24, 29–37.

Schulz, K. F., Altman, D. G. & Moher, D. 2010. CONSORT 2010 statement: Updated guidelines for reporting parallel group randomised trials. *British Medical Journal*, 340.

Son, H. M., Kim, D. H., Kim, E., Jung, S. Y., Kim, A. R. & Kim, T. H. 2013. A qualitative study of the experiences of patients with knee osteoarthritis undergoing moxibustion. *Acupuncture in Medicine*, 31, 39–44.

Spitaels, D., Vankrunkelsven, P., Desfosses, J., Luyten, F., Verschueren, S., Van Assche, D., Aertgeerts, B. & Hermens, R. 2017. Barriers for guideline adherence in knee osteoarthritis care: A qualitative study from the patients' perspective. *Journal of Evaluation in Clinical Practice*, 23, 165–172.

Suarez-Almazor, M. E., Richardson, M., Kroll, T. L. & Sharf, B. F. 2010. A qualitative analysis of decision-making for total knee replacement in patients with osteoarthritis. *JCR: Journal of Clinical Rheumatology*, 16, 158–163.

Tallon, D., Chard, J. & Dieppe, P. 2000. Exploring the priorities of patients with osteoarthritis of the knee. *Arthritis Care & Research*, 13, 312–319.

Thorstensson, C. A., Roos, E. M., Petersson, I. F. & Arvidsson, B. 2006. How do middle-aged patients conceive exercise as a form of treatment for knee osteoarthritis? *Disability and Rehabilitation*, 28, 51–59.

Tong, A., Flemming, K., McInnes, E., Oliver, S. & Craig, J. 2012. Enhancing transparency in reporting the synthesis of qualitative research: ENTREQ. *BMC Medical Research Methodology*, 12, 181.

Toye, F., Room, J. & Barker, K. L. 2017. Do I really want to be going on a bloody diet? Gendered narratives in older men with painful knee osteoarthritis. *Disability & Rehabilitation*, 40, 1914–1920.

Toye, F. M., Barlow, J., Wright, C. & Lamb, S. E. 2006. Personal meanings in the construction of need for total knee replacement surgery. *Social Science & Medicine*, 63, 43–53.

Victor, C. R., Ross, F. & Axford, J. 2004. Capturing lay perspectives in a randomized control trial of a health promotion intervention for people with osteoarthritis of the knee. *Journal of Evaluation in Clinical Practice*, 10, 63–70.

Wallis, J. A., Webster, K. E., Levinger, P., Singh, P. J., Fong, C. & Taylor, N. F. 2017a. Perceptions about participation in a 12-week walking program for people with severe knee osteoarthritis: A qualitative analysis. *Disability & Rehabilitation*, doi:10.1080/09638288.2017.1408710 [EPub ah4ead of print].

Wallis, J. A., Webster, K. E., Levinger, P., Singh, P. J., Fong, C. & Taylor, N. F. 2017b. A walking program for people with severe knee osteoarthritis did not reduce pain but may have benefits for cardiovascular health: A phase II randomised controlled trial. *Osteoarthritis and Cartilage*, 25, 1969–1979.

Wallis, J. A., Webster, K. E., Levinger, P. & Taylor, N. F. 2013. What proportion of people with hip and knee osteoarthritis meet physical activity guidelines? A systematic review and meta-analysis. *Osteoarthritis and Cartilage*, 21, 1648–1659.

Wen-Ling, Y., Yun-Fang, T., Kuo-Yao, H., Weichih Chen, D. & Ching-Yen, C. 2017. Factors related to the indecision of older adults with knee osteoarthritis about receiving physician-recommended total knee arthroplasty. *Disability & Rehabilitation*, 39, 2302–2307.

Wilson, R. & Abbott, J. H. 2018. Development and validation of a new population-based simulation model of osteoarthritis in New Zealand. *Osteoarthritis and Cartilage*, 26, 531–539.

Woolhead, G., Donovan, J., Chard, J. & Dieppe, P. 2002. Who should have priority for a knee joint replacement? *Rheumatology*, 41, 390–394.

Xie, F., Li, S. C., Fong, K. Y., Lo, N. N., Yeo, S. J., Yang, K. Y. & Thumboo, J. 2006. What health domains and items are important to patients with knee osteoarthritis? A focus group study in a multiethnic urban Asian population. *Osteoarthritis and Cartilage*, 14, 224–230.

9

Shaping Rehabilitation after Spinal Cord Injury: The Impact of Qualitative Research

Kristin E. Musselman, Hardeep Singh and Janelle Unger

CONTENTS

Introduction to Spinal Cord Injury and Disease

Compared with other neurological conditions, the incidence of spinal cord injury or disease (SCI/D) is low, but it is a costly condition that results in significant disability. SCI/D results from a combination of direct damage to the spinal cord and secondary reactions to the damage, such as ischemia, inflammation, ion derangement, and apoptosis (Somers 2009). This leads to cell death and demyelination, impeding transmission of some or all afferent and efferent information between areas below and above the damage. Motor, sensory, and autonomic functions are commonly affected. Further, the lack of sensation and/or mobility following SCI/D results in a number of significant sequelae, including contractures, pressure injuries, osteoporosis, muscle atrophy, pain, and cardiovascular deconditioning (McKinley et al. 1999, 2002; Giangregorio and McCartney 2006; Sipski and Richards 2006; Tan et al. 2013; Brienza et al. 2018). Depression (Khazaeipour et al. 2015) and cognitive impairment (Craig et al. 2017) may also be experienced, and many individuals with SCI/D have low levels of participation in social relationships, employment, and recreation (Dijkers 2005; Hammell 2007a).

SCI may result from a traumatic event causing a sudden onset of damage, for example, the cause may be a fall, motor vehicle accident, sports accident, or act of violence. The global prevalence of traumatic SCI is estimated to be 10.5 cases per 100,000 people, with about 768,473 new cases occurring each year (Kumar et al. 2018). In contrast, the onset of damage to the spinal cord may also be more gradual, as in the case of tumours, infections, or degeneration of the spinal column. Non-traumatic SCI/D is a heterogeneous group of conditions that can be challenging to identify (New et al. 2017). As a result, good quality epidemiological data on non-traumatic SCI/D are lacking (New et al. 2017). Non-traumatic SCI/D is estimated to be two to three times more common than traumatic SCI (Nesathurai 2013), with a recent Australian study estimating the prevalence to be 36.7 cases per 100,000 people (New et al. 2013).

Although SCI/D is a low prevalence condition, it is expensive. The total annual cost of SCI/D in the United States is 21.5 billion dollars, with direct costs accounting for 14.0–18.1 billion dollars and indirect costs (e.g., loss of wages) accounting for 3.83–7.0 billion dollars (Ma et al. 2014). The 'lifetime economic burden' of SCI/D increases with increasing severity of SCI/D, ranging from 1.5 million Canadian dollars for incomplete paraplegia to 3.0 million Canadian dollars for complete tetraplegia (Krueger et al. 2013). With respect to the cost of specific health services, the cost of inpatient rehabilitation exceeds the cost of other services, such as emergency care, acute inpatient, complex continuing care, physician visits, and home care services (Munce et al. 2013). Moreover, access to these services extends beyond the initial spinal damage. Each year individuals with SCI/D have more than double the number of hospital visits than the general population and the lengths of stay of individuals with SCI/D are three times longer (Dryden et al. 2004). With respect to indirect costs, at 1 year after the onset of SCI/D, the employment rate amongst individuals with SCI/D is only about 12%, increasing to about 35% in the chronic stages of injury (Ottomanelli and Lind 2009; Ma et al. 2014). This long-term employment rate is considerably lower than the reported 57% employment rate prior to onset of SCI/D (Ma et al. 2014). Compared with other neurological conditions, individuals with SCI/D are significantly younger, yet they have the largest proportion with low education (20%), and the largest proportion living on a household income of less than $25,000 USD/year (Matsuda et al. 2015). Thus, SCI/D comes with great economic, as well as personal, cost.

The clinical presentation of SCI/D is heterogeneous and primarily influenced by the areas of the spinal cord that are damaged (i.e., neurological level of injury) and the severity of that damage. Many individuals with SCI/D will experience autonomic dysfunction, as normal sympathetic-parasympathetic balance is disrupted (Somers 2009). Injury to the cervical and thoracic spinal cord results in an upper motor neuron injury, characterised by paralysis, hyperreflexia, spasticity, sensory impairments, and a spastic bladder and bowel. Respiration is considerably impaired in individuals with damage to the fifth cervical segment or higher, but also compromised in those with damage to the lower cervical and thoracic cord due to the role of intercostal and abdominal muscles in respiration. Lesions below the second lumbar vertebral body result in primarily lower motor neuron signs, such as flaccid weakness, hyporeflexia, sensory impairments, and a flaccid bladder and bowel, whilst injury to the first and second lumbar vertebral bodies result in a mix of upper and lower motor neuron signs (Nesathurai 2013). The neurological level of injury is an important determinant of independence in self-care, individuals with damage to the first thoracic level or lower are typically able to complete self-care activities independently (Ma et al. 2014), regardless of the severity of their injury.

The severity of damage to the spinal cord also impacts the degree of impairment and resulting restrictions in function. The American Spinal Injury Association Impairment Scale (AIS) characterises the severity of damage to the motor and sensory systems. An AIS A SCI/D indicates the most severe damage, there is no preservation of sensory or motor function below the neurological level of injury, including the fourth and fifth sacral segments. With AIS B SCI/D there is some sensory, but no motor, function present below the injury level. In contrast, AIS C and D SCI/D are motor incomplete injuries, meaning some motor and sensory functions are preserved below the level of injury, with the difference between these two grades dependent upon the strength of the affected muscles. Severity of SCI/D is an important determinant of mobility status after SCI/D (Marino et al. 1999; Burns et al. 2012; Scivoletto et al. 2014). Whilst individuals initially diagnosed with AIS A injuries rarely regain walking function, 20%–50% of those with AIS B injuries and 75% of those with AIS C or D injuries will regain some walking function by 1 year post-injury (Burns et al. 2012).

In sum, SCI/D is a rare, but expensive, health condition that is characterised by sensory, motor, and autonomic dysfunction, often resulting in life-long disability. There is considerable heterogeneity in the clinical presentation of SCI/D, hence, each individual's experiences and rehabilitation needs following SCI/D are unique.

Evidence-Based and Person-Centred Care in SCI/D Rehabilitation

The medical care and rehabilitation of individuals with SCI/D are life-long processes. In recent decades there has been a shift towards adoption of a person- or client-centred approach to the delivery of healthcare services, in which the client is viewed as an equal and active participant in the planning and monitoring of his/her care (Ministry of Health and Long Term Care 2000; Cott 2004). A person-centred approach is both holistic (i.e., targets biological, psychological, and social aspects of health) and specific to the individual (i.e., considers his/her values and preferences) (Leplege et al. 2007; Epstein and Street 2011). Person-centred care addresses everyday challenges, preparing clients for community living and the specific life roles they assume (Leplege et al. 2007). The role of healthcare professionals within person-centred care is to inform and empower their clients such that the clients are well-positioned to make healthcare decisions (Leplege et al. 2007). Person-centred care facilitates a personalised approach to rehabilitation, which is well-suited for a heterogeneous condition like SCI/D. This approach improves outcomes, reduces costs, and prepares individuals with SCI/D to manage their own care once discharged from inpatient rehabilitation (Ministry of Health and Long Term Care 2000; Cott 2004; Delaney 2017).

Although there is increasing emphasis on a person-centred approach in the rehabilitation of people with SCI/D, an evidence-based approach is also valued. Currently, evidence-based care is informed by research findings derived largely from quantitative studies (Carpenter and Suto 2008) in which a homogeneous group of study participants, and standardised study interventions and outcomes, are desired. For example, Spinal Cord Injury Research Evidence (SCIRE) is a Canadian initiative to review and rate original research in the areas of acute care and rehabilitation for SCI/D (SCIRE 2018). Five levels of evidence, modified from Sackett et al. (2000), are used to rate the strength of the evidence. Randomised controlled trials provide the strongest evidence, whilst case reports, clinician consensus, and observational studies provide the lowest (SCIRE 2018). The SCIRE organisation (SCIRE 2018) and Sackett et al. (1996) acknowledge the importance of clinical experience in making evidence-based decisions, yet the levels of evidence offer little to no detail on how the client's perspectives factor into evidence-based care.

Standardised, quantitative outcomes are valued not only in research studies, but clinical environments as well. In recent years large databases of quantitative outcomes have been collected during the acute care and rehabilitation of SCI/D, for example, the European Multicenter Study about Spinal Cord Injury (EMSCI) and the Rick Hansen Spinal Cord

Injury Registry (RHSCIR) in Canada. Whilst these data are helpful for informing healthcare practices and policies, reliance on such positivist approaches results in an incomplete body of evidence that neglects the perspectives of the clients, caregivers, and healthcare professionals (Carpenter and Suto 2008).

In theory, evidence-based practice should consider the strongest research evidence, along with clinical expertise and each client's unique values, perceptions, and experiences (Carpenter and Suto 2008), however, the latter two are currently under-valued. Qualitative research can address this gap. Qualitative methodologies contribute to the evaluation of clinically relevant questions that are meaningful to individuals with SCI/D and the clinicians who work with them. Clinicians naturally adopt qualitative inquiry, monitoring change in their client's function through dialogue, and open-ended questions. For individuals with SCI/D, who spend a limited amount of time as inpatients, it is important that rehabilitation is productive. Keeping in mind that the overall goal of rehabilitation is to equip clients with the skills needed for community integration, it is important that the information and training provided is useful, relevant, and meaningful to individuals with SCI/D. Qualitative studies can help healthcare professionals set priorities for rehabilitation. Moreover, since qualitative research is able to embrace the heterogeneity of SCI/D, rather than trying to control and reduce it, qualitative methodologies may be particularly well-suited for the development and evaluation of interventions, services, and policies in SCI/D rehabilitation.

Translation of SCI/D Research Evidence into Clinical Practice

Advancements in the medical care and rehabilitation of individuals with SCI/D require not only person-centred and evidence-based methods, but successful implementation of these methods into practice. Implementation refers to 'systematic efforts to encourage adoption' (Graham et al. 2006). The challenge of implementing research findings in practice was highlighted at a recent gathering of international experts in SCI/D, which included individuals with SCI, researchers, clinicians, and representatives from SCI/D funding organisations (Rick Hansen Institute 2016). Similarly, we recently completed an environmental scan of current research studies that promote neurorecovery in SCI/D and demonstrated a gap between the interventions being researched and the characteristics known to facilitate clinical implementation of new research findings (Musselman et al. 2018b). For example, interventions feasible to use in hospitals and clinics, appropriate for the current healthcare context, and meaningful to the client, are more likely to be adopted (Pearson et al. 2005; Musselman et al. 2018b). When considering how to lessen this gap, one of our recommendations was to incorporate more qualitative methodologies into SCI/D research, enabling the perspectives of individuals with SCI, clinicians, and other stakeholders to guide the research process and subsequent implementation (Musselman et al. 2018b).

The process of translating evidence-based research findings into clinical practice is frequently depicted by the Knowledge to Action (KTA) framework (see Figure 9.1). The KTA framework has been adapted for a variety of health service settings and is one of the most commonly cited conceptual frameworks for knowledge translation (Field et al. 2014). This framework includes two dynamic components that influence one another: knowledge creation and the action cycle (Graham et al. 2006). Knowledge creation reflects the process of generating knowledge, largely through research-based activities. This process is depicted

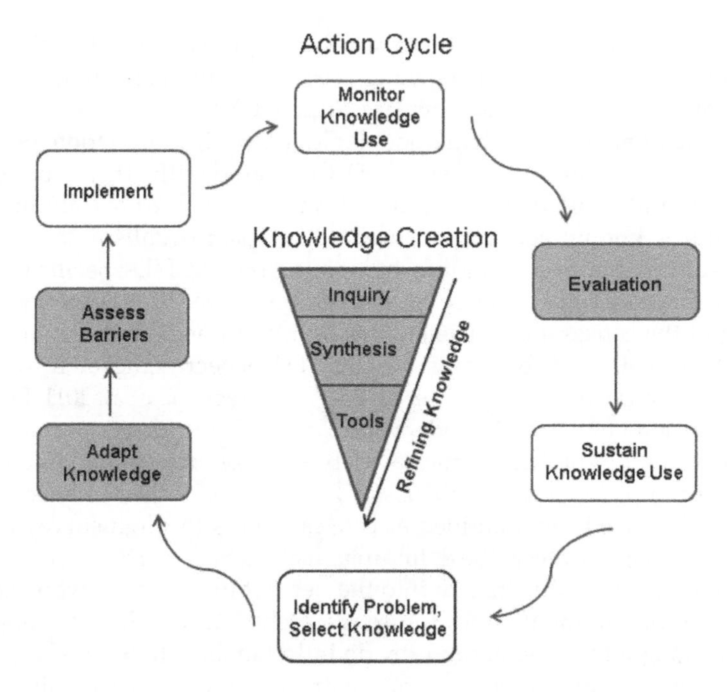

FIGURE 9.1
KTA framework. Grey shading indicates phases within the Knowledge Creation or Action Cycle where qualitative research methodologies have been applied to advance evidence-based and person-centred care in SCI/D rehabilitation. (Adapted from Graham, I. et al., *J. Contin. Educ. Health Prof.*, 26, 13–24, 2006.)

as a funnel, with knowledge becoming more refined, and likely more useful to stakeholders, as it passes through the phases of inquiry, synthesis, and tool or product development. As knowledge enters the action cycle, it is tailored to the needs of those who will use it and applied in their environment. The outcomes of the implementation initiative(s) are evaluated, and these results are used to refine the implementation process. Newly generated knowledge is adopted as the cycle continues (Graham et al. 2006).

To maintain a person-centred and evidence-based approach to SCI/D rehabilitation, qualitative research methodologies are being increasingly used throughout knowledge creation and the action cycle/implementation (see grey-shaded phases in Figure 9.1). In the remainder of this chapter, we will demonstrate how qualitative research methodologies highlight the perspectives of individuals with SCI/D and other stakeholders throughout the processes of knowledge creation and implementation, ultimately resulting in person-centred and evidence-based care.

Knowledge Creation for SCI/D Rehabilitation: Inquiry

Knowledge creation begins with the inquiry phase, when one is trying to determine what issues or problems exist and why. The inquiry phase of knowledge creation can be thought of as 'first-generation knowledge' (Graham et al. 2006) in which the research questions are exploratory in nature, examining relationships and seeking information to guide future research directions. Qualitative research designs are well-suited to facilitate the process of inquiry. Detailed insight into an issue or problem may be achieved through qualitative methods, which involve an ongoing process of refining the research questions as understanding of the issue or problem increases (Agee 2009).

We have used qualitative research methodologies to lay the foundation for our research examining falls and fall prevention after SCI/D. Compared with other neurological populations (Batchelor et al. 2010; Allen et al. 2013; Cameron et al. 2014; Canning et al. 2014), surprisingly little is known about the causes and impact of falls amongst individuals with SCI/D, resulting in a paucity of information to guide SCI/D-specific fall prevention initiatives. As a first step towards effective fall prevention for SCI/D, we sought a greater understanding of the causes and consequences of falls amongst individuals with SCI/D. The majority of data collected about falls after SCI/D has been achieved through quantitative means, such as surveys (Brotherton et al. 2007; Amatachaya et al. 2011; Phonthee et al. 2013a, 2013b; Matsuda et al. 2015; Saunders and Krause 2015). Since quantitative research questions are based on hypotheses, study variables are predetermined (Hammell 2007a), resulting in an incomplete picture of the issue. For example, a 'loss of balance' and 'environmental hazards' have been identified as causes of falls through survey methodology (Phonthee et al. 2013b), however, these findings lack clarity. Further, surveys and other quantitative methods offer little insight into the perceptions of those who experience the falls. To develop a solid foundation for future research on a complex, multi-factorial issue such as falls, we sought to understand: Why do individuals with SCI/D believe they fall? What factors do they perceive to place them at a greater or lesser risk of falling? How does the risk of falling impact their lives?

To learn about the issue of falls from the experts – people with SCI/D who live with the experience and risk of falling – we are using qualitative methodologies, specifically photo-elicitation interviewing (Harper 2002; Clark-Ibáñez 2004; Musselman et al. 2018a) and photovoice (Wang and Burris 1997; Wang 1999, 2006; La Vela et al. 2018). Photo-elicitation interviewing and photovoice are emerging qualitative methodologies in health-related research (Lal et al. 2012). These methods use photographs, interviews, and group discussion to explore a group's strengths and concerns surrounding an issue (Wang and Burris 1997). We asked participants with ASI C or D SCI/D to take pictures that: (1) identified factors that influenced, positively or negatively, their risk of falling and (2) described how the risk of falling affected their mobility and physical activity (Musselman et al. 2018a). The photos provided visual data to support the stories and information being shared by the participants and facilitated dialogue between the interviewer and interviewee.

We found that the participants primarily perceived environmental factors (e.g., stairs, unmaintained sidewalks, snow, and ice) as placing them at risk of falls, along with some biological (e.g., reduced strength, fatigue) and behavioural (e.g., taking risks) factors (see Figure 9.2) (Musselman et al. 2018a). These findings were not surprising and generally aligned with the results of previous quantitative studies (Brotherton et al. 2007; Nelson et al. 2010; Phonthee et al. 2013b; Amatachaya et al. 2015). However, some categories and themes that emerged through thematic analysis of the data were unexpected. For example, despite the focus of the study on mobility and physical activity, participants spoke of the impact of fall risk on their emotional well-being. Moreover, participants explained that they learnt to reduce their risk of falling and injury through previous experience with falls. We had not thought to ask a priori about emotional well-being and/or how the experience of falling may be helpful, but the qualitative research approach enabled these issues to be discovered. The detailed information and insight that we obtained into the issue of falls and fall risk after incomplete SCI/D would not have been possible through quantitative research methods.

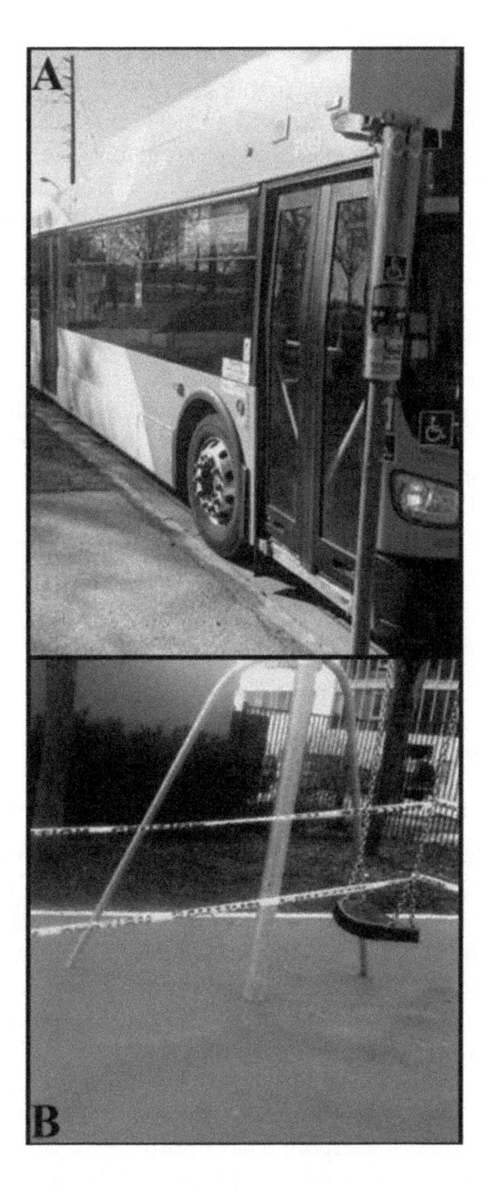

FIGURE 9.2
Photos representing situations that increase fall risk, taken by individuals with motor incomplete SCI/D. (a) One participant with central cord syndrome explained how taking the bus, which was her primary means of transportation, placed her at risk of falls. *If you don't have that ability to reach for [the grab handles], then your likelihood to fall is greater.* Because her upper extremities were more affected than her lower extremities, her balance impairments were not evident, and she often had difficulty getting a seat on a crowded bus. Taking the bus was stressful for her: *...the first thing that I look for is how full is the bus and will I get a seat? If it's too full then I won't go on [that] bus...if you miss that one bus you kind of impact yourself for whatever you have scheduled later.* This photo demonstrates the intersection of environmental and biological factors contributing to fall risk. (b) One participant took a picture of the playground that he visits with his 3-year-old daughter. He has fallen several times at this park, whose artificial ground has been in need of repair for some time. The participant did not want to stop taking his daughter to the playground though: *I wouldn't stop myself to not go to a park or any environment. Just be more aware of certain things, what my ability is and what I can do.* He chooses to take a risk in this situation. This photo demonstrates the intersection of environmental and behavioural factors contributing to fall risk.

Through photo-elicitation interviewing, individuals with SCI/D were able to inform us about the important issues that warrant further study. For example, since individuals with SCI/D spoke about feelings of frustration and anxiety as related to falls, we are now completing a mixed-methods study that examines the impact of falls on the quality of life and autonomy of wheelchair users and ambulators with SCI/D. Another example concerns a new approach to balance training after SCI/D. Since individuals with SCI/D reported learning how not to fall through falling, we are evaluating the efficacy of a balance training program that enables participants with AIS C or D SCI/D to experience falling in a safe environment (Unger et al. 2018a).

There are numerous examples of how exploratory qualitative research methods have been used by researchers during the inquiry phase of knowledge creation (see Table 9.1). This preliminary research is guiding the direction of future SCI/D rehabilitation research and intervention development concerning issues such as physical activity promotion (Papathomas et al. 2015), management of chronic pain (Norman et al. 2010), and needs of SCI/D caregivers (Espino et al. 2018). Hence, exploratory qualitative research enables individuals with SCI/D, caregivers, and other stakeholders to identify meaningful issues. This foundational knowledge is crucial for the development of appropriate and effective interventions, products, measurement tools, and policies in rehabilitation.

Knowledge Creation for SCI/D Rehabilitation: Synthesis

Following the inquiry phase, 'second-generation knowledge' (Graham et al. 2006) is produced through the aggregation and appraisal of findings from the inquiry phase using rigorous methods, such as systematic reviews, meta-analyses, and meta-syntheses. The synthesis of research findings enables identification of common results and/or principles across studies that likely vary in geographical location and/or research context (Graham et al. 2006). This level of evaluation often produces what is considered the highest level of evidence by knowledge sharing initiatives.

Although aggregating the results of quantitative studies is commonplace in rehabilitation research, the use of review methodology for qualitative studies is becoming more common (Estabrooks et al. 1994; Carpenter and Suto 2008). Unlike quantitative reviews, qualitative syntheses aim to create new interpretations through thematic analysis across studies (Finfgeld 2003), in addition to identifying similarities and differences in the findings of included studies. Amongst the first meta-syntheses completed in the area of SCI/D rehabilitation are the works by Hammell (2007a, 2007b). One of these meta-syntheses examined the experiences of inpatient rehabilitation from the perspectives of individuals with SCI/D (Hammell 2007b). This synthesis of eight qualitative studies highlighted the dimensions that contribute to a positive inpatient rehabilitation experience, such as working with caring staff, interacting with SCI/D peers, and practicing skills that match the skills needed in the 'real world' (Hammell 2007b).

Similarly, we recently used thematic synthesis methodology to complete a meta-synthesis examining the experiences of individuals with SCI/D participating in 26 different physical rehabilitation interventions (Unger et al. 2018c). Thirty-one studies were included in our meta-synthesis. This number is an almost four-fold increase from the review completed by Hammell (2007b) a decade earlier, reflecting the increased uptake of qualitative methods in

TABLE 9.1

Examples of Qualitative Studies Reflecting the Inquiry Stage of Knowledge Creation

Citation	Study Aim (A), Methods (M), and Participants (P)	Key Findings	Recommendation(s) for Future Research
Chan (2000)	**A:** Explore the impact of SCI/D upon the family & marital relationship **M:** Semi-structured interviews analysed using content analysis **P:** Individuals with SCI/D (n = 66), spouses (n = 40)	• Spousal relationship & family dynamics were altered • Culture & environment had an influence on spousal & family roles • Greater strain in relationship during early stage of SCI/D • Mutual understanding, support, & open communication were important components of lasting relationships	• Investigate intervention framework based on perspectives of both partners • Qualitative research to broaden understandings of the impact of SCI/D on partner relationships
Mahoney et al. (2007)	**A:** Understand daily experiences of individuals with SCI/D who experience spasticity **M:** Semi-structured interviews, observations, field notes **P:** Individuals with SCI/D who experience spasticity (n = 24)	• Spasticity impacts multiple domains of an individual's life including the physical, emotional, economic, interpersonal, management, & cognitive • Perspectives on spasticity management of insiders (individuals experiencing spasticity) can vary from outsiders (e.g., clinician)	• Understand the perspective of consumers to broaden frames of reference & inform interventions • Qualitative findings to guide instrument development to measure impact of spasticity • Shift in thinking from a 'fix it' model to a more individualised intervention in spasticity management
Norman et al. (2010)	**A:** Explore questions that individuals with SCI/D have about their chronic pain and their preferred methods to seek information **M:** Semi-structured interviews analysed using content analysis **P:** Individuals with SCI/D (n = 12)	• Unmet information needs about chronic pain were identified • Questions about chronic pain were related to: the cause, management, communication, getting information, others' experiences, & expectations	• Develop comprehensive, innovative chronic pain interventions that address information gaps • Tailor current/future interventions to preferred information seeking method • Knowledge translation efforts in SCI/D-pain research should consider engaging individuals with SCI/D as trainers & educators • Qualitative research to understand whether information needs of men with chronic pain differ from those of women

(Continued)

TABLE 9.1 (*Continued*)

Examples of Qualitative Studies Reflecting the Inquiry Stage of Knowledge Creation

Citation	Study Aim (A), Methods (M), and Participants (P)	Key Findings	Recommendation(s) for Future Research
Kuipers et al. (2011)	**A:** Explore how adults with SCI/D describe their local communities **M:** Telephone interviews analysed using thematic analysis **P:** Individuals with SCI/D (n = 269)	• Three aspects of community were significant to an individual's understanding of their community: social integration, independent living, & occupation • Diversity in responses existed amongst participants	• Investigate the diversity in perspectives amongst individuals with SCI/D about community integration • Consider individual perspectives in community rehabilitation interventions • Understand macro & societal level influences in community integration such as advocacy & policy change
Aune (2013)	**A:** Explore how women with traumatic SCI/D manage their daily lives after becoming mothers & societal barriers experienced **M:** Semi-structured interviews **P:** Mothers with SCI/D (n = 4)	• New mothers with SCI/D perceived health professionals lacked knowledge of their needs • Environmental barriers related to inaccessible public spaces & societal attitudes were challenges faced by mothers • Over time & with experience mothers felt more confident in their abilities	• Investigate interventions to meet better needs of mothers with SCI/D • Qualitative research to include the perspective from fathers with disabilities & changing family role when one parent has a disability
Papathomas et al. (2015)	**A:** Identify physical activity narratives **M:** Open-ended, semi-structured interviews analysed using narrative analysis **P:** Physically active individuals with SCI/D (n = 30)	• After SCI/D, exercise was: A restitution, medicine, & progressive redemption • Restitution may motivate physical activity in early stages of rehabilitation • Exercise as medicine may be a life-long motivator to continued physical activity participation • Exercise as progressive redemption may motivate individuals to work towards goals of improving function/ overcoming barriers (i.e., environmental)	• Qualitative data collection to further explore this topic in more detail (e.g., examine whether time of injury impacts perspectives, & whether differences exist based on age, sex, & type of SCI/D) • Explore whether these narratives can be used to promote engagement in physical activity

(*Continued*)

TABLE 9.1 (*Continued*)

Examples of Qualitative Studies Reflecting the Inquiry Stage of Knowledge Creation

Citation	Study Aim (A), Methods (M), and Participants (P)	Key Findings	Recommendation(s) for Future Research
Eglseder and Demchick (2017)	**A:** To identify the lived experiences of intimate partners of individuals with SCI/D related to sexuality **M:** Education & Resource Needs checklist & semi-structured interviews, analysed using a within-case analysis **P:** Partner of an individual with SCI/D (n = 4)	• Partners of people with SCI/D found aspects of SCI/D negatively impacted intimacy (e.g., taking a caregiver role, physical characteristics, & fear of causing injury) • Extreme discomfort was felt with resuming sexual activity • Unmet needs with sexual education & resource identified	• Qualitative research to explore gender & sexual preference differences of intimate partners of individuals with SCI/D • Further evaluation of discomfort related to sexual activity after SCI/D to inform future practice • Investigate informational needs/training for healthcare providers related to sexuality • Explore effectiveness of individualised education programs, mindfulness sexual interventions, & adaptations to enhance sexual comfort
Conti et al. (2016)	**A:** Explore experiences of informal caregivers during discharge transitions from SCI/D units **M:** Semi-structured interviews analysed using phenomenological methodology **P:** Caregivers of individuals with SCI/D recently discharged from SCI/D unit (n = 11)	• Caregivers had implicit & explicit unmet needs during discharge transitions from SCI/D unit • Caregivers should be involved in discharge planning	• Understand problem-solving abilities of people with disability to enhance the self-efficacy of patients & caregivers • Consideration for caregiver involvement in current/future rehabilitation interventions & discharge planning
Espino et al. (2018)	**A:** Explore unmet needs & preferences for support of caregivers of youth with SCI/D **M:** Focus groups **P:** Caregivers of youth with SCI/D living in USA (n = 26)	• Unmet needs early post-SCI/D were related to coping, navigating paediatric SCI/D services, & managing life after discharge • Unmet needs in community included navigating community services & managing care routines in the home	• Investigate interventions targeting unmet needs (e.g., methods to provide comprehensive info to caregivers on navigating health system & community resources, community support programs linking caregivers to peer support) • Qualitative data collection including more diverse care settings

SCI/D rehabilitation research (VanderKaay et al. 2018). The four themes identified through our meta-synthesis (i.e., '(1) benefits of physical rehabilitation, (2) challenges of physical rehabilitation, (3) need for support, and (4) issue of control') resulted in recommendations for future rehabilitation practices and policies that drive person-centred care (see Table 9.2) (Unger et al. 2018c).

Divanoglou and Georgiou (2017) provide another example of a meta-synthesis resulting in recommendations for rehabilitation practice. They completed a meta-synthesis of qualitative studies in order to determine the perceived effectiveness of community-based

TABLE 9.2

Recommendations for Healthcare Professionals Working in SCI/D Rehabilitation Derived from Meta-syntheses

Unger et al. (2018c)

To assist clients to realise the benefits of rehabilitation:

- Focus on abilities rather than disability
- Provide opportunities to succeed to enhance confidence
- Encourage participation in activities valued by the client
- Find and use motivational factors
- Use verbal encouragement often and demonstrate dedication to rehabilitation
- Keep rehabilitation program meaningful

To assist clients in addressing the challenges of rehabilitation:

- Identify and advise about coping strategies
- Encourage discussion about and provide help through negative emotions
- Discuss realistic goals for recovery
- Education about condition, recovery trajectory, and timeline
- Maintain environment of respect and autonomy
- Work with individuals to plan community transition and address concerns
- Modify programs based on individual experiences

To effectively provide clients with support:

- Continually provide support and encouragement, include caregivers in rehabilitation
- Work together in a partnership
- Implement peer support and mentorship programs

To effectively provide clients with control:

- Plan to avoid taking control away from individual
- Allow decision-making to be done by the individual
- Encourage individuals to take control as they may not feel they are in a position to do so
- Maintain open and honest communication about goals
- Support choices made by clients and work together to achieve goals

Divanoglou and Georgiou (2017)

To create an effective peer-mentoring program:

- Include opportunities for both formal and informal mentorship in a dynamic, supportive, and flexible environment to increase self-efficacy through peer observation
- Include peer mentors at different stages of recovery and with various injury characteristics and socio-cultural backgrounds to act as credible resources and increase relatedness with individuals
- Facilitate peer mentorship to fill service gaps and promote factors that encourage positive outcomes in all aspects of life post-SCI

Williams et al. (2014)

To facilitate a physically active lifestyle in clients:

- Understand relationships between benefits, barriers, and facilitators of physical activity
- Understand how SCI/D disrupts sense of self and exercise can redefine identity
- Identify 'credible messengers' to share information about exercise (i.e., benefits, how, and where to exercise)

peer-mentorship programs for individuals with SCI/D. Individual qualitative studies involving interviews with mentees indicated that peer-mentoring increased the mentee's motivation, hope, self-confidence, and well-being (Beauchamp et al. 2016), and that the unique support provided through peer-mentorship was a major support for the adjustment to life after a SCI/D (Veith et al. 2006). The synthesis by Divanoglou and Georgiou (2017) is timely as there is an increasing interest in the role of peer-mentorship in SCI/D rehabilitation as a cost-effective and person-centred approach to education. This meta-synthesis resulted in three analytical themes that describe the characteristics of effective peer-mentorship, which may be interpreted as recommendations for community-based peer-mentorship programs (see Table 9.2) (Divanoglou and Georgiou 2017). The meta-synthesis strengthens the evidence provided by individual qualitative studies and supports the translation of knowledge about peer-mentorship into clinical practice.

Table 9.2 includes one other example of how a qualitative meta-synthesis can result in tangible recommendations for SCI/D rehabilitation services. The meta-synthesis by Williams and colleagues (2014) summarised the existing qualitative research that examined the benefits, barriers, and facilitators of physical activity as perceived by individuals with SCI/D (Williams et al. 2014). Through this review of 18 qualitative studies, eight key concepts were identified and translated into three recommendations for healthcare professionals aiming to promote physical activity amongst their clients with SCI/D (see Table 9.2). The findings of meta-syntheses, such as those completed by Hammell (2007b), Unger et al. (2018c), Divanoglou and Georgiou (2017), and Williams et al. (2014), provide SCI/D rehabilitation professionals and services with tangible recommendations that can be implemented into practice to strengthen the delivery of evidence-based and person-centred care.

Knowledge Creation for SCI/D Rehabilitation: Tool or Product Development

Findings from meta-analyses and meta-syntheses are used to create best practice guidelines, care pathways, clinical-decision making tools, and rehabilitation products. These healthcare products reflect 'third-generation knowledge' (Graham et al. 2006) that is displayed in a user-friendly manner with the intention of influencing relevant stakeholders, whether individuals with SCI/D, their families, healthcare professionals, or makers of healthcare policy. Engaging the perspectives of relevant stakeholders in the development of knowledge tools or products is beneficial, as consulting end-users will lessen the gap between knowledge creation and clinical implementation (Boninger et al. 2012; Musselman et al. 2018a).

For several decades, focus groups and interviews have been used to consult end-users on the design of rehabilitation products and tools (e.g., Dijkers et al. 1991). More recently, end-users have been included throughout the design process, with qualitative methods being used for the collection and analysis of their perspectives. For example, Allin and colleagues (2018) adopted a participatory design process in order to create an online self-management program for individuals with SCI/D. The researchers first completed qualitative (i.e., semi-structured interviews) and quantitative (i.e., online survey) studies to explore the desired characteristics of a self-management program from the perspectives of individuals with SCI/D, their families and managers from acute care and rehabilitation hospitals (Munce et al. 2014a, 2014b). They learnt that individuals with SCI/D would like self-management programs to be SCI-specific, peer-run, and online (Munce et al. 2014a, 2014b). With this knowledge, a participatory design process was initiated involving researchers (n = 7) and individuals with SCI/D (n = 9), who together acted as co-designers and key informants to develop the online self-management tool (Allin et al. 2018). To document the participatory design process, the group meetings were audio recorded and the transcripts analysed through inductive thematic analysis. The co-designers with SCI/D identified issues to consider throughout the design process, such as evaluating the credibility of online information and valuing the expertise of the SCI/D community. It was concluded that these contributions benefited the design of the self-management tool, which is now being used and evaluated by Canadians with SCI/D (Allin et al. 2018).

Putting Knowledge into Action

Once knowledge tools or products are established, there is a focus on clinical implementation. The action cycle consists of the activities required to successfully implement the evidence-based and person-centred knowledge that has been refined through the process of knowledge creation (Graham et al. 2006). The phases of the action cycle are dynamic and influence each other, so although the phases are presented in a specified order (see Figure 9.1), there is flexibility and variability in how the action cycle proceeds.

In our experience, qualitative research can positively influence the translation of knowledge from research to clinical environments at three phases within the action cycle: adapting knowledge, assessing barriers, and evaluating outcomes (see grey shaded phases in Figure 9.1). To illustrate this point, we will use examples from our recent experiences with customising, implementing, evaluating, and refining approaches to the assessment and training of walking function in a SCI/D rehabilitation environment.

Action Cycle: Adapting Knowledge and Assessing Barriers

Adapting knowledge involves considering the added-value, usefulness, and appropriateness of the knowledge, tool, or product, as well as modifying it for one's local healthcare environment (Graham et al. 2006). An assessment of the barriers to knowledge uptake may occur in tandem or following adaptation of the knowledge and should also include the identification of facilitators that can be leveraged for the knowledge translation effort. Quantitative methods, such as surveys with Likert scales, are often used to identify the barriers and facilitators of knowledge use (Canadian Institutes of Health Research 2010). When we used a mixed-methods approach to identify the barriers to clinical use of functional electrical stimulation, however, we found that the qualitative data provided more detailed insight into the perceived barriers and facilitators than a quantitative rating scale (Auchstaetter et al. 2016).

To illustrate the role qualitative methodologies may play in the adaptation of knowledge and assessment of barriers, we will use the implementation of a clinical decision-making tool, the SCI Standing and Walking Assessment Tool (SWAT), as an example. The SWAT resulted from an identified gap in clinical care; a scoping review of the state of SCI/D rehabilitation practice in Canada identified a lack of guidelines for the assessment of walking after SCI/D (Craven et al. 2012). To address this gap, the Canadian Standing and Walking Measures Group was created consisting of SCI/D rehabilitation researchers, expert clinicians, and representatives from the Rick Hansen Institute (Walden et al. 2018). Through synthesis of pre-existing literature and clinical expertise, the group developed the SWAT (Verrier et al. 2014). The SWAT is a staging tool intended for use by physical therapists (see Figure 9.3). It standardises the timing and content of walking assessment during inpatient SCI/D rehabilitation. Using the SWAT, physical therapists determine a client's stage of walking ability, which then indicates which measures of balance (e.g., Berg Balance Scale, Mini-Balance Evaluation Systems Test) and walking (e.g., Ten-meter Walk Test, Six-minute Walk Test, modified Timed Up and Go) to complete. Following its development, the SWAT was implemented by physical therapists at nine rehabilitation hospitals in Canada (Walden et al. 2018). To support implementation, the Canadian Standing and Walking Measures Group sought to understand the acceptance, challenges, and facilitators of using the SWAT at each rehabilitation facility, the 'Adapt Knowledge' and 'Assess Barriers' stages of the KTA framework (see Figure 9.1). To achieve this understanding, we completed focus groups with physical therapists from each rehabilitation site who were using the SWAT in their clinical practice (Musselman et al. 2017). Semi-structured interview questions queried the clinicians' perceptions and experiences with the SWAT stages, specifically, the appropriateness of the content and the barriers and facilitators to the tool use (Musselman et al. 2017). Although some facilitators and barriers were site-specific, there were also similarities across rehabilitation sites. For example, a facilitator was the appreciation of objective standardised outcome measures (see Figure 9.3). Another was the flexibility to adapt the process of staging to fit one's local environment. Physical therapists spoke of customised strategies to integrate SWAT staging into their clinical routines. High caseloads, short inpatient lengths of stay, and a lack of time were common systems-level barriers experienced by the therapists. A lack of familiarity with the staging tool was also identified as a barrier by many participants.

Through identification of the barriers to clinical implementation of the SWAT, the Canadian Standing and Walking Measures Group identified strategies to address these barriers. For example, a standardised training workshop on how to administer the SWAT was developed and delivered (Musselman et al. 2017), and webinars concerning the SWAT outcome measures were provided to the therapists in order to address the lack of familiarity with the tool. This study is an example of how qualitative research can be used to facilitate the processes of adapting knowledge for a given clinical environment, as well as addressing the barriers to knowledge uptake, which are both important phases of the action cycle.

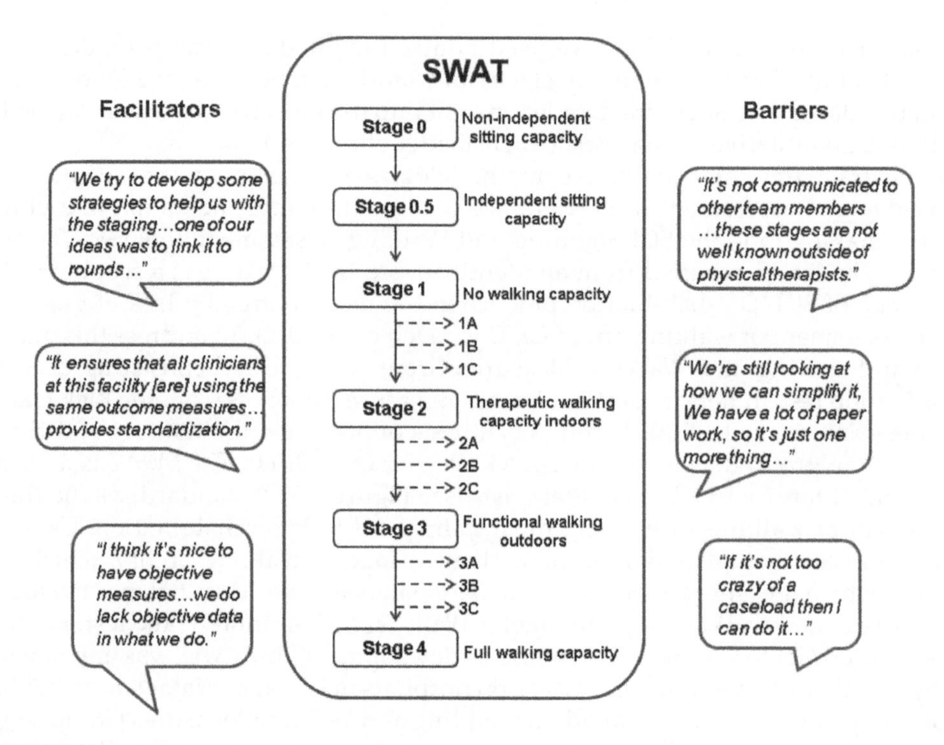

FIGURE 9.3
The SCI Standing and Walking Assessment Tool (SWAT) (middle). Quotes reflecting facilitators and barriers of clinical implementation of SWAT on left and right sides, respectively. Descriptors for sub-stages are as follows: 1A = no lower extremity movement; 1B = voluntary non-functional lower extremity movement; 1C = voluntary functional lower extremity movement; 2A = maximum assist; 2B = moderate assist; 2C = minimum assist; 3A = supervised household ambulator; 3B independent household ambulator; and 3C = community ambulator.

Action Cycle: Evaluating Outcomes

After knowledge has been adapted for a specific clinical environment and implemented by the end-users, the outcomes of this implementation are evaluated. The evaluation phase of the action cycle involves determining whether the implemented knowledge, tool, or product has resulted in a positive impact on the health of the target population, the clinicians, and/or the healthcare system (Graham et al. 2006). Standardised, quantitative measures of physical function, quality of life, and health economics may be used for this purpose, however, understanding of the impact is limited to the variables measured. Qualitative research methodologies enable documentation of unexpected benefits as well as those perceived to be meaningful to the study participants.

Retraining the ability to walk, also known as locomotor training, after SCI/D is a topic that has been extensively researched over the past three to four decades. Many studies demonstrated improvements in standardised measures of walking ability after individuals with motor incomplete SCI/D participated in intensive locomotor training programs (Lam et al. 2007; Yang and Musselman 2012). Typically, these programs include a combination of body weight-supported treadmill training and overground walking practice, however, functional electrical stimulation and robotic devices, such as the Lokomat®, have been used as therapy adjuncts to facilitate walking practice. Evidence to support the benefit of locomotor training after motor incomplete SCI was sufficiently strong that the NeuroRecovery Network was established in the United States to standardise the delivery of locomotor training, collect national-level data, and provide individuals with traumatic spinal injuries with an evidenced-based intervention for the rehabilitation of walking (Harkema et al. 2012). At our facility in Canada, we implemented a modified version of the NeuroRecovery Network locomotor training program, called personalised adapted locomotor training (PALT) (Singh et al. 2018c). Like the NeuroRecovery Network program, PALT consisted of body weight-supported treadmill training combined with overground practice in each session, however, in PALT, the content of overground training was customised to each client's goals and rehabilitative needs. Overground training may have involved therapy targeting walking, balance, transfers, trunk control, or upper limb function. This emphasis on customisation of therapy content enabled a person-centred approach.

Although evaluation of the impact of locomotor training programs has traditionally been completed with quantitative measures, a few evaluation studies have adopted qualitative methodologies as well (Nymark et al. 1998; Hannold et al. 2006; Bowden et al. 2008). In our experience with PALT, we found that a full understanding of the benefits of the program was not achieved until data derived from both qualitative and quantitative methods were obtained. We evaluated the outcomes of the PALT program in seven individuals with subacute AIS C or D SCI/D. Of these first seven participants of PALT, all but one showed clinically relevant improvements in walking speed and endurance (Chan et al. 2017). Through the semi-structured interviews, participants reported physical and psychological benefits that extended beyond the function of walking (Singh et al. 2018c). They reported that the PALT program facilitated their transition from inpatient rehabilitation to community living and gave them the confidence to self-manage their rehabilitation. Similarly, the participant that did not regain walking function through PALT reported that the program gave her confidence in her ability to cope with life after SCI/D:

> It gave me a lot of confidence, doing all of these sessions. Before I started I was really nervous about how am I going to cope at home, even if I do have my husband there? He can't be there 24-7, that's not healthy for him, so how on earth am I going to dress myself or be able to reach to get something, or do the dishes or whatever? After the program, I have no qualms about going home. I feel much stronger, I feel more confident.

Through PALT, this participant gained more independence in transfers, dressing and self-care, and required less assistance from her caregivers. These insights would not have been revealed through the quantitative data alone.

We followed up with the PALT participants 1 year after they completed the program. The quantitative measures of walking ability showed retention of walking gains, however, data from the semi-structured interviews highlighted some struggles since discharge from PALT (Singh et al. 2018b). For example, there were reports of depressed mood, falls causing injury, and difficulty accessing rehabilitation services in the community, either due to cost or the perceived poor quality of these services. Although participants reported that some aspects of their lives were going well (e.g., three participants had returned to work), there was a consistent view amongst participants that recovery is never complete. These qualitative analyses enabled reflection on the impact of PALT on the lives and well-being of participants, providing a more in-depth understanding of the intervention's effects.

The two qualitative evaluations of the PALT program also highlighted opportunities for program improvement based on the experiences and perspectives of the participants (Singh et al. 2018b, 2018c). Tangible recommendations for the PALT program are outlined in

TABLE 9.3

Recommendations for PALT

During PALT
Provide education on self-management of rehabilitation • E.g., instruction on how to exercise in community gym • Comprehensive home exercise program
Provide greater focus on transferring skills practiced in PALT to regular environments • E.g., practice walking outdoors
Provide education on fall prevention • E.g., discuss behavioural strategies and relevant assistive equipment to reduce fall risk
Provide a gradual discharge from PALT • E.g., gradually reduce frequency of sessions from 4 sessions/week to discharge over the month prior to discharge
Provide a flexible program structure • E.g., vary proportion of session spent on treadmill vs overground according to client's needs and preferences
After PALT
Provide routine follow-up after discharge to monitor psychological and physical health • E.g., follow-up phone calls to monitor progress and screen for declines in mental health
Link client to community resources, as appropriate • E.g., wheelchair accessible gym, community physical therapists/exercise trainers

Source: Singh, H. et al., *Spinal Cord Ser. Cases*, 4, 6, 2018; *Disabil. Rehabil.*, 40, 820–828, 2018.

Table 9.3. These recommendations likely apply to locomotor training programs for individuals with SCI/D in general. We have implemented some of these recommendations in an effort to improve the training experience for individuals with SCI/D. We recently reported a case study involving PALT for an individual with paralysis due to West Nile neuroinvasive disease (Unger et al. 2018b). The knowledge gained from the semi-structured interviews with previous PALT participants was applied in this case. For example, the structure of the PALT program was flexible, the order of treadmill training and overground therapy varied depending on the preference of the client each day, and some training sessions involved only one training mode. Further, the amount of time spent in overground training increased mid-way through the program as the client regained the ability to ambulate independently and her goals for PALT changed (Unger et al. 2018b).

There are other examples of how qualitative research contributes to the evaluation of intervention outcomes in SCI/D rehabilitation. Curtis and colleagues (2015) evaluated participant (n = 6) experiences and satisfaction with a modified yoga program using a mixed methods approach: self-report questionnaires and individual semi-structured interviews analysed through content analysis. Insignificant changes in health and well-being were found in the surveys after program completion, however, the qualitative results revealed that the intervention was positively regarded by participants, as it supported personal growth beyond symptom reduction. Participants provided specific recommendations for program improvement, for example, regarding the frequency and duration of classes and variety of postures. Hence, qualitative data provide evidence of the effectiveness of an intervention or program that has been implemented and suggest areas for program improvement to support continued implementation.

The evaluation of implementation initiatives applies to healthcare policy as well as rehabilitation interventions. Recently, we studied hospital administrators' experiences with fall prevention policies in SCI/D rehabilitation environments in an effort to evaluate the policies' strengths and shortcomings (Singh et al. 2018a). Transcripts from semi-structured interviews were analysed with interpretive description. Identified strengths included improved client safety, increased staff awareness of fall prevention, and learning opportunities for clients, however, administrators reported challenges such as balancing the prevention of falls with the need to increase mobility, inconsistent compliance with the fall prevention policy on the part of the front-line staff, and some clients' impulsive behaviour. To translate this knowledge, we presented a summary of our findings and recommendations to administrators and policymakers. Presenting research findings in the form of recommendations informed by the study findings and previous literature may lead to greater uptake in clinical practice. In our experience with this study, administrators were eager to receive the executive summary to integrate our research findings into quality improvement of their policies. Ongoing evaluation and quality improvement were brought up as important components to fall prevention in SCI rehabilitation.

Future Directions of Qualitative Research to Inform SCI/D Rehabilitation

The generation of qualitative research is rapidly increasing in the area of rehabilitation (VanderKaay et al. 2018). As this research field grows, there is an opportunity to expand and refine its role in evidence-based and person-centred care. We expect the nature of qualitative research into SCI/D rehabilitation to evolve in several ways. First, we expect researchers will engage a variety of stakeholders early in the research process (Musselman et al. 2018b). By involving individuals with SCI, caregivers, healthcare professionals, funders, and policymakers, a broader perspective on an issue will be obtained. This broader perspective may more effectively meet the needs of those delivering and receiving health services.

Second, we expect that clinicians, healthcare administrators, and policymakers may require some guidance in how to interpret qualitative research findings and when and how to implement the findings. Prior to implementing qualitative research into practice, healthcare stakeholders should consider how thoroughly the findings are described and how comprehensive and relevant the conclusions are (Giacomini and Cook 2000). Clinicians should also think about their individual practice and clients (Giacomini and Cook 2000): Is the study appropriate in their specific healthcare context? Can the study findings help them to optimise care? Do the study findings help them to understand their interactions and relationships with clients and their families?

Third, we expect that multiple data sources will be increasingly used in qualitative SCI/D research. Data triangulation is an approach used to strengthen and enhance the reliability of findings in qualitative research studies (Denzin 1978; Patton 1999). Researchers gather multiple qualitative data sources (e.g., interviews, observations, documents) to test for the consistency of the findings across sources (Patton 1999). We employed data source triangulation in the study examining administrators' experiences with fall prevention policies (Singh et al. 2018a). We combined semi-structured individual interviews with a document review (i.e., hospitals' falls policies) to strengthen the reliability of our findings. By combining these two data sources, a more comprehensive understanding of the problem was investigated. The inconsistencies amongst the data sources provided us with opportunities to probe further, and we identified gaps in policy (through the document review) and in clinical practice (through interviews). Data source triangulation is a means to enhance SCI/D qualitative research, particularly in evaluations of programs, processes, and interventions.

Fourth, we expect to see increased integration of qualitative and quantitative research findings. In this chapter, we have illustrated how qualitative methods can address limitations of quantitative research, however, limitations of qualitative research exist as well. Qualitative research studies typically involve a small number of study participants, which limits the generalisability of the study results (Hammell 2007a). As well, there may be perceptions of researcher bias being present in qualitative data due to the interpretive and subjective nature of qualitative data analysis (Hammell 2007a). In contrast, well-designed quantitative research studies are adequately powered to address the study objectives and utilise objective approaches to data analysis. Hence, qualitative and quantitative research methods complement one another, and we expect usage of mixed-methods in SCI/D rehabilitation research to rise (VanderKaay et al. 2018).

Fifth, we expect to see greater innovation in the translation of research knowledge into clinical practice. Effective knowledge translation involves communicating research knowledge in a way that is tailored to the appropriate audience, and arts-based approaches are feasible methods to convey research knowledge (Canadian Institute for Health Research 2012, 2016). Arts-based approaches in knowledge translation are becoming increasingly popular in rehabilitation and health research (Rieger and Schultz 2014; VanderKaay et al. 2018), as these can be quick and easy avenues to share knowledge, stories, and emotions explored through qualitative research. In our own study using photovoice methodology, participants share their stories through photographs to relevant stakeholders (i.e., others with SCI/D, clinicians, and administrators working in SCI/D rehabilitation) to raise awareness of the impact of falls on the everyday lives of those with SCI/D. Through this event, we also hope to influence clinical practice change in rehabilitation to include a greater focus on fall prevention. This is now acknowledged by the Canadian Institute for Health Research (2012), which cites arts-based approaches as a feasible option for the dissemination of research findings.

In summary, qualitative research findings make valuable contributions to the rehabilitative care of a heterogeneous and complex condition like SCI/D. As qualitative methods are increasingly used throughout the translation of knowledge to action, an evidence-based and person-centred approach to care will be achieved.

References

Agee, J. (2009). 'Developing qualitative research questions: A reflective process', *International Journal of Qualitative Studies in Education*, 22 (4), pp. 431–447.

Allen, N., Schwarzel, A., and Canning, C. (2013). 'Recurrent falls in Parkinson's disease: A systematic review', *Parkinson's Disease*, 2013 (906274), pp. 1–16.

Allin, S., Shepherd, J., Tomasone, J., Munce, S., Linassi, G., Hossain, S. N., and Jaglal, S. (2018). 'Participatory design of an online self-management tool for users with spinal cord injury: Qualitative study', *JMIR Rehabilitation and Assistive Technologies*, 5 (1), p. e.6.

Amatachaya, S., Pramodhyakul, W., Wattanapan, P., and Eungpinichpong, W. (2015). 'Ability of obstacle crossing is not associated with falls in independent ambulatory patients with spinal cord injury', *Spinal Cord*, 53 (8), pp. 598–603.

Amatachaya, S., Wannapakhe, J., Arrayawichanon, P., Siritarathiwat, W., and Wattanapun, P. (2011). 'Functional abilities, incidences of complications and falls of patients with spinal cord injury 6 months after discharge', *Spinal Cord*, 49 (4), pp. 520–524.

Auchstaetter, N., Luc, J., Lukye, S., Lynd, K., Schemenauer, S., Whittaker, M., and Musselman, K. E. (2016). 'Physical therapists' use of functional electrical stimulation for clients with stroke: Frequency, barriers, and facilitators', *Physical Therapy*, 96 (7), pp. 995–1005.

Aune, G. (2013). 'Everyday challenges for mothers with spinal cord injury: A qualitative study', *Scandinavian Journal of Disability Research*, 15 (2), pp. 185–198.

Batchelor, F., Hill, K., Mackintosh, S., and Said, C. (2010). 'What works in falls prevention after stroke?: A systematic review and meta-analysis', *Stroke*, 41 (8), pp. 1715–1722.

Beauchamp, M. R., Scarlett, L. J., Ruissen, G. R., Connelly, C. E., McBride, C. B., Casemore, S., and Martin Ginis, K. A. (2016). 'Peer mentoring of adults with spinal cord injury: A transformational leadership perspective', *Disability & Rehabilitation*, 38 (19), pp. 1884–1892.

Boninger, M., French, J., Abbas, J., Nagy, L., Ferguson-Pell, M., Taylor, S., Rodgers, M. et al. (2012). 'Technology for mobility in SCI 10 years from now', *Spinal Cord*, 50 (5), pp. 358–363.

Bowden, M., Hannold, E., Nair, P., Fuller, L., and Behrman, A. (2008). 'Beyond gait speed: A case report of a multidimensional approach to locomotor rehabilitation outcomes in incomplete spinal cord injury', *Journal of Neurologic Physical Therapy*, 32 (3), pp. 129–138.

Brienza, D., Krishnan, S., Karg, P., Sowa, G., and Allegretti, A. (2018). 'Predictors of pressure ulcer incidence following traumatic spinal cord injury: A secondary analysis of a prospective longitudinal study', *Spinal Cord*, 56 (1), pp. 28–34.

Brotherton, S., Krause, J., and Nietert, P. (2007). 'Falls in individuals with incomplete spinal cord injury', *Spinal Cord*, 45 (1), pp. 37–40.

Burns, A., Marino, R., Flanders, A., and Flett, H. (2012). 'Clinical diagnosis and prognosis following spinal cord injury', *Handbook of Clinical Neurology*, 109 (3), pp. 47–62.

Cameron, M., Coote, S., and Sosnoff, J. (2014). 'Whom to target for falls-prevention trials', *International Journal of MS Care*, 16 (4), pp. 203–207.

Canadian Institutes of Health Research. (2010). *Assessing Barriers and Facilitators to Knowledge Use.* Available at: http://www.cihr-irsc.gc.ca/e/42293.html (Accessed 9 May 2018).

Canadian Institute of Health Research. (2012). *Guide to Knowledge Translation Planning at CIHR: Integrated and End-of-Grant Approaches.* Available at: http://www.cihr-irsc.gc.ca/e/documents/kt_lm_ktplan-en.pdf (Accessed 9 May 2018).

Canadian Institute of Health Research. (2016). *Knowledge Translation.* Available at: http://www.cihrirsc.gc.ca/e/29418.html#2 (Accessed 9 May 2018).

Canning, C., Paul, S., and Nieuwboer, A. (2014). 'Prevention of falls in Parkinson's disease: A review of fall risk factors and the role of physical interventions', *Neurodegenerative Disease Management*, 4 (3), pp. 203–221.

Carpenter, C., and Suto, M. (2008). *Qualitative Research for Occupational and Physical Therapists: A Practical Guide.* Oxford, UK: Blackwell Publishing.

Chan, K., Verrier, M., Craven, B. C., Alappat, C., Flett, H., Furlan, J. C., and Musselman K. (2017). 'Effects of personalized adapted locomotor training (PALT) on walking function in individuals in the subacute stage after spinal cord injury: A prospective case series', *Journal of Spinal Cord Medicine*, 40, pp. 813–869.

Chan, R. (2000). 'How does spinal cord injury affect marital relationship? A story from both sides of the couple', *Disability and Rehabilitation*, 22 (17), pp. 764–775.

Clark-IbáÑez, M. (2004). 'Framing the social world with photo-elicitation interviews', *American Behavioral Scientist*, 47 (12), pp. 1507–1527.

Conti, A., Garrino, L., Montanari, P., and Dimonte, V. (2016). 'Informal caregivers' needs on discharge from the spinal cord unit: Analysis of perceptions and lived experiences', *Disability and Rehabilitation*, 38 (2), pp. 159–167.

Cott, C. (2004). 'Client-centred rehabilitation: Client perspectives', *Disability and Rehabilitation*, 26 (24), pp. 1411–1422.

Craig, A., Guest, R., Tran, Y., and Middleton, J. (2017). 'Cognitive impairment and mood states after spinal cord injury', *Journal of Neurotrauma*, 34 (6), pp. 1156–1163.

Craven, C., Verrier, M., Balioussis, C., Wolfe, D., Hsieh, J., Noonan, V., Rasheed, A., and Cherban, E. (2012). *Rehabilitation Environmental Scan Atlas: Capturing Capacity in Canadian SCI Rehabilitation*. Vancouver, Canada: Rick Hansen Institute.

Curtis, K., Hitzig, S., Leong, N., Wicks, C., Ditor, D., and Katz, J. (2015). 'Evaluation of a modified yoga program for persons with spinal cord injury', *Therapeutic Recreation Journal*, 49 (2), pp. 97–117.

Delaney, L. J. (2017). 'Patient-centred care as an approach to improving health care in Australia', *Collegian*, 25 (1), pp. 119–123.

Denzin, N. K. (1978). *Sociological Methods*. New York: McGraw-Hill.

Dijkers, M. P. (2005). 'Quality of life of individuals with spinal cord injury: A review of conceptualization, measurement, and research findings', *The Journal of Rehabilitation Research and Development*, 42 (3 Suppl 1), pp. 87–110.

Dijkers, M. P., deBear, P. C., Erlandson, R. F., Kristy, K., Geer, D. M., and Nichols, A. (1991). 'Patient and staff acceptance of robotic technology in occupational therapy: A pilot study', *The Journal of Rehabilitation Research and Development*, 28 (2), pp. 33–44.

Divanoglou, A., and Georgiou, M. (2017). 'Perceived effectiveness and mechanisms of community peer-based programmes for spinal cord injuries – A systematic review of qualitative findings', *Spinal Cord*, 5 (3), pp. 225–234.

Dryden, D., Saunders, L., Rowe, B., May, L., Yiannakoulias, N., Svenson, L., Schopflocher, D., and Voaklander, D. (2004). 'Utilization of health services following spinal cord injury: A 6-year follow-up study', *Spinal Cord*, 42 (9), pp. 513–525.

Eglseder, K., and Demchick, B. (2017). 'Sexuality and spinal cord injury: The lived experiences of intimate partners', *OTJR: Occupation, Participation, & Health*, 37 (3), pp. 125–131.

Epstein, R. M., and Street, R. L. (2011). 'The values and value of patient-centered care', *Annals of Family Medicine*, 9 (2), pp. 100–103.

Espino, S., Kelly, E., Rivelli, A., Zebracki, K., and Vogel, L. (2018). 'It is a marathon rather than a sprint: An initial exploration of unmet needs and support preferences of caregivers of children with SCI', *Spinal Cord*, 56 (3), pp. 284–294.

Estabrooks, C., Field, P., and Morse, J. (1994). 'Aggregating qualitative findings: An approach to theory development', *Qualitative Health Research*, 4 (4), pp. 503–511.

Field, B., Booth, A., Ilott, I., and Gerrish, K. (2014). 'Using the Knowledge to Action framework in practice: A citation analysis and systematic review', *Implementation Science*, 9 (1), pp. 174–186.

Finfgeld, D. (2003). 'Metasynthesis: The state of the art – So far', *Qualitative Health Research*, 13 (7), pp. 893–904.

Giacomini, M. K., Cook, D. J., and Evidence-Based Medicine Working Group. (2000). 'Users' guides to the medical literature: XXIII. Qualitative research in health care B. What are the results and how do they help me care for my patients?' *The Journal of the American Medical Association*, 284 (4), pp. 478–482.

Giangregorio, L., and McCartney, N. (2006). 'Bone loss and muscle atrophy in spinal cord injury: Epidemiology, fracture prediction, and rehabilitation strategies', *The Journal of Spinal Cord Medicine*, 29 (5), pp. 489–500.

Graham, I., Logan, J., Harrison, M., Straus, S., Tetroe, J., Caswell, W., and Robinson, N. (2006). 'Lost in knowledge translation: Time for a map?' *Journal of Continuing Education in the Health Professions*, 26 (1), pp. 13–24.

Hammell, K. W. (2007a). 'Quality of life after spinal cord injury: A meta-synthesis of qualitative findings', *Spinal Cord*, 45 (2), pp. 124–139.

Hammell, K. W. (2007b). 'Experience of rehabilitation following spinal cord injury: A meta-synthesis of qualitative findings', *Spinal Cord*, 45 (4), pp. 260–274.

Hannold, E., Young, M., Rittman, M., Bowden, M., and Behrman, A. (2006). 'Locomotor training: Experiencing the changing body', *The Journal of Rehabilitation Research and Development*, 43 (7), pp. 905–916.

Harkema, S., Schmidt-Read, M., Lorenz, D., Edgerton, V., and Behrman, A. (2012). 'Balance and ambulation improvements in individuals with chronic incomplete spinal cord injury using locomotor training-based rehabilitation', *Archives of Physical Medicine and Rehabilitation*, 93 (9), pp. 1508–1517.

Harper, D. (2002). 'Talking about pictures: A case for photo elicitation', *Visual Studies*, 17 (1), pp. 13–26.

Khazaeipour, Z., Taheri-Otaghsara, S., and Naghdi, M. (2015). 'Depression following spinal cord injury: Its relationship to demographic and socioeconomic indicators', *Topics in Spinal Cord Injury Rehabilitation*, 21 (2), pp. 149–155.

Krueger, H., Noonan, V., Trenaman, L., Joshi, P., and Rivers, C. (2013). 'The economic burden of traumatic spinal cord injury in Canada', *Chronic Diseases and Injuries in Canada*, 33 (3), pp. 113–122. Available at: https://www.canada.ca/en/public-health/services/reports-publications/health-promotion-chronic-disease-prevention-canada-research-policy-practice/vol-33-no-3-2013/economic-burden-traumatic-spinal-cord-injury-canada.html (Accessed 9 May 2018).

Kuipers, P., Kendall, M., Amsters, D., Pershouse, K., and Schuurs, S. (2011). 'Descriptions of community by people with spinal cord injuries', *International Journal of Rehabilitation Research*, 34 (2), pp. 167–174.

Kumar, R., Lim, J., Mekary, R., Rattani, A., Dewan, M., Sharif, S., Osorio-Fonseca, E., and Park, K. (2018). 'Traumatic spinal injury: Global epidemiology and worldwide volume', *World Neurosurgery*, 113, pp. e345–e363.

La Vela, S., Balbale, S., and Hill, J. (2018). 'Experience and utility of using the participatory research method, photovoice, in individuals with spinal cord injury', *Topics in Spinal Cord Injury Rehabilitation*, 24, pp. 295–305.

Lal, S., Jarus, T., and Suto, M. (2012). 'A scoping review of the photovoice method: Implications for occupational therapy research', *Canadian Journal of Occupational Therapy*, 79 (3), pp. 181–190.

Lam, T., Eng, J., Wolfe, D., Hsieh, J., and Whittaker, M. (2007). 'A systematic review of the efficacy of gait rehabilitation strategies for spinal cord injury', *Topics in Spinal Cord Injury Rehabilitation*, 13 (1), pp. 32–57.

Leplege, A., Gzil, F., Cammelli, M., Lefeve, C., Pachoud, B., and Ville, I. (2007). 'Person-centredness: Conceptual and historical perspectives', *Disability and Rehabilitation*, 29 (20–21), pp. 1555–1565.

Ma, V. Y., Chan, L., and Carruthers K. J. (2014). 'The incidence, prevalence, costs and impact on disability of common conditions requiring rehabilitation in the US: Stroke, spinal cord injury, traumatic brain injury, multiple sclerosis, osteoarthritis, rheumatoid arthritis, limb loss, and back pain', *Archives of Physical Medicine and Rehabilitation*, 95 (5), pp. 986–995.

Mahoney, J., Engebretson, J., Cook, K., Hart, K., Robinson-Whelen, S., and Sherwood, A. (2007). 'Spasticity experience domains in persons with spinal cord injury', *Archives of Physical Medicine and Rehabilitation*, 88 (3), pp. 287–294.

Marino, R., Ditunno, J., Donovan, W., and Maynard, F. (1999). 'Neurologic recovery after traumatic spinal cord injury: Data from the model spinal cord injury systems', *Archives of Physical Medicine and Rehabilitation*, 80 (11), pp. 1391–1396.

Matsuda, P., Verrall, A., Finlayson, M., Molton, I., and Jensen, M. (2015). 'Falls among adults aging with disability', *Archives of Physical Medicine and Rehabilitation*, 96 (3), pp. 464–471.

McKinley, W., Gittler, M., Kirshblum, S., Stiens, S., and Groah, S. (2002). '2. Medical complications after spinal cord injury: Identification and management', *Archives of Physical Medicine and Rehabilitation*, 83, pp. S58–S64.

McKinley, W., Jackson, A., Cardenas, D., and De Vivo, M. (1999). 'Long-term medical complications after traumatic spinal cord injury: A regional model systems analysis', *Archives of Physical Medicine and Rehabilitation*, 80 (11), pp. 1402–1410.

Ministry of Health and Long Term Care. (2000). *Provincial rehabilitation reference group. Managing the seams: Making the rehabilitation system work for people.* Toronto, Ontario: Ministry of Health and Long-Term Care. Available at: http://www.rehabcarealliance.ca/uploads/File/knowledge-exchange/Managing_the_Seams_sept_2000.doc (Accessed 9 May 2018).

Munce, S., Fehlings, M., Straus, S., Nugaeva, N., Jang, E., Webster, F., and Jaglal, S. (2014a). Views of people with traumatic spinal cord injury about the components of self-management programs and program delivery: A Canadian pilot study. *BMC Neurology*, 14 (1), p. 48.

Munce, S., Webster, F., Fehlings, M., Straus, S., Jang, E., and Jaglal, S. (2014b). Perceived facilitators and barriers to self-management in individuals with traumatic spinal cord injury: A qualitative descriptive study. *BMC Neurology*, 14 (1), p. 48.

Munce, S., Wodchis, W., Guilcher, S., Couris, C., Verrier, M., Fung, K., Craven, B., and Jaglal, S. (2013). 'Direct costs of adult traumatic spinal cord injury in Ontario', *Spinal Cord*, 51 (1), pp. 64–69.

Musselman, K. E., Arnold, C., Pujol, C., Lynd, K., and Oosman, S. (2018a). 'Falls, mobility and physical activity after spinal cord injury: An exploratory study using photo-elicitation interviewing', *Spinal Cord Series and Cases*, 4 (1), p. 39.

Musselman, K. E., Lemay, J. F., McCullum, S. A., Guy, K., and Walden, K. (2017). 'Assessment of upright mobility after spinal cord injury: A 'how-to' guide to the Canadian spinal cord injury standing and walking assessment tool', *Journal of Spinal Cord Medicine*, 40, pp. 813–869.

Musselman, K. E., Shah, M., and Zariffa, J. (2018b). 'Rehabilitation technologies and interventions for individuals with spinal cord injury: Translational potential of current trends', *Journal of NeuroEngineering and Rehabilitation*, 15 (1), pp. 40–48.

Nelson, A., Groer, S., Palacios, P., Mitchell, D., Sabharwal, S., Kirby, R., Gavin-Dreschnack, D., and Powell-Cope, G. (2010). 'Wheelchair-related falls in veterans with spinal cord injury residing in the community: A prospective cohort study', *Archives of Physical Medicine and Rehabilitation*, 91 (8), pp. 1166–1173.

Nesathurai, S. (2013). *The Rehabilitation of People with Spinal Cord Injury*. Whitinsville, MA: AAP Publishing.

New, P., Farry, A., Baxter, D., and Noonan, V. (2013). 'Prevalence of non-traumatic spinal cord injury in Victoria, Australia', *Spinal Cord*, 51 (2), pp. 99–102.

New, P., Guilcher, S., Jaglal, S., Biering-Sørensen, F., Noonan, V., and Ho, C. (2017). 'Trends, challenges, and opportunities regarding research in non-traumatic spinal cord dysfunction', *Topics in Spinal Cord Injury Rehabilitation*, 23 (4), pp. 313–323.

Norman, C., Bender, J., Macdonald, J., Dunn, M., Dunne, S., Siu, B., Hitzig, S., Jadad, A., and Hunter, J. (2010). 'Questions that individuals with spinal cord injury have regarding their chronic pain: A qualitative study', *Disability and Rehabilitation*, 32 (2), pp. 114–124.

Nymark, J., DeForge, D., Barbeau, H., Badour, M., Bercovitch, S., Tomas, J., Goudreau, L., and MacDonald, J. (1998). 'Body weight support treadmill gait training in the subacute recovery phase of incomplete spinal cord injury', *Neurorehabilitation and Neural Repair*, 12 (3), pp. 119–136.

Ottomanelli, L., and Lind, L. (2009). 'Review of critical factors related to employment after spinal cord injury: Implications for research and vocational services', *The Journal of Spinal Cord Medicine*, 32 (5), pp. 503–531.

Papathomas, A., Williams, T., and Smith, B. (2015). 'Understanding physical activity participation in spinal cord injured populations: Three narrative types for consideration', *International Journal of Qualitative Studies on Health and Well-being*, 10 (1), p. 27295.

Patton, M. Q. (1999). 'Enhancing the quality and credibility of qualitative analysis', *HSR: Health Services Research*, 34 (5), pp. 1189–1208.

Pearson, A., Wiechula, R., Court, A., and Lockwood, C. (2005). 'The JBI model of evidence-based healthcare', *International Journal of Evidence-Based Healthcare*, 3 (8), pp. 207–215.

Phonthee, S., Saengsuwan, J., and Amatachaya, S. (2013a). 'Falls in independent ambulatory patients with spinal cord injury: Incidence, associated factors and levels of ability', *Spinal Cord*, 51 (5), pp. 365–368.

Phonthee, S., Saengsuwan, J., Siritaratiwat, W., and Amatachaya, S. (2013b). 'Incidence and factors associated with falls in independent ambulatory individuals with spinal cord injury: A 6-month prospective study', *Physical Therapy*, 93 (8), pp. 1061–1072.

Rick Hansen Institute. (2016). *Advancing spinal cord injury research into improved outcomes: Praxis 2016*. Available at: http://www.rickhanseninstitute.org/resource/publications-media/news/526-advancing-spinal-cord-injury-research-into-improved-outcomes-praxis-2016 (Accessed 25 April 2018).

Rieger, K., and Schultz, A. S. (2014). 'Exploring arts-based knowledge translation: Sharing research findings through performing the patterns, rehearsing the results, staging the synthesis', *Worldviews on Evidence-Based Nursing*, 11 (2), pp. 133–139.

Sackett, D., Rosenberg, W., Gray, J., Haynes, R., and Richardson, W. (1996). 'Evidence based medicine: What it is and what it isn't', *British Medical Journal*, 312 (7023), pp. 71–72.

Sackett, D., Straus, S., Richardson, W., Rosenberg, W., and Haynes, B. (2000). *Evidence-Based Medicine: How to Practice and Teach EBM*, 2nd ed. Edinburgh, UK: Churchill Livingstone.

Saunders, L., and Krause, J. (2015). 'Injuries and falls in an aging cohort with spinal cord injury: SCI aging study', *Topics in Spinal Cord Injury Rehabilitation*, 21 (3), pp. 201–207.

SCIRE. (2018). *SCIRE Project*. Available at: https://scireproject.com/ (Accessed 25 April 2018).

Scivoletto, G., Tamburella, F., Laurenza, L., Torre, M., and Molinari, M. (2014). 'Who is going to walk? A review of the factors influencing walking recovery after spinal cord injury', *Frontiers in Human Neuroscience*, 8 (141), pp. 1–11.

Singh, H., Craven, B. C., Flett, H., Kerry, C., Jaglal, S., Silver, M., and Musselman, K. E. (2018a). 'Views on fall prevention, management and training from the perspective of administrators of Canadian SCI rehabilitation centres', *2018 Meeting of the International Spinal Cord Society*, Sydney, Australia.

Singh, H., Sam, J., Verrier, M., Flett, H., Craven, B., and Musselman, K. (2018b). 'Life after personalized adaptive locomotor training: A qualitative follow-up study', *Spinal Cord Series and Cases*, 4 (1), p. 6.

Singh, H., Shah, M., Flett, H., Craven, B., Verrier, M., and Musselman, K. (2018c). 'Perspectives of individuals with sub-acute spinal cord injury after personalized adapted locomotor training', *Disability and Rehabilitation*, 40 (7), pp. 820–828.

Sipski, M., and Richards, J. (2006). 'Spinal cord injury rehabilitation', *American Journal of Physical Medicine & Rehabilitation*, 85 (4), pp. 310–342.

Somers, M. (2009). *Spinal Cord Injury*. Upper Saddle River, NJ: Pearson Education.

Tan, C. O., Battaglino, R. A., and Morse, L. R. (2013). 'Spinal cord injury and osteoporosis: Causes, mechanisms, and rehabilitation strategies', *International Journal of Physical Medicine and Rehabilitation*, 1, p. 127.

Unger, J., Chan, K., Scovil, C., Craven, B. C., Mansfield, A., Masani, K., and Musselman, K. E. (2018a). 'Intensive balance training for adults with incomplete spinal cord injuries: Protocol for an assessor-blinded randomized clinical trial', *Physical Therapy*.

Unger, J., Jervis Rademeyer, H., Furlan, J., Pujol, C., Dawe, J., and Musselman, K. E. (2018b). 'Personalized adapted locomotor training for an individual with sequelae of West Nile virus infection: A mixed method case report', *Physiotherapy Theory and Practice*, pp. 1–11.

Unger, J., Singh, H., Mansfield, A., Hitzig, S., Lenton, E., and Musselman, K. (2018c). 'The experiences of physical rehabilitation in individuals with spinal cord injuries: A qualitative thematic synthesis', *Disability and Rehabilitation*, pp. 1–18.

VanderKaay, S., Moll, S. E., Gewurtz, R. E., Jindal, P., Loyola-Sanchez. A., Packham, T. L., and Lim, C. Y. (2018). 'Qualitative research in rehabilitation science: Opportunities, challenges, and future directions', *Disability & Rehabilitation*, 40 (6), pp. 705–713.

Veith, E. M., Sherman, J. E., Pellino, T. A., and Yasui, N. Y. (2006). 'Qualitative analysis of the peer-mentoring relationship among individuals with spinal cord injury', *Rehabilitation Psychology*, 51 (4), pp. 289–298.

Verrier, M., Gagnon, D., Musselman, K., and the Canadian Standing and Walking Measures Group. (2014). *Toolkit for SCI Standing and Walking Assessment*. Available at: http://sci2.rickhansen-institute.org/standing-walking/rhscir-toolkit/sci2-standingandwalking-toolkit-online-html (Accessed 20 April 2018).

Walden, K., Musselman, K., Verrier, M., Gagnon, D., Lemay, J. F., Guy, K., and Canadian Standing and Walking Measures Group. (2018). 'Development and implementation of a universal standing and walking assessment tool (SWAT) for spinal cord injury during the rehabilitation process', *2018 Meeting of the American Spinal Injury Association*, Rochester, Minnesota, 2–4 May 2018.

Wang, C. (1999). 'Photovoice: A participatory action research strategy applied to women's health', *Journal of Women's Health*, 8 (2), pp. 185–192.

Wang, C. (2006). 'Youth participation in photovoice as a strategy for community change', *Journal of Community Practice*, 14 (1–2), pp. 147–161.

Wang, C., and Burris, M. (1997). 'Photovoice: Concept, methodology, and use for participatory needs assessment', *Health Education & Behavior*, 24 (3), pp. 369–387.

Williams, T. L., Smith, B., and Papathomas, A. (2014). 'The barriers, benefits and facilitators of leisure time physical activity among people with spinal cord injury: A meta-synthesis of qualitative findings', *Health Psychology Review*, 8 (4), 404–425.

Yang, J. F., and Musselman, K. E. (2012). 'Training to achieve over ground walking after spinal cord injury: A review of who, what, when and how', *Journal of Spinal Cord Medicine*, 35 (5), pp. 293–304.

10

Hand Injuries and Disorders during the Life Cycle; Consequences, Adaptation and Therapeutic Approach

Ingela K. Carlsson, Anette Chemnitz and Lars B. Dahlin

CONTENTS

Introduction

Qualitative research is crucial and has enriched the field of hand surgery and hand rehabilitation. Different qualitative methods can describe the complex nature of human experience in health and disease and contribute to a deeper understanding of how patients perceive the impact of hand injuries and disorders on all levels outlined in the International Classification of Functioning, Disability and Health (ICF) (World Health Organization 2001). The experience related to the consequences of a congenital condition, disease or trauma, the adaptation to lost capabilities, valued occupations or life roles, the importance of personal resources, and support has been highlighted in various qualitative studies in the field of hand surgery and rehabilitation, as well as the need for healthcare professionals to embrace a holistic approach when supporting patients' adaptation. Furthermore, qualitative research has deepened the knowledge concerning influencing factors for patient and caregiver interaction and patient-centred practice. By embracing new insights and a deepened understanding in how a hand injury/disease may influence a person's whole life, the therapeutic approach can be developed in accordance with patients' needs.

The results from qualitative research have also been used as a knowledge base when creating patient rated outcome questionnaires (PROMs) and formed a base for quantitative studies in larger populations, including national health quality registries (hakir.se).

To explore patients own experiences may also shed new light on findings from earlier quantitative studies and serve as an inspiration when finding new ways of addressing research (Carroll and Rothe 2010). It has been pointed out that human experience cannot be understood by reductionism, i.e., meaning, only by identifying and examining its parts. Meaning in human experience is derived from an understanding of individuals in their social environment. Whatever we learn is going to be shaped by our own constructed perspective when we learn about patients experiences (Chan and Spencer 2004). Quantitative and qualitative studies produce different levels of meaning, but integrating these approaches can benefit in defining a more complete picture of complexity and meaning in, e.g., living with a hand injury or hand disorder. Our aim is to illustrate a selection of areas in which qualitative studies have contributed to an important and deepened knowledge base in the field of hand surgery and hand rehabilitation. Unless otherwise stated, the following chapter includes the results from solely qualitative studies, which represent different methods of analyses, such as phenomenology, grounded theory, content analyses, or mixed methods or articles reflecting over qualitative research.

Emotional Reactions and Stress Factors

Different emotional reactions, such as anger, frustration, guilt, jealousy, and blame, have been expressed by parents of children with a *congenital upper limb difference*. These initial grief-related emotions were primarily related to an initial sense of a loss of 'normality' for the children's lives. Worries about how the child would cope with challenges, such as teasing and curiosity, occurred and an uncertainty about how to maximise and promote children's development of self-esteem (Murray et al. 2007). Receiving the diagnosis of a *brachial plexus birth injury* (*BPBI*) in a child can also create much anger and a lifelong distress in parents and has been described to have an impact also on siblings, as explored in a large national quantitative study using registries (Psouni et al. 2018). Therefore, treatment of conditions leading to lifelong disabilities, such as BPBI and *cerebral palsy*, should include the whole family (Beck 2009, Bellew and Kay 2003).

Persistent nightmares and flashbacks caused by the shock of trauma have been described in long-term follow-up of *nerve injuries sustained in adolescence*. Depressive symptoms, e.g., sadness, darkness, hopelessness, a sense of bitterness, frustration, and anger, are mentioned, but also a sense of grief over the hand and the life as it used to be before the trauma. This could even give rise to an identity crisis expressed as *'I became the injury'* (Chemnitz et al. 2013). Struggling with symptoms, such as anxiety, depression, and post-traumatic stress disorder, are also expressed in which the lived experience of a hand nerve disorder are in focus and explored in a constructed grounded theory study (Ashwood et al. 2017). Recalling the events of a *burn injury* to the hand gives rise to similar emotions typical of post-traumatic response in an early acute phase of the injury (Dunpath et al. 2015). Patients suffering from an acquired *upper limb amputation* may also suffer long-term psycho-social problems (Saradjian et al. 2008) as concluded in a qualitative metasyntheses article. Greater use of psychological interventions and education, involvement of patients' social support, and use of psychotherapy were here highlighted as key implications for rehabilitation (Murray and Forshaw 2013). The emotional reaction linked to the loss of a limb has been compared to a similar grief process of losing a spouse, including an initial shock, denial, and numbness followed by anxiety and depression, before the person was able to adjust (Parkes 1975).

Several stress factors in the early stage of an *acute traumatic hand injury* have also been explored (Gustafsson et al. 2000). The trauma experience includes examples of involuntary recollection and re-experience of the trauma, impaired functioning, practical problems with daily activities, dependency on others, involuntary inactivity, uncertainty about function in the future, and pain experience (Gustafsson et al. 2000).

Depressive mood state is described for patients suffering from *rheumatoid arthritis* (*RA*), especially apparent when symptoms are more persistent, but also in the early stage of the disease when feelings of uncertainty about the future exist. Anger is also expressed when experiencing occupational limitations or when pain and fatigue cause a sense of helplessness. A sense of fear or insecurity about the future or disease process is also expressed (Lutze and Archenholtz 2007). Misuse of drugs in combination with worse mental health has been highlighted amongst patients with BPBI based on extensive data from national registries (Psouni et al. 2018), an interesting topic to further explore in depth in a qualitative study.

To embrace a holistic approach addressing crisis reactions, emotional needs, and stress factors as described in the qualitative studies mentioned above, may be paramount to the patients' recovery and future outlook. To screen for early symptoms of post-traumatic stress provide an empathetic and understanding approach, and early psychological support for those in need is highly emphasised. The support given should also include the needs for close family members. Patients with access to few coping strategies should be recognised.

Appearance-Related Concerns and Body Image

Appearance-related concerns, and their psycho-social consequences, are important to consider following different hand disorders or injuries (Dunpath et al. 2015, Kelley et al. 2016, Saradjian et al. 2008). Hands are difficult to conceal, always visible to the patients, and to those with whom they interact. Hands have personal significance, are important for an individual's self-concept, and affect how we are perceived by others. Hands are also important for human interaction, non-verbal communication, and social integration. The long-term psychosocial effect of being visibly different is described in an inductive, semi-structured interview study of a group of patients being born with a *congenital malformation* in the upper extremity. The emotional reactions to the visible difference vary from total acceptance and a sense of pride in being special, to deep distress and social withdrawal (Carlsson et al. 2018). Changes in appearance gained through upper extremity surgery in patients with a *hemiplegic hand* in *cerebral palsy* are highly valued. How participants viewed aspects of appearance varied with age and changes could affect self-esteem. The overall impression, such as body position when walking, sitting, and performing activities, after upper extremity surgery is of major importance as highlighted both in quantitative and qualitative research (Dahlin et al. 1998, Skold et al. 2007).

Struggling with a visibly different 'claw' hand deformity and the scars from the injury are also mentioned as the feeling of self-consciousness associated with an *ulnar nerve injury* (Ashwood et al. 2017). Appearance-related concerns following an *amputation injury* to the upper limb may affect self-image and confidence in social situations. A greater emotional sensitivity may also lead to a hyper-vigilance to reactions from others, especially in the early stages, as found in interpretive phenomenological analyses (Saradjian et al. 2008).

However, the severity or extent of a disfigurement is not always related to the degree of emotional distress and appearance-related concerns. It is rather the perception of how noticeable the difference is to others that seems to be more relevant. A habitual pattern of hiding the hand is frequently described. On the other hand, some choose to expose the injured or malformed hand to open up to questions from others. Hiding the hand is considered to draw more attention to it and could therefore be considered counterproductive (Carlsson et al. 2018). Patients with forearm *amputations* and their views of prosthesis use and sensory feedback show that appearance is important for identity and blending into society and sometimes the main reason for wearing prosthesis. The feeling of agency, i.e., feeling authorship of bodily ownership, is present, but not that of body ownership, which is defined as the experience of body parts as one's own. The lack of sensory feedback is considered as an important factor, still blocking the achievement of body ownership (Wijk and Carlsson 2015).

The visible difference after an *amputation of a limb* may have a profound psychological impact as well as affecting the person's perception of body image. Mirror viewing can be used as a tool when adapting to a new body and includes viewing one's own body in a mirror, and viewing the affected or missing limb, in different sizes of mirrors. The effect has recently been explored in focus groups of patients suffering from amputation to the arm or leg. The phenomenological interpretation yielded a description of mirror trajectory, which contains the experience of a profound initial shock, followed by feelings of anguish. Recognising self is possible in a full-length mirror and includes a focus on missing parts, positive thoughts, and whole body symmetry. The acceptance of a new normal is facilitated by mirror viewing, but to integrate the amputation into a sense of identity is explained as a long-term, cyclic process. It is stressed that nurses or therapists need to have the right attitude and adequate training to be able to prepare and deal with the emotions that the patient may experience, and when needed, refer the patient to a psychologist (Freysteinson et al. 2017).

The need for healthcare professionals to address appearance-related concerns is highlighted in qualitative research, adding new insights into the long-term emotional distress and social consequences of a visible difference.

Activity, Participation, and Health-Related Quality of Life

The impact of a hand injury or disorder on activity and participation has been a frequent focus in qualitative research (Ammann et al. 2012, Bromann Bukhave et al. 2014, Carlsson et al. 2018, Chemnitz et al. 2013, Engstrand et al. 2016, Hansen et al. 2017, Wilburn et al. 2013). In ICF, *body functions* are the physiological functions of the body, *activity* is defined as the execution of a task or action by an individual, and *participation* is involvement in a life situation (World Health Organization 2001). However, the terms activity and participation are highly interrelated. Patients with *osteoarthritis in the hand* experience participation restrictions in their everyday lives and activity limitations as an aspect of participation, which implies that participation in everyday life seems complex. Important for subjective meaning-making is, what to participate in, how to participate, and with whom (Bromann Bukhave et al. 2014). To extract definitions of the term participation, a deductive content analyses was used, followed by interviews with patients and experts. It is concluded that the domains, included in the ICF, are not comprehensive enough to conceptualise participation. This limitation can hinder measuring disability and health (Farzad et al. 2017). There has lately been a frequent use of the additional concept, 'social participation'. A change in ICF's definition of participation towards social roles has also been suggested in a discussion article, which makes a synonymous use of the two concepts possible (Piskur et al. 2014). Within occupational therapy practice and in the Canadian Model of Occupational Performance and Engagement (CMOP-E), the word occupation is the core concept. Occupations (self-care, productivity, leisure) are defined as groups of activities and tasks in everyday life. Occupational performance is the result of a dynamic interwoven relationship between the person, the environment, and the occupation and refers to carrying out of an occupation. The regular and predictable ways of doing this are considered occupational patterns (Townsend and Polatajko 2007). Although, some differences in terminology exist, both ICF and CMOP-E point to the importance of the interaction of person and environment for human functioning (Townsend and Polatajko 2007). The use of different terminology is reflected in qualitative research, aiming at describing consequences for the individual in their daily life.

Qualitative research improves our understanding and knowledge about the quality of life for the whole family, not only for the single patient. Adolescents suffering from a *BPBI* report a good overall quality of life, whereas the parents, struggling with feelings of guilt, do not share the same experiences as their child (Squitieri et al. 2013). Evaluation of interventions can be more comprehensive by including the close family as well as the patient.

Children, who are treated for *congenital hand differences*, and their parents describe difficulties with personal care, school activities, and household tasks. Complex anomalies are associated with greater disability and limitations in sports and music. It is discouraging for the children to experience the difference in abilities compared with their peers, but with increasing age, an adaptive behaviour is demonstrated. It is emphasised that early hand therapy guided towards areas of concern may enhance functional adaptation (Kelley et al. 2016).

To fall behind with schoolwork and experience limitations in practical school subjects, such as drawing, crafts, and physical training, is a reality for some of the patients with a *nerve injury sustained in adolescence*. The consequences can also influence the participants' choice of profession. For those who cannot follow their chosen path, a sense of sorrow is expressed. For others, the injury causes no hindrance. Playing a guitar or tennis are leisure activities no longer possible, since numbness, muscular cramp, or tiredness affect the performance. Fishing, hunting, or playing hockey is problematic for those with cold sensitivity, whilst others experience no problems with skating or skiing (Chemnitz et al. 2013). Activity limitations affected by an irreversible *ulnar nerve paralysis* are, e.g., holding soap, eating, buttoning, holding a glass, and lifting small objects. Affected areas are mobility – carrying, moving and handling objects, self-care, domestic life; major life areas – employment and community, social and civic life (McCormick et al. 2008).

Practical and psychological aspects of enhanced independency after grip reconstructive surgery in patients with *tetraplegia* is described in an interview study. Surgical interventions have an impact on all domains in the ICF and self-efficacy in hand control is pointed out as an essential factor to promote during the rehabilitation process (Wangdell et al. 2013).

Facing an inability to perform most occupations independently in the *early post-operative phase of a hand injury* causes frustration and tempered mood. Single-handedness, whilst wearing a splint on the injured hand, affects independence. Furthermore, the time consuming experience when trying to perform activities is an incisive and disillusioning experience. After a long period of occupational disruption, a strong will for normality is evoked. Being able to drive is regarded as an example of return to 'normal independence' (Ammann et al. 2012).

Patients suffering from symptoms of severe *cold sensitivity* following a *traumatic hand injury* experience that the engagement in meaningful occupations at work, at home, or during leisure and social activities are influenced or limited. Handling groceries from the refrigerator or freezer, cutleries, glass, vacuum cleaner, door handle, steering wheel, or key board trigger cold-induced symptoms. The exposure to water, when hanging up wet laundry, peeling potatoes, or cleaning the windows, causes problems. Even night sleep and social activities can be affected because of exposure to temperature, draft, ventilation, or air conditioning. Participating in outdoor activities, such as hunting, skiing, transportation, washing the car, bedding plants, or doing repair work, causes long-lasting discomfort, which exacerbate problems with overall hand function. Outdoor jobs, involving extensive cold exposure, and mittens or gloves hinders dexterity or fine motor skills. The exposure to cold objects or cold from air ducts can limit work capacity for those working indoors (Carlsson et al. 2010).

For patients with *Dupuytren's disease with contracture in the hand,* limitations of activity includes shaking hands, gripping/holding/opening, carrying, lifting, personal care, dressing, writing, jobs around the house, employment, and hobbies (Engstrand et al. 2016, Wilburn et al. 2013). Patient and expert interviews were used to generate similar items included in the Unité Rhumatologique des Affections de la Main (URAM) scale (Beaudreuil et al. 2011). Unstructured interviews subjected to content analysis and themes related to the needs-based model of quality of life show that the impact of Dupuytren's disease on quality of life fall into the categories of physiological, safety/security, social, affection, esteem, and cognitive needs. (Wilburn et al. 2013).

To be as active as possible in leisure activities is important for patients with RA, although limitations in the choice of activities are experienced. Most activities take more time and leave less time for leisure. The need of finding a balance between activity and rest and between active and passive activities is expressed. To find satisfaction in activities that they do manage to carry out is necessary and important for self-confidence. Being dependent of others is hard to accept. Participating in a social context, sharing activities with friends is also expressed as a necessity (Wikstrom et al. 2005).

A detailed knowledge about which activity limitations and participation restriction patients with various hand-related diagnosis generally may face can guide the surgeon, therapists, and patient when setting realistic treatment goals. It may also serve as basic knowledge when identifying effective problem-solving strategies, e.g., creating specific information booklets containing ergonomic advice, compensatory measures, such as change of handedness, assistive devices, or alterations in occupational performance or occupational patterns.

Impact on Relations and Life Roles

Having a child with a *BPBI* requires long-term care and will impact the whole family. The psychological burden for caregivers is recognised by qualitative analysis, and the parental experiences do not seem to correlate to the severity of the injury (Bellew and Kay 2003). Other factors, such as lack of adequate information initially or mistrust of the healthcare system, influence how the parents adapt to the situation and deal with time-consuming long-term therapy and surgeries as described in a phenomenological study (Beck 2009).

Approaching the other sex can be a scary adolescent experience for some when being born with a *congenital anomaly,* even when treated with empathy and respect.

However, over time, when the visibly different hand is accepted internally, that feeling diminish. *'A girl I met held my hand and felt that something was different, but she didn't care, she just squeezed my hand tight, calmed my fear, accepted it, and then I felt that my self-confidence came back to me knowing that girls could like me despite my hand'* (Carlsson et al. 2018).

Intimacy is affected in a variety of ways as expressed by patients following a *nerve injury in adolescence* and consequently also the role as a spouse. The altered or loss of sensibility causes an awareness of the use of the uninjured hand whilst caressing or holding hands. To choose the 'right side' in bed affects spontaneity and intimacy for some participants (Chemnitz et al. 2013). The physical and psychological consequences of a *disease or trauma* to the hand may cause stress and an increased risk of conflicts between partners. On the other hand, support and empathy from spouses may also lead to positive changes and a closer, more intensive relationship (Coenen et al. 2013).

Profound degree of change in ability to perform satisfactorily in life roles, such as a spouse, caregiver, and worker, is described after an *acute hand injury* (Schier and Chan 2007). This is also a consequence as experienced by patients living with severe *cold sensitivity* following a *severe hand injury*. Occupations that are normally performed as part of the role as a spouse are avoided because of symptoms from cold exposure. This leads to a shift in roles, when, e.g., taking care of wet laundry, cleaning, or gardening. Outdoor activities, such as fishing or walking in the woods and fields, are activities that enrich life and play an important part in social interaction with friends and family. Inability to take an active part in such activities with, e.g., own children give rise to a sense of inadequacy and alter the perception of being an active parent. A struggle to maintain self-image, when facing dependency and altered life roles, requires inner strength and reorientation. Loss of work tasks because of cold exposure is distressing for some patients, since a sense of completeness in the work role is lost. However, other patients simply consider changes as rational measures for earning a living (Carlsson et al. 2010).

A change in role position in the family is also described by patients with RA when experiencing inabilities to perform daily activities. To lose a work role is especially painful for male participants. Female patients are more concerned about inabilities to carry out household chores, whilst male patients with RA complain over loss of ability to perform heavier tasks in the family (Lutze and Archenholtz 2007).

Taking into consideration, the patients' different life roles and occupational patterns are important when supporting patients' adaptation. Embracing a top-down philosophy, which starts with an inquiry into role competency and meaningfulness and continues by determining which particular tasks that define each of the roles may here facilitate a more holistic approach (Weinstock-Zlotnick and Hinojosa 2004).

Adaptation to Challenges in Daily Life

Adaptation to challenges in daily life is richly described in qualitative studies and for different groups of hand injuries or disorders (Ashwood et al. 2017, Carlsson et al. 2010, 2018, Cederlund et al. 2010, Gustafsson et al. 2002). Both emotion-based and problem-based coping strategies are represented and vary depending on the challenges patients are facing. To compensate for altered or loss of sensibility, decreased grip strength and dexterity, numbness, pain, and cold sensitivity, patients with *nerve injuries* use adaptive strategies, such as vision, non-injured hand/fingers, tricks, assistive devices, and warm gloves/water.

Social support, dissociation, minimisation, avoidance, acceptance, and to hide or cover up are important strategies when facing emotional reactions to the trauma. During the period of education, assistive devices, information, and support by teachers and schoolmates play an important role, as well as oral, instead of written, tasks or examination. When it came to professional life, it is important to have realistic career plans. Some avoid difficult occupations, whilst others develop new skills or change their performance pattern. Whilst managing daily life and the role as a spouse or parent, an open communication, asking for help, and the use of assistive devices is helpful. To develop new interests or avoid leisure activities that increase or risk symptom severity, is also highlighted (Chemnitz et al. 2013).

For patients with a *nerve disorder* in the hand, there is a process of struggling and overcoming followed by an internal process of psychological adaptation or acceptance. Eventually, a transforming process takes place when being changed as a result of the journey they experience. The influence of the nerve disorder is related to patients' type of personality and pre-existing coping strategies. Furthermore, the process of struggling and overcoming is not only experienced by the patient, but also partners, family, and employers are affected, which emphasises the social nature of adaptation (Ashwood et al. 2017).

Several different coping strategies are also used to manage specific stress factors following *acute hand injuries*, such as comparing with something worse, positive thinking, relaying on personal capacity, distancing, distracting attention, accepting the situation, seeking social support, maintaining control, solving practical problems by oneself, pain relieving strategies, and active processing of the trauma experience (Gustafsson et al. 2002). To enable performance in daily occupations 3 months after a *severe or major hand injury*, the following strategies are described, changing performance of daily occupations, actively processing trauma experience, changing occupational patterns, receiving assistance, using emotional strategies, and keeping up a social network (Cederlund et al. 2010). Patients suffering from severe *cold sensitivity* after a *severe hand injury* describe a flexible use of relieving strategies because various occupations or situations require different approaches. Compensatory aids or equipment, the use of own body, a changed grip pattern, or actions to influence the environment can ease cold-induced symptoms or discomfort. Changing occupational performance and/or occupational pattern is a conscious or habitual way of achieving a balance between goals, abilities, and environmental demands. Taking control and trying to master occupational challenges during cold exposure are understood as key factors in the process of adaptation, although enduring the consequences, whilst pushing one's limit, is sometimes the only option (Carlsson et al. 2010).

An ongoing awareness of difference in ability and appearance is experienced after an *amputation injury* to the upper limb. A functional adaptation and psychosocial adjustment occur and the use of prosthesis as well as a positive coping style facilitate this process. A sense of worth is regained by minimising the sense of difference when being able to participate in meaningful activities and roles. Future research is probably needed to embrace a wider view on the use and satisfaction of prosthesis. To what extent the prosthesis allows the wearer to fulfil a role may be more important than evaluating cosmesis in isolation (Saradjian et al. 2008).

The disrupted life during the rehabilitative phase after a *flexor tendon injury* is frustrating and coped with in different ways. The impact on individuals life is captured in three themes; struggling-adapting, retreating-battling, and denying-accepting. Every little task takes longer time when being one-handed. When the hampering effect of the large splint finally is over, the relief is replaced with more exercises and pain to overcome disability.

The lived experience is challenging emotionally, practically, and socially. Impaired functioning mean a reorganisation of activities of daily life and relationships (Fitzpatrick and Finlay 2008).

Patients with RA express that it is necessary to adjust or 'dose' the activity level according to their level of energy. Some changes are temporary, whilst others are more permanent depending on the fluctuation of the disease. To stretch one's limit and being able to do special things is worth the risk, even though they have to pay for it afterwards. Having the pleasure of being 'normal' is also a reason mentioned. To accept being on sick leave or giving up work or leisure activities is a difficult process. However, a sense of relief can appear after a period of trying to keep up or modifying activities (Lutze and Archenholtz 2007). To choose leisure activities 'within the range' of capability and plan when, where, and how to carry out them are also expressed as a necessity for patients with RA (Wikstrom et al. 2005).

An understanding of patient's own resources and experiences in solving challenges in daily life may guide healthcare professionals in providing adequate support. A holistic approach, including screening of occupational roles, habits, and psycho-social needs is essential to gain the information needed to support patients in achieving a sense of control and self-mastery – key factors for adaptation.

Decision-Making Process and Patients Expectations

Traumatic *brachial plexus injuries (BPI)* in adults can lead to severe disabilities, and the restoration of function may not be the only concern for the patient. The decision-making process and the long-term satisfaction with decision in patients with BPI with completely avulsed spinal nerve roots has been analysed qualitatively (Franzblau et al. 2015). Suggested surgical procedures for such extensive BPI can raise questions of potential risks as well as costs and influence the patient's treatment choices. Surgery cannot restore all lost functions, but providing the patient with realistic expectations prior to surgery is crucial, also concerning pain management and ability to return to work as highlighted in a mixed method study (Franzblau et al. 2014). Concomitant injuries and the time frame after the injury are other important decision factors, which all need to be addressed in order to choose the unique treatment for each patient (Franzblau et al. 2015).

Patient factors that influence the decision to undergo *upper extremity reconstruction* are explored in a grounded theory study, including patients with *tetraplegia*. The results yield a conceptual model that describes common characteristics for those patients who underwent *upper extremity reconstruction*. They follow a stepwise shared sequence of steps, such as functional dissatisfaction, awareness of *upper extremity reconstruction*, and acceptance of surgery. Three checkpoints determine the patients' ability to meet the criteria: access to coping strategies, access to information, and acceptability of surgery. Either extremely positive or negative coping prevent patients from moving from the checkpoint of coping towards the information phase. Both personal and contextual factors influencing the patients' positive or negative coping are stressed. Highly positive coping with a rebuild of identity post-injury decreases the patients' incentive to search for additional treatment. A dominance of negative behaviour causes a sense of worthlessness and changed self-concept, which also hinders a search for further treatment. Depending on contextual factors, such as physical environment, social support, and financial resources, coping is either reinforced or combated. Many of the contextual factors that support a strong coping also facilitate the access to information. Being aware of the surgical options, grip strength is a main priority to enable task performance and family participation (Harris et al. 2017).

The decision-making process to undergo a *joint arthroplasty surgery* is also described in a semi-structured interview study of patients with rheumatoid arthritis. Improved hand function is the primary reason for surgery for a majority of the patients. Some patients are concerned with the aesthetics, whereas others do not feel that aesthetics is a good reason for surgery. Invasiveness of the surgical procedure, variability of outcomes, and the required post-operative rehabilitation influence the decision not to undergo surgery. Most patients make their final decision for surgery without involvement from their physician. The authors conclude that the decision to undergo surgery can be personal. Furthermore, it is stressed that a collaborative counselling between the rheumatologist and hand surgeons is important to ensure that patients make knowledgeable decisions. An increased understanding of the decision-making process may also allow the physicians to tailor treatment options in accordance with patients' values and goals (Mathews et al. 2016).

Shared decision-making is also a valuable factor to consider when advancing a more patient-centred approach in medical care. A semi-structured interview of *older patients* (≥ 62 years old), who had sustained a *distal radius fracture* within the last 5 years, focusing on the perceived versus the desired role of the provider, indicated a varied level of shared decision-making with the hand surgeon. The perceived role of the surgeon does not always correspond to the desired role. The recommendation concerning technical aspects of treatment from the hand specialist is trusted by a majority of subjects. However, the participants want to provide input related to outcomes or functionality. Although there is contradictory evidence, most adult patients wish to have a shared approach in their treatment decisions. Detailing specific technical aspects of care is of less importance than exchanging information and outcomes of different treatment options. The desired role of the patient should be evaluated at the start of surgeon-patient interaction to provide high quality care and treatment decisions (Huetteman et al. 2018).

The close connection between being involved in decision-making and the need for knowledge throughout the whole care process has been emphasised in an interview study concerning the patients' needs during surgical intervention for Dupuytrens's disease (Turesson et al. 2017). The expectations before surgical intervention for *Dupuytren's disease* include the trajectory of illness, the expectations of results based on surgeon's competence, the care process, and readiness for treatment (Engstrand et al. 2016).

Patient Satisfaction and Appraisal of Results

Patient satisfaction is an important outcome factor for healthcare providers. However, the relationship between the patients' and hand surgeons' satisfaction with outcome is not always straightforward, as showed in in-depth, open-ended interviews. A discrepancy in what patients' and clinicians mean with a satisfactory outcome can exist. The patients' perspective of satisfaction show that it is experienced as a relative lack of tension between the patient's sense of self and the affected hand, meaning that satisfaction is having a hand that could be lived with unselfconsciously. It was concluded that emotional and social effects of intervention and the influence of context should be considered in future measures of satisfaction with treatment outcome. It is also suggested that interventions directed towards facilitating patients' experience of body-self unity can promote satisfaction with treatment outcome (Hudak et al. 2004).

Qualitative evaluation after upper extremity surgery in young persons with *haemiplegia* shows that the hand is easier to use and is used more. The surgery facilitates activities of daily living (ADL) and promotes independence (Skold et al. 2007) as well as fulfilment of personal expectations based on specific open questions to the patients preoperatively (Dahlin et al. 1998), i.e., important parameters that might be difficult to estimate in a quantitative analysis. In another study of the parent's experiences of treatment with botulinum toxin in children with *cerebral palsy,* the authors conclude that the treatment can facilitate motor functions, such as using the hand. However, the injections are also perceived as troublesome, negative, and sometimes even traumatic. Since the treatment has to be repeated, involved healthcare professionals must deal with these concerns from the children and their parents (Lorin and Forsberg 2016). However, one has to take the age of the patient into consideration when judging these concerns, since treatment of patients with *cerebral palsy* with botulinum toxin usually starts at an earlier age than when surgery is indicated as pointed out in suggestions for national treatment guidelines (Arner et al. 2008).

The most important criteria for measuring success of surgery following *carpal tunnel syndrome* is relief of symptoms, such as tingling, numbness, sleep disturbance, and resumptions of important activities. The patients also express a hope that surgery may address the negative impact that *carpal tunnel syndrome* has on their quality of life. It is stressed that the assessment of outcomes of surgical decompression of *carpal tunnel syndrome* needs to include measures of symptom resolution, but also activity limitations and participation restrictions (Jerosch-Herold et al. 2008).

For patients with surgical intervention of *Dupuytren's disease,* a previous positive experience of healthcare can be related to involvement in decisions, a smooth and rational care process, and staff competence. The ability to extend the fingers and absence of pain during and after surgery are positive experiences connected to hand function. Previous negative experiences related to treatment are seeing many different doctors, being sent back and forth between different healthcare providers, postponed surgery at short notice, lack of information or follow-up, or post-operative pain. Negative factors related to hand function are recurrence of contractures, scar issues, or impaired sensibility (Engstrand et al. 2016).

The role of hand therapy in the rehabilitation process in patients with a dominant side *wrist fracture* shows that occupational therapy input increases the patients' motivation, and that the therapy is particularly valued for those who attended rehabilitation sessions in the department. The authors recommend that early and continued patient education is provided by the therapist and that relatives are engaged when appropriate. Patient and family anxieties may then be alleviated and realistic expectations of recovery facilitated. Although objective measurements generally have an engaging effect for patients, the assessment and treatment needs to be relevant to their ADL to ensure motivation for therapy (Bamford and Walker 2010).

The focus of hand therapy following a *flexor tendon repair* remains on promoting healing of the body structures and maintaining the functions of these structures. The precautions of flexor tendon repair require patients to function one-handed for several weeks. Kaskutas and Powell reported, in a mixed method study, that a majority of patients with flexor tendon repair brake their precautions to be able to perform necessary tasks. However, patients who receive interventions directed towards performance of meaningful activities and participation in life roles perceive these advices as useful. To add instructions in one-handed methods, use of adaptive equipment and exploration of accommodations needed at work are therefore important in addition to ensure the integrity and function of the healing tendon (Kaskutas and Powell 2013). To provide dedicated therapy time on how to change handedness is also important for *nerve disorders* when struggling with sensory-motor deficits (Ashwood et al. 2017). The impact of unilateral hand training on observed and self-reported functional performance has been explored in a group of *upper extremity trauma*. The unilateral hand training includes participant education focusing on activity modification and compensatory strategies to perform daily activities one-handed, provision of a one-handed backpack with adaptive equipment, and a home exercise program for the unaffected upper extremity. Participants are forced to alter or avoid most activities, have an increased dependency on others, and take longer time to perform activities, but felt that unilateral hand training decreases the impact on upper extremity trauma on function. The results encourage a change in culture in hand therapy (Troianello et al. 2017).

A focus on occupation, when providing treatment, means that the individual hand patient is viewed as more than physical impairments. This approach also facilitates holism, which enables the therapists to meet the complex needs of the patients. A group of interviewed therapists expressed the psychosocial benefits of occupation-based interventions (*occupations are used as both the means, that make use of purposeful activities as the method, as well as the endpoint, which refers to the goal of the intervention*), as it makes patients responsible, engaged, and motivated. Successful accomplishment of goals in occupational performance also makes recovery relevant and easily discerned by the patient (Che Daud et al. 2016, Colaianni et al. 2015). It has been pointed out that therapists that provide holistic care must consciously keep holism in mind as work demands compete with the ability to provide such care in a cost containment environment (Dale et al. 2002).

Three themes emerged when studying the experience of medical and rehabilitation interventions for *traumatic hand injuries* in rural and remote North Queensland. They are medical interventions, experience of rehabilitation, and travel and technology. A lack of local knowledge is expressed and concerns that delays in medical interventions resulted in ongoing impairment. The exercise program given is modified to fit into daily routines. A limited understanding of problems related to rural and remote life styles from Metropolitan therapists appears. Local therapists also have limited experience in hand injuries and are not always available. Distance and cost of travels to appointments are of significant concern, and the use of telehealth or tele rehabilitation have a mixed response. The authors suggest that rural and remote therapists with limited competence in hand rehabilitation should find a mentor to ensure that clinical practice concerns can be addressed. Furthermore, that alternative models of rehabilitation, e.g., telehealth, shared care, or outreach services should be adapted to the skills of the local therapist and the needs as well as the preferences of the patient (Kingston et al. 2015).

Adherence – Client-Centred Practice

Adherence is described as an 'active, voluntary, and collaborative involvement by the patient in a mutually acceptable course of behaviour to produce a preventative or therapeutic result'. A large proportion of patients do not adhere to long-term treatment

(World Health Organization 2003), which may have a negative effect on outcome and healthcare costs (Nieuwlaat et al. 2014). Examples of reasons for non-adherence are lack of understanding of benefits of treatment, social support, belief in one's own ability to make a change, or perceiving the treatment as being too time-consuming (WHO 2003, Nieuwlaat et al. 2014).

According to a multidimensional model by the World Health Organization, predictors of adherence are multifactorial and include five interdependent dimensions related to; patient, condition, socio-economic factors, healthcare system, and therapy (World Health Organization 2003). The experiences from rehabilitation of the upper extremity, expectations, and treatment adherence are focused in patients who reported discrepancy between functional gains and overall improvement. The qualitative analyses confirms the relevance of the model of the World Health Organization. Patients view themselves as laypersons, where dedication, knowledge, and trust of therapist are important for adherence. The therapist ability to clarify the injury, collaboratively make goals, explain rehabilitative interventions, and help the patient back into life as quickly as possible is highlighted. The perception on what is clinically relevant change may differ between the therapist and the patient. Early clarification on the rate of recovery is therefore important as well as an empathetic approach in order to build trust and establish a patient-centred care (Smith-Forbes et al. 2016).

Sustained adherence to a progressive strengthening and stretching exercise program for people with RA (SARAH trial) has been explored at 4 months and 12 months after initiation of the program. The interview data showed that crucial for adherence is the ability to establish a routine. This is sometimes influenced by practical issues, such as modifying the exercises or fitting the exercises into life. The therapeutic encounter, perceived benefits of exercise, positive attitude of mind, confidence, and unpredictability, e.g., dealing with the stage of disease, represent a facilitator or barrier for adherence. It is stressed that behavioural change components, e.g., exercise planner, daily dairy sheets, and joint goal setting, are helpful to establish routines, flexible enough to fit in with the person's life (Nichols et al. 2017).

The patients' experiences of early sensory relearning following a *median and/or ulnar nerve repair* are described in a mixed method, Q-methodology study. This concept includes abstract thinking whilst, e.g., imagining a sense of a specific texture when there is no sensibility in the hand before reinnervation. A large proportion of the patients have difficulties in creating an illusion of touch, lack motivation to complete the sensory relearning, and need more support. It is suggested that the training should be related to everyday occupations and the patient's life situation to enhance motivation and meaningfulness – important factors for adherence (Vikstrom et al. 2017).

The perceptions of client-centred practice amongst patients with *hand-related disorders* have been illustrated in a recent Danish study, where patients, who are engaged in rehabilitation at six different outpatient clinics, consider information paramount in understanding their situation and to feel empowered and motivated. To participate in decision-making is important for a meaningful rehabilitation. Moreover, the rehabilitation should be individualised, taking patients personalities and life situations into account. Central for client-centred approach is patient participation in decision-making, client-centred education, evaluation of outcomes from the patient perspective, emotional support, cooperation and coordination, and enabling occupation. These qualitative results may now form a base in the development of a Danish questionnaire focusing on outpatients' experience of client-centredness (Hansen et al. 2017).

Discussion

Qualitative research has the potential to enhance practice by addressing important concerns, such as the hand patient's subjective experience of disability, patient-care giver interaction, clinical reasoning, and decision-making as described in a reflective overview of qualitative research in rehabilitation science (VanderKaay et al. 2018). An increased understanding of and knowledge in the patients' expectations, resources, life situation, needs, and desired role may allow healthcare professionals within the field of hand surgery to tailor treatment options in accordance with the patients' values and goals. Furthermore, outcome may be improved by a deeper understanding of important factors for adherence. Dedication, knowledge, and trust of the care-taker are highly valued aspects. The ability to present information in an understandable way seems paramount for patients' ability to comprehend their situation and to feel empowered and motivated. Pedagogic components, such as amount and rate of flow of information, learning strategies, as well as ways to enhance motivation and meaningfulness, need to be further studied.

When evaluating functioning, health, and treatment effects, the choice of PROMs should match the domains and construct in terms of the ICF that is relevant to the specific clinical subgroup. As pointed out in a combined qualitative study and systematic review, important and relevant aspects of functioning and environmental factors are only to a limited extent captured in PROMs today. Emotional functions, i.e., anger, anxiety related to every day demands and coping ability, potential deterioration or fear of increased pain, as well as positive emotional states, e.g., being satisfied and hopeful, are aspects which were described as highly important for the patients. Skin-related functions, aesthetic changes, stress, loss of autonomy, and interpersonal interaction are other examples of missing or rarely occurring aspects in PROMs. The role of environmental factors, such as support from family, friends, peers, and colleagues or adaptive products, also needs further attention (Coenen et al. 2013). Furthermore, the process and structure of care needs to be evaluated in order to provide a broader perspective on outcome (Engstrand et al. 2016). The gap in current measures can be addressed when developing new measures or by altering existing measures (Coenen et al. 2013). Current and future qualitative research can then play an important role in providing the patients' perspective.

Overview

In conclusion, some areas of concern have been illustrated in the present overview, which are important from the patient's point of view. A congenital condition, a disease, or trauma to the hand or arm may entail consequences during the whole life cycle of the patient and on all levels outlined in the ICF. By embracing the results from qualitative research, healthcare professionals have the opportunity to gain new insights into the views of the treated patient's experiences and needs. The results achieved from qualitative research can serve not only as valid and important information for the patient-care giver interactions and the treatment of the patient, but also as a knowledge base to broaden the content included in PROMs. Questionnaires that contain valid items from the patient point of view are crucial for the quality of quantitative research and the motivation to reply to PROMs included in national quality registries. Future challenges for qualitative research include advances in methodology and a careful and broad inclusion of relevant patients illustrating the complexity. Increased use of mixed methods may here play an important role when investigating composite research questions. Critical evaluation of the trustworthiness of qualitative findings requires detailed information about credibility, dependability, confirmability, and transferability. Qualitative research can then contribute to an important and deepened knowledge base in the field of hand surgery and hand rehabilitation and the care of patients with a congenital condition, a hand disorder, or a hand trauma may thereby be improved.

References

Ammann, B., Satink, T. & Andresen, M. 2012. Experiencing occupations with chronic hand disability: Narratives of hand-injured adults. *Hand Ther*, 17, 87–94.

Arner, M., Himmelmann, K., Ponten, E., Stankovic, N., Hansson, T. & Dahlin, L. B. 2008. Upper extremity botulinum toxin treatment in cerebral palsy. Treatment guidelines the first step towards national cooperation. *Lakartidningen*, 105, 3009–3013.

Ashwood, M., Jerosch-Herold, C. & Shepstone, L. 2017. Learning to live with a hand nerve disorder: A constructed grounded theory. *J Hand Ther*, doi:10.1016/j.jht.2017.10.015.

Bamford, R. & Walker, D.-M. 2010. A qualitative investigation into the rehabilitation experience of patients following wrist fracture. *Hand Ther*, 15, 54.

Beaudreuil, J., Allard, A., Zerkak, D., Gerber, R. A., Cappelleri, J. C., Quintero, N., Lasbleiz, S., Bernabe, B., Orcel, P., Bardin, T. & Group, U. S. 2011. Unite Rhumatologique des Affections de la Main (URAM) scale: Development and validation of a tool to assess Dupuytren's disease-specific disability. *Arthritis Care Res (Hoboken)*, 63, 1448–1455.

Beck, C. T. 2009. The arm: There is no escaping the reality for mothers of children with obstetric brachial plexus injuries. *Nurs Res*, 58, 237–245.

Bellew, M. & Kay, S. P. 2003. Early parental experiences of obstetric brachial plexus palsy. *J Hand Surg Br*, 28, 339–346.

Bromann Bukhave, E., La Cour, K. & Huniche, L. 2014. The meaning of activity and participation in everyday life when living with hand osteoarthritis. *Scand J Occup Ther*, 21, 24–30.

Carlsson, I. K., Dahlin, L. B. & Rosberg, H. E. 2018. Congenital thumb anomalies and the consequences for daily life: Patients' long-term experience after corrective surgery. A qualitative study. *Disabil Rehabil*, 40, 69–75.

Carlsson, I. K., Edberg, A. K. & Wann-Hansson, C. 2010. Hand-injured patients' experiences of cold sensitivity and the consequences and adaptation for daily life: A qualitative study. *J Hand Ther*, 23, 53–61.

Carroll, L. J. & Rothe, J. P. 2010. Levels of reconstruction as complementarity in mixed methods research: A social theory-based conceptual framework for integrating qualitative and quantitative research. *Int J Environ Res Public Health*, 7, 3478–3488.

Cederlund, R., Thoren-Jonsson, A. L. & Dahlin, L. B. 2010. Coping strategies in daily occupations 3 months after a severe or major hand injury. *Occup Ther Int*, 17, 1–9.

Chan, J. & Spencer, J. 2004. The usefulness of qualitative knowledge development in hand therapy. *J Hand Ther*, 17, 1–5.

Che Daud, A. Z., Yau, M. K., Barnett, F. & Judd, J. 2016. Occupation-based intervention in hand injury rehabilitation: Experiences of occupational therapists in Malaysia. *Scand J Occup Ther*, 23, 57–66.

Chemnitz, A., Dahlin, L. B. & Carlsson, I. K. 2013. Consequences and adaptation in daily life – patients' experiences three decades after a nerve injury sustained in adolescence. *BMC Musculoskelet Disord*, 14, 252.

Coenen, M., Kus, S., Rudolf, K. D., Muller, G., Berno, S., Dereskewitz, C. & Macdermid, J. 2013. Do patient-reported outcome measures capture functioning aspects and environmental factors important to individuals with injuries or disorders of the hand? *J Hand Ther*, 26, 332–342.

Colaianni, D. J., Provident, I., Dibartola, L. M. & Wheeler, S. 2015. A phenomenology of occupation-based hand therapy. *Aust Occup Ther J*, 62, 177–186.

Dahlin, L. B., Komoto-Tufvesson, Y. & Salgeback, S. 1998. Surgery of the spastic hand in cerebral palsy. Improvement in stereognosis and hand function after surgery. *J Hand Surg Br*, 23, 334–339.

Dale, L. M., Fabrizio, A. J., Adhlakha, P., Mahon, M. K., Mcgraw, E. E., Neyenhaus, R. D., Sledd, T. & Zaber, J. M. 2002. Occupational therapists working in hand therapy: The practice of holism in a cost containment environment. *Work*, 19, 35–45.

Dunpath, T., Chetty, V. & Van Der Reyden, D. 2015. The experience of acute burns of the hand – Patients perspectives. *Disabil Rehabil*, 37, 892–898.

Engstrand, C., Kvist, J. & Krevers, B. 2016. Patients' perspective on surgical intervention for Dupuytren's disease – Experiences, expectations and appraisal of results. *Disabil Rehabil*, 38, 2538–2549.

Farzad, M., Layeghi, F., Hosseini, S. A., Hamidreza, K. & Asgari, A. 2017. Are the domains considered by ICF comprehensive enough to conceptualize participation in the patient with hand injuries? *J Hand Microsurg*, 9, 139–153.

Fitzpatrick, N. & Finlay, L. 2008. "Frustrating disability": The lived experience of coping with the rehabilitation phase following flexor tendon surgery. *Int J Qual Stud Health Well-Being*, 3, 143–154.

Franzblau, L. E., Maynard, M., Chung, K. C. & Yang, L. J. 2015. Medical treatment decision making after total avulsion brachial plexus injury: A qualitative study. *J Neurosurg*, 122, 1413–1420.

Franzblau, L. E., Shauver, M. J. & Chung, K. C. 2014. Patient satisfaction and self-reported outcomes after complete brachial plexus avulsion injury. *J Hand Surg Am*, 39, 948–955 e4.

Freysteinson, W., Thomas, L., Sebastian-Deutsch, A., Douglas, D., Melton, D., Celia, T., Reeves, K. & Bowyer, P. 2017. A Study of the amputee experience of viewing self in the mirror. *Rehabil Nurs*, 42, 22–32.

Gustafsson, M., Persson, L. O. & Amilon, A. 2000. A qualitative study of stress factors in the early stage of acute traumatic hand injury. *J Adv Nurs*, 32, 1333–1340.

Gustafsson, M., Persson, L. O. & Amilon, A. 2002. A qualitative study of coping in the early stage of acute traumatic hand injury. *J Clin Nurs*, 11, 594–602.

Hansen, A. O., Kristensen, H. K., Cederlund, R., Lauridsen, H. H. & Tromborg, H. 2017. Client-centred practice from the perspective of Danish patients with hand-related disorders. *Disabil Rehabil*, 1–11.

Harris, C. A., Muller, J. M., Shauver, M. J. & Chung, K. C. 2017. Checkpoints to progression: Qualitative analysis of the personal and contextual factors that influence selection of upper extremity reconstruction among patients with tetraplegia. *J Hand Surg Am*, 42, 495–505 e11.

Hudak, P. L., Mckeever, P. D. & Wright, J. G. 2004. Understanding the meaning of satisfaction with treatment outcome. *Med Care*, 42, 718–725.

Huetteman, H. E., Shauver, M. J., Nasser, J. S. & Chung, K. C. 2018. The desired role of health care providers in guiding older patients with distal radius fractures: A qualitative analysis. *J Hand Surg Am*, 43, 312–320.

Jerosch-Herold, C., Mason, R. & Chojnowski, A. J. 2008. A qualitative study of the experiences and expectations of surgery in patients with carpal tunnel syndrome. *J Hand Ther*, 21, 54–61.

Kaskutas, V. & Powell, R. 2013. The impact of flexor tendon rehabilitation restrictions on individuals' independence with daily activities: Implications for hand therapists. *J Hand Ther*, 26, 22–28.

Kelley, B. P., Franzblau, L. E., Chung, K. C., Carlozzi, N. & Waljee, J. F. 2016. Hand function and appearance following reconstruction for congenital hand differences: A qualitative analysis of children and parents. *Plast Reconstr Surg*, 138, 73e–81e.

Kingston, G. A., Judd, J. & Gray, M. A. 2015. The experience of medical and rehabilitation intervention for traumatic hand injuries in rural and remote North Queensland: A qualitative study. *Disabil Rehabil*, 37, 423–429.

Lorin, K. & Forsberg, A. 2016. Treatment with botulinum toxin in children with cerebral palsy: A qualitative study of parents' experiences. *Child Care Health Dev*, 42, 494–503.

Lutze, U. & Archenholtz, B. 2007. The impact of arthritis on daily life with the patient perspective in focus. *Scand J Caring Sci*, 21, 64–70.

Mathews, A. L., Burns, P. B. & Chung, K. C. 2016. How rheumatoid arthritis patients make decisions regarding hand reconstruction: A qualitative study from the silicone arthroplasty in rheumatoid arthritis project. *Plast Reconstr Surg*, 137, 1507–1514.

Mccormick, C. A., Rath, S., Patra, P. N., Pereira, J. & Wilkinson, M. 2008. A qualitative study of common functional problems experienced by people with complete ulnar nerve paralysis. *Lepr Rev*, 79, 154–161.

Murray, C. D., Kelley-Soderholm, E. L. & Murray, T. L. 2007. Strengths, challenges, and relational processes in families of children with congenital upper limb differences. *Fam Syst Health*, 25, 276–292.

Murray, C. D. & Forshaw, M. J. 2013. The experience of amputation and prosthesis use for adults: A metasynthesis. *Disabil Rehabil*, 35, 1133–1142.

Nichols, V. P., Williamson, E., Toye, F. & Lamb, S. E. 2017. A longitudinal, qualitative study exploring sustained adherence to a hand exercise programme for rheumatoid arthritis evaluated in the SARAH trial. *Disabil Rehabil*, 39, 1856–1863.

Nieuwlaat, R., Wilczynski, N., Navarro, T., Hobson, N., Jeffery, R., Keepanasseril, A., Agoritsas et al. 2014. Interventions for enhancing medication adherence. *Cochrane Database Syst Rev*, CD000011.

Parkes, C. M. 1975. Psycho-social transitions: Comparison between reactions to loss of a limb and loss of a spouse. *Br J Psychiatry: J Mental Sci*, 127, 204–210.

Piskur, B., Daniels, R., Jongmans, M. J., Ketelaar, M., Smeets, R. J., Norton, M. & Beurskens, A. J. 2014. Participation and social participation: Are they distinct concepts? *Clin Rehabil*, 28, 211–220.

Psouni, E., Perez Vicente, R., Dahlin, L. B. & Merlo, J. 2018. Psychotropic drug use as indicator of mental health in adolescents affected by a plexus injury at birth: A large population-based study in Sweden. *PLoS One*, 13, e0193635.

Saradjian, A., Thompson, A. R. & Datta, D. 2008. The experience of men using an upper limb prosthesis following amputation: Positive coping and minimizing feeling different. *Disabil Rehabil*, 30, 871–883.

Schier, J. S. & Chan, J. 2007. Changes in life roles after hand injury. *J Hand Ther*, 20, 57–68.

Skold, A., Josephsson, S., Fitinghoff, H. & Eliasson, A. C. 2007. Experiences of use of the cerebral palsy hemiplegic hand in young persons treated with upper extremity surgery. *J Hand Ther*, 20, 262–272.

Smith-Forbes, E. V., Howell, D. M., Willoughby, J., Armstrong, H., Pitts, D. G. & Uhl, T. L. 2016. Adherence of individuals in upper extremity rehabilitation: A qualitative study. *Arch Phys Med Rehabil*, 97, 1262–1268 e1.

Squitieri, L., Larson, B. P., Chang, K. W., Yang, L. J. & Chung, K. C. 2013. Understanding quality of life and patient expectations among adolescents with neonatal brachial plexus palsy: A qualitative and quantitative pilot study. *J Hand Surg Am*, 38, 2387–2397 e2.

Townsend, E. A. & Polatajko, H. J. 2007. *Enabling occupation II: Advancing an Occupational Therapy Vision for Health, Well-being, & Justice through Occupation*, Ottawa, Ontario, Canada, Canadian Association of Occupational Therapists.

Troianello, T., Yancosek, K. & Rhee, P. C. 2017. Unilateral hand training on functional performance in patients with upper extremity trauma. *J Hand Ther.* doi:10.1016/j.jht,2017.10.002.

Turesson, C., Kvist, J. & Krevers, B. 2017. Patients' needs during a surgical intervention process for Dupuytren's disease. *Disabil Rehabil*, 21, 1–8.

Vanderkaay, S., Moll, S. E., Gewurtz, R. E., Jindal, P., Loyola-Sanchez, A., Packham, T. L. & Lim, C. Y. 2018. Qualitative research in rehabilitation science: Opportunities, challenges, and future directions. *Disabil Rehabil*, 40, 705–713.

Vikstrom, P., Carlsson, I., Rosen, B. & Bjorkman, A. 2017. Patients' views on early sensory relearning following nerve repair-a Q-methodology study. *J Hand Ther.* doi:10.1016/j.jht.2017.07.003.

Wangdell, J., Carlsson, G. & Friden, J. 2013. Enhanced independence: Experiences after regaining grip function in people with tetraplegia. *Disabil Rehabil*, 35, 1968–1974.

Weinstock-Zlotnick, G. & Hinojosa, J. 2004. Bottom-up or top-down evaluation: Is one better than the other? *Am J Occup Ther*, 58, 594–599.

Wijk, U. & Carlsson, I. 2015. Forearm amputees' views of prosthesis use and sensory feedback. *J Hand Ther*, 28, 269–277.

Wikstrom, I., Jacobsson, L. T. & Arvidsson, B. 2005. How people with rheumatoid arthritis perceive leisure activities: A qualitative study. *Musculoskeletal Care*, 3, 74–84.

Wilburn, J., Mckenna, S. P., Perry-Hinsley, D. & Bayat, A. 2013. The impact of Dupuytren disease on patient activity and quality of life. *J Hand Surg Am*, 38, 1209–1214.

World Health Organization 2001. *International Classification of Functioning, Disability and Health*, Geneva, Switzerland, World Health Organization.

World Health Organization. 2003. *Adherence to Long-term Therapies: Evidence for Action*, Geneva, Switzerland, World Health Organization.

11

Giving People with Aphasia a Voice through Qualitative Research

Linda Worrall

CONTENTS

Qualitative enquiries created a new era in the history of aphasia research. It provided a voice for people with aphasia and their families and enriched our understanding of aphasia. It helped service providers understand what it is like to have aphasia and understand how they experience everyday life with aphasia.

Aphasia occurs because of an impairment to the language processing pathways of the brain. It can occur after a stroke, an aneurysm, a brain tumour, or a head injury from a car accident or gunshot wound. The damage can be so severe that neither understanding nor expressing words and sentences is possible. Alternatively, the aphasia can be so mild that occasional words are substituted for another. Depending on the area of damage, understanding or expression can be differentially affected.

History shows a progression of understanding of aphasia from the antiquities in which the mind-body link was being explored through to the current day where neuroimaging enables us to see the association between the brain and language (Tesak & Code 2008). Naturally, a medical model predominated in the early aphasia literature in which localised lesions of the brain were attributed to types of aphasia. Then, linguistics and neuropsychology made their mark on our understanding of aphasia. From the 1980's, rehabilitation sciences had an impact, particularly since the therapists delivering aphasia therapy were based in rehabilitation wards and centres.

Qualitative research revolutionised our understanding of aphasia in the late 1990's. The impetus came from the group of British researchers who established the organisation 'Connect UK'. Whilst Connect had a physical presence in the centre of London, its reach to other parts of the United Kingdom was important, and their influence in the international aphasia community was significant. They used qualitative research to publish a seminal text 'Talking about Aphasia; Living with Loss of Language after Stroke' (Parr et al. 1997), which described the lives and concerns of 50 people with aphasia.

How Can People with Aphasia Participate in Qualitative Research?

Qualitative research uses data collection methods that involve language such as interviews or surveys whilst the research process itself (e.g., appointments, consent forms) is via written text. People with aphasia have difficulty with all forms of communication (oral as well as written), so reading and writing are affected as well as talking. Many stroke researchers therefore do not include participants with aphasia in their research (Ali et al. 2014). This excludes up to a third of the stroke population. Hence, conclusions drawn from stroke studies that exclude people with aphasia may be biased towards non-aphasic stroke survivors.

All researchers should be prepared to use supported communication strategies (Kagan et al. 2001; Simmons-Mackie et al. 2013) to collect valid responses from participants with aphasia. These include acknowledging the competency of the person with aphasia at the beginning of the interview ('I know you know'), asking short and simple questions (no embedded phrases or clauses, no compound sentences or reversed questions), writing keywords down in front of the person with aphasia to help their understanding, helping the person express themselves by having relevant photos and pictures present, and allowing the participant more time to respond. Some people with aphasia prefer a family member present to help find the words to convey their message. Sending the questions to the participants and the family prior to the interview can help them discuss their responses at home and be primed to respond at the interview. Videotaping in addition to audiotaping has the benefit of allowing non-verbal behaviour to be noted in the transcript since this can reveal the meaning of the utterance (Luck & Rose 2007). For people with severe aphasia, enabling them to agree or disagree with statements in an interview (e.g., other people have said …, is this your experience?) can help them to contribute to the interview (Lanyon et al. 2018a).

Some researchers have found novel ways of gaining more in-depth responses from participants with aphasia. Brown et al. (2013) used self-generated photography to help people with aphasia convey abstract concepts in her study of what it means to live successfully with aphasia. At the end of one interview, participants were asked to take photos of what they considered to represent successfully living with aphasia using a disposable camera or their own camera. At the next interview, the participants described how the photos related to successfully living with aphasia. Both interviews provided a richer understanding of what people with aphasia considered to be living successfully with aphasia.

Davidson et al. (2008) used stimulated recall to probe the perceptions of participants with aphasia about the interactional component of communication. As part of a qualitative collective case study, she asked three people with aphasia to choose typical social situations in which conversations took place with two regular communication partners. The conversations were videotaped and then the participant with aphasia was interviewed about the interaction whilst watching the video of the conversation with the researcher. This provided greater detail and depth to the responses of the participants because they could comment directly on real conversations that they were involved in.

How Has Qualitative Research Enhanced Aphasia Rehabilitation?

Interviews

As noted earlier, Parr et al. (1997) provided one of the first glimpses into the lived experience of aphasia. The chapter headings of their book use the uncorrected words of people with aphasia and provide an insight into some of the results. For example, to describe the early experience of stroke and aphasia the chapter title is 'Is frightened. Is frightened.' Describing their need for more information about aphasia is the quote 'Everything seems a secret', whilst the chapter on learning to live with aphasia is 'I'm fed up of saying I'm sorry'. Any person who reads the book can't help but react to the powerful messages conveyed by the people with aphasia who were interviewed.

Worrall et al. (2010b) repeated the Parr et al. (1997) study by interviewing 50 people with aphasia but with a research question focussed on what people with aphasia want. In addition, this study interviewed the family members of the participants as well as their treating speech pathologists to determine if there was a match between the goals of the client, the family member, and the therapist. Qualitative description was used to describe what people with aphasia want (Worrall et al. 2010b), what family members wanted both for the people with aphasia as well as themselves (Howe et al. 2012), and what speech pathologists reported their goals were for the client (Sherratt et al. 2011). Comparing the interviews from the three groups, tensions were identified (Worrall et al. 2010a) in the areas of relationships, hope, contextual influences, goal translation and communication, and translation of identity. The overall conclusion of the study was that the tensions could be partly resolved through a greater emphasis on relationship-centred care by aphasia therapists. Whilst a strong relationship is core to most healthcare interactions, interactions to develop relationships are significantly compromised by aphasia so additional efforts are needed to ensure that a strong healthcare relationship is built between the person with aphasia, the family members, and the healthcare professional.

Both the Parr et al. (1997) study and Worrall et al. (2010) study adopted a phenomenological approach using in-depth semi-structured interviews as the method. Similar methodology to gain the 'insider's perspective' has been used to describe the construct of successfully living with aphasia (Brown et al 2010; Grohn et al. 2014), quality of life (Cruice et al. 2009), engagement in healthcare (Bright et al. 2017), what aphasia means in other cultures such as Maori (McLellan et al. 2013), barriers to participation in the community (Howe et al. 2007) and in the hospital (O'Halloran et al. 2012), participation in aphasia groups (Lanyon et al. 2017, 2018a, 2018b), or the preferences of people with aphasia for service provision in psychological healthcare (Baker et al., 2018).

Whilst gaining the insider perspective of people with aphasia has been an important contribution of qualitative research in aphasia, insights from other stakeholders (e.g., family members, healthcare professionals) has also alerted researchers to gaps in service provision (Baker et al., 2018; Shrubsole et al. 2018a) or perceptions of evidence-based practice by speech pathologists in acute care (Foster et al. 2013, 2014, 2015). Whilst these studies have used interviews as a method of data collection, other research questions require a different approach.

Observations

Observations with a focussed ethnographic approach have also been an important adjunct to interviews. Observational methodology is suitable for real-life situations where the researcher wants to observe what happens in the natural context, rather than relying on a person's retrospective description of an event. For example, Howe et al. (2008) used participant observation to observe people with aphasia in the community (at the shops, at the doctors, at social events) to identify potential barriers and facilitators to community participation. The primary investigator predominantly adopted a passive participant role so that she could observe natural communication as it occurred. This often provided her with a different perspective to the client about the success of the communication. That is, she observed communicative interactions that she considered to be unsuccessful, but that the participants with aphasia did not consider to be problematic. Triangulation of the data can therefore provide some interesting insights.

O'Halloran et al. (2007) observed communication activities of people with a communication disability in hospital, including those with aphasia, to identify the communication needs of hospital inpatients. The goal of this research was to identify items for the Inpatient Functional Communication Interview (O'Halloran et al. 2004), however, this initial observational study provided an insight into how people with aphasia and people with other communication disabilities are able to communicate their healthcare needs. A second observational study was conducted to investigate the environmental factors that influenced communication in hospital (O'Halloran et al. 2011). Whilst context was a major facilitator for communication, this study identified barriers to communication such as the healthcare providers' attitude to communicating, the physical environment, and hospital policies and procedures. The impact of aphasia on communicating important healthcare needs whilst in hospital was therefore highlighted in this study.

Nominal Group Technique

A type of group discussion that is often used in our program of research is the nominal group technique (Delbecq et al. 1975). The nominal group technique has a structured and staged approach to group discussions that results in a prioritised list being generated at the end of the group discussion. The first stage is a 'round robin' individual response to the question. Each person is provided with time to privately reflect on the research question and prepare a response. For people with moderate or severe aphasia, they often need a support person beside them helping them to achieve this. The advantage of this approach for people with aphasia is that the round robin of contributions allows them to have their say without one more verbal group member dominating the discussion. Each response is written on a board for all to see. This process of writing responses on the board is a strategy also used in supported communication so it facilitates the comprehension of all responses by the participants. The process of clarification and grouping of each response in the next stage is also helpful for people with aphasia, as it cements the meaning of each response. The final round where each participant votes on the responses generates a ranked list of items. People with aphasia are provided with three sticky notes that has a 1, 2, or 3 written on each. They place their number 1 sticky note on an item to indicate that this is what they vote as the highest priority. Then they proceed to vote for other items on the board with their two other sticky notes. This simple numerical voting system enables them to indicate their preferences without needing to use words. In addition, an advantage for the researcher is that transcription of the whole focus group conversation is not needed. The ranked list on the board is the only result that is important. It is the in-situ synthesis of the group so themes are not only identified by group members, but also prioritised.

Wallace (2017c) used this approach to seek the perspectives of people with aphasia and their families on what outcomes were important to them. The research was conducted internationally in different languages because it was only the ranked list at the end that needed to be translated. A manual and demonstration video were used to ensure consistency. Group discussions were audio or video recorded to allow for data checking. The ranked lists from each site across the world were combined into a single list of the concepts that people with aphasia and their family members considered to be important outcomes.

Qualitative Research Has Described Therapeutic Practices in Aphasia Rehabilitation

Surveys

Online surveys using software such as SurveyMonkey or Checkbox can be disseminated more widely than paper-based surveys and can save the respondent and the researcher time. Surveys typically have a free text section in addition to forced choice responses. The free text can be analysed using simple content analysis and in some software, analysis of free text is automated as well as analysis of the forced choice sections. Free text analysis using qualitative methods may serve to elaborate on the quantitative responses in the survey.

Rose et al. (2010) used a structured verbal survey to explore whether people with aphasia considered it important to receive written stroke and aphasia information, and what their preferences were for health information media and timing of provision. Forty adults with aphasia were purposefully selected using maximum variation sampling for a variety of variables including time post stroke, aphasia severity, and reading ability. Rose et al. presented questions in a multimodal format (i.e., both spoken and written) to maximise comprehension. The written survey was formatted using aphasia-friendly principles, which included simplified language, large sans-serif font, white spacing, and relevant pictures. By administering the survey in a face-to-face manner, she was able to repeat and rephrase questions and to clarify and confirm participant responses. She chose to use this structured approach because the questions were specific (e.g., *What is your first choice (from the presented options) for how to be given stroke and aphasia information soon after your stroke?*), and it enabled her to use both open-ended questions and fixed response formats (e.g., dichotomous yes/no and visual analogue scales) to assist participations with severe to mild aphasia to participate (aphasia quotient: range, 6.58–93.1; $M \pm SD = 75 \pm 20.5$). Hence, a semi-structured in-depth interview was not appropriate for the research questions being asked. During the survey, participants were also shown examples of written health information that they could tangibly hold and refer to when responding to questions, for example, ordering them according to preference. The menu of possibilities provided in the fixed-choice response formats also meant that further exploration of concepts, as is typical when using a semi-structured interview methodology, was not needed. In addition, this descriptive methodology permitted the audio recording of responses to open-ended items and other spontaneous elaborations which were transcribed verbatim and categorised according to the principles of qualitative content analysis. This added depth to the descriptive data obtained, in that a summary of the qualitative responses including illustrative quotes followed the reporting of descriptive data. Therefore, despite the reading and language difficulties associated with aphasia, this research identified that participants considered written information to be important, and that people with aphasia desired both written stroke and aphasia information particularly from one-month post stroke.

The impact of aphasia has therefore been detailed using predominantly qualitative methods. A group of researchers involved in the Collaboration of Aphasia Trialists (http://www.aphasiatrials.org/) identified that these findings should be included in the definition of aphasia. Berg et al. (2016) designed a serial mixed methods study which sought to develop a consensus from aphasia researchers on the definition of aphasia through online surveys. They proposed a definition and asked whether the respondent agreed or not with the definition. They also had a free text field where respondents could state their reasons for not agreeing with the definition. A simple content analysis revealed that there were two main concerns with the definition. In future rounds of the online survey, the two collated concerns were voted upon by all respondents with the surety that all perspectives were considered. Hence, the qualitative analysis contributed significantly to the overall aim of obtaining a consensus definition.

Email Interviews

Email interviews (McCoyd & Kerson 2006) are like face-to-face interviews, but allow the respondent the flexibility to answer questions when they have time free. For the researcher, there is no need for transcription, and the responses are generally more considered when written. This format of interview also allows greater anonymity so the respondent may be more willing to reveal aspects of their practice that they would be reticent to do in a face-to-face interview. Worrall et al. (2018) sought the perspective of speech pathologists about the use of mobile technology for measuring functional communication in aphasia using email interviews. A sample of 11 experienced speech pathologists were recruited and an interview schedule of six questions was developed. Two questions were sent to the clinicians in each email. When the responses were emailed back, the interviewer probed and clarified the responses as they would have in a face-to-face interview. Any complex answers were paraphrased back to the participant for confirmation so that the meaning was clear. A further two questions were then emailed. This process continued until all questions were answered by all participants. Content analysis was used since the questions were quite specific and respondents provided relatively succinct responses. Respondents enjoyed the opportunity to reflect on their practice, and the email interview format worked well for busy clinicians. Oral interviews and observation may have provided greater depth of understanding of the issue in this research, however, the emailed responses gave a clear message without the need for further data in this early stage of the research.

Focus Groups

Focus groups are another way of collecting data in a time limited way. Clinicians are often able to allocate an hour to participate in a focus group on a topic that is relevant to their practice. Focus groups allow participants to hear from other team members and discussions can trigger responses from other focus group members. Baker et al. (2018) have used focus groups to efficiently collect data from multidisciplinary teams in metropolitan and non-metropolitan stroke rehabilitation hospital and community settings. The focus group topic was about managing depression in aphasia after stroke and needed input from all professions. The group discussion also enabled the team to discuss this complex multilayered topic, and whilst the purpose was to collect data, the discussion also created greater awareness of the issue by the team.

Delphi Technique

The Delphi technique is the process of collecting data from a group with the aim of achieving group consensus. When disseminated via the Internet, the term has become the eDelphi process.

Wallace et al. (2017b) conducted an eDelphi study with aphasia therapists and their managers and then aphasia researchers Wallace et al. (2016) about outcomes that were important to measure in aphasia research. The process for clinicians and their managers began with an open-ended question, and these were analysed using content analysis. In the next round, respondents rated the importance of the items generated in the first round. Those items that achieved the predefined consensus criteria were sent back to participants and re-rated. The study provided a list of outcomes that were considered important by aphasia therapists and their managers. In the study of researchers, the same eDelphi process was used and consensus was also achieved for some outcomes. The important outcomes from all stakeholder groups were then combined using the classification scheme of the International Classification of Functioning Disability and Health (Wallace et al. 2017a). This research program is now determining which measures within each construct should be used in aphasia research (Wallace et al., 2018).

Qualitative Research Is an Important Precursor to the Development of Self-report Measures

The patient's perspective is the core component of patient-centred care. Self-report measures are frequently used at all stages of aphasia rehabilitation from goal setting to outcome measurement. Previously, the items for the measure were generated by the authors' own opinions about what should be measured or through theoretical concepts. More recently, rigorous qualitative research has used the patient's own words to develop item sets. This has ensured the validity of the tool from the perspective of the patient.

Grawburg et al. (2019) used this process to develop the Significant Other Scale for Aphasia (Significant Other Scale-Aphasia). The scale seeks to measure the disability experienced by significant others when their family member acquires a communication disability. Grawburg et al. (2013) interviewed the significant others of people with aphasia to determine the positive and negative aphasia-related changes to their lives after their family member acquired aphasia. The results not only provided a holistic view of the impact of aphasia on significant others, but the themes also became the items for the Significant Other Scale-Aphasia measure. Whilst psychometric analysis continues to refine the measure, the initial generation of items using qualitative research has captured the most important content for the measure – the perspective of the respondents themselves.

Qualitative Research Can Help to Explain the Results of Large Randomised Controlled Trials

Qualitative research has often been used to explain the results of quantitative research, but the need for qualitative investigations alongside large randomised controlled trials (RCTs) is becoming increasingly important. The science of aphasia rehabilitation is relatively young, and high-level quality evidence for the effectiveness of therapies remains a challenge. In addition, the requirements of clinical trials in complex interventions such as aphasia therapy is rapidly developing with a growing recognition that RCTs' need earlier phased studies to examine the feasibility and potential effect of the trial as well as refining all aspects of the potential trial such as the intervention, the appropriateness of randomisation, the sensitivity of outcome measures to change, and the specificity of the selection criteria.

Process evaluation should be a major component of all stages of trials. Process evaluation determines whether the trial was delivered per protocol. Qualitative research is a major part of process evaluation. In the field of aphasia rehabilitation trials, data collected from all stakeholders (participants, researchers, therapists, managers) are an important component. Their perception of the trial is an important indicator of whether the trial proceeds to implementation into clinical practice or perhaps to a larger trial.

An example of this in aphasia rehabilitation is from an early stage trial investigating the effect of a tailored implementation intervention on speech pathologist uptake of recommendations from clinical guidelines (Shrubsole et al., 2018b). The trial itself was a feasibility study of a cluster randomised controlled trial. As part of the process evaluation, Hickey et al. (2019) conducted focus groups with the speech pathologists involved in the study at each site or cluster. This revealed differences between sites in the extent of trial participation. Organisational readiness was a key factor in the differences. The authors propose that organisation readiness be measured as part of the selection criteria for upscaling the trial. If the focus groups had not occurred, this key factor would not have emerged as a consideration for the next trial.

Overall, Qualitative Research Has Enhanced Healthcare and Rehabilitation for People with Aphasia and Their Families

In summary, people with aphasia can and should participate in qualitative research. Interviews, observations, and nominal group techniques have been the primary methodologies. Each methodology needs to be adapted to meet the communication needs of participants with aphasia. Qualitative research has enhanced the understanding of what it is like to live with aphasia.

Qualitative research has also been frequently used to gain insights from health professionals into healthcare practices surrounding people with aphasia. Surveys, email interviews, focus groups, and Delphi techniques have been the methodology of choice because they are time efficient for busy clinicians. This has progressed aphasia rehabilitation to greater person-centredness, better understanding of how the hospital and community environment may need to change to accommodate the communication disability of aphasia, and greater cohesion of service delivery. The person with aphasia and their family now have a voice about the impact that aphasia has had on them. It has also provided them with a forum for directing services that meet their needs.

Qualitative Research Impacts on All Stakeholders in Aphasia

Many people with aphasia state that lack of awareness of aphasia is the most important barrier to living well after their stroke. Stories of the experiences of people with aphasia and their family are powerful tools to create greater aphasia awareness in the media, the social media, in health profession education, on the type of research questions academics ask, and how educators teach speech pathology students about aphasia.

Aphasia is difficult to describe, because language is generally taken for granted. Videos of people with aphasia or the participation of people with aphasia in awareness raising events is highly beneficial. Listening to the conversation of a person with aphasia helps people understand what aphasia is and how it might affect their lives. It solicits empathy and helps to overcome stereotypical attitudes that associate language impairment with 'mental impairment'. People with aphasia go to great pains to say they are not stupid. Hence, research that includes people with aphasia has greater impact.

An example of how qualitative research has had an impact on speech pathologists is the research of Worrall et al. 2010 on the goals of people with aphasia. When oral presentations about the project occur, quotes are used to illustrate themes. The illustrative quotes are kept intact with no aphasic errors corrected or omissions inserted. Speech pathologists can see that these are real quotes of real people with aphasia and identify strongly with the type of language impairment used in the quotes. The quotes are often things they have heard their own clients say in practice so the realism of the data has an emotional impact on therapists. Moreover, as qualitative research tends to ask questions about how people with aphasia experience something, and tends also to offer details about the 'why' and 'how' questions that clinicians may have, the type of findings gathered provide quite different perspectives to quantitative research. This can lead to ideas about how best to approach intervention in a client-centred way. An example of this is the shared, monitored, accessible, relevant, transparent, evolving and relationship-centred (SMARTER) goal setting framework (Hersh et al. 2012), which was developed from the stories of people with aphasia and their families collected in the goals in aphasia project (GAP) (Worrall et al. 2010a). This framework included ideas about the need for goal setting to be collaborative, accessible, flexible, and relationship-centred. As this model was a translation of research results into clinical use, the framework immediately has greater face validity and meaning to therapists. Qualitative research seeks to build on the expertise of people with aphasia as research partners rather than subjects, and so their voices can positively shape how therapists approach their work.

Some of the qualitative research in aphasia have exposed failures of the health system and given service users a stronger voice to promote quality improvement. Tomkins et al. (2013), for example, described themes of satisfaction and dissatisfaction expressed by people with aphasia about services they received. People with aphasia are rarely asked for their opinion about the services they have received within the healthcare system because most patient experience surveys are written. Patient experience surveys are either not given to people with aphasia because of the assumption that they can't respond, the items on the survey are not always relevant to their concerns about communication breakdown with staff, or the person with aphasia themselves will not expose their language disability by trying to complete the survey. The implementation of aphasia-friendly processes within hospitals (e.g., mealtime menus, speech pathology reports, appointment letters) has thus begun to emerge, and aphasia-friendly patient experience surveys are another step towards enabling people with aphasia to have more say about the services they receive.

The Future of Qualitative Research in Aphasia

Qualitative publicly available digital data are beginning to emerge as a source of service user data for analysis. The emergence of social media platforms such as Facebook and YouTube are rich sources of qualitative data that are making the unheard voice of the service user more prominent. For example, the Aphasia Recovery Connection Facebook site provides a safe forum for people with aphasia and their families to ask questions, receive encouragement, and feel part of a community. People with aphasia don't often post because of their language impairment, but if they do, this is an avenue of expression for them. Family members often post their own questions or post on behalf of the person with aphasia. The forum is a log of unmet needs and qualitative researchers might delve into the online forum to let service providers know what services are not being provided. Another source of online data are YouTube videos. There has been an increase in the number of videos of people with aphasia on YouTube. The most popular is the annual video post of Sarah Scott who developed aphasia when she was 18 years of age. This video has been seen by 1.7 million viewers. They frequently leave comments on the video about their reactions to the videos or how they use the videos to help people learn about aphasia. If aphasia awareness is so important to people with aphasia, then being highly visible in the social media channels and provoking positive reactions to aphasia is important, then qualitative research in the future can help identify what needs to be done.

A future challenge of qualitative research is to include people with severe aphasia in the participant sample. Capturing valid responses and opinions of people with a severe aphasia is especially challenging, and new flexible methodologies need to be developed that assist in that process.

A further challenge is to obtain qualitative data about abstract topics that need metalinguistic skills that people with aphasia may not have. Topics such as how the health service can better engage them or how aphasia affects their psychological health are difficult for most people, let alone people who have aphasia. These are important topics in aphasia rehabilitation that may not be measurable and can only be investigated via qualitative methods.

The insistence that qualitative methods inform the development of measures used in aphasia rehabilitation may lead to more valid measures where patient opinion is important. Not only will patient-reported outcome measures have greater person-centredness and relevance to the person completing the measure, but also reflect more valid constructs.

The efficacy of aphasia rehabilitation has had a chequered past. Cochrane reviews of speech and language therapy for aphasia failed to show a difference between speech pathology-provided intervention and no treatment or volunteer-provided treatment (Greener et al. 1999). Similar results still occur today, and so mixed messages about the effectiveness of aphasia rehabilitation are still prevalent. Integrating qualitative research into RCT designs through process evaluation will give insights into why some RCTs showed positive results and some others did not.

A major enhancement of aphasia rehabilitation practices would be to give people with aphasia a voice by using qualitative methods to seek feedback on services. Focus groups of past patients are an easy method for obtaining feedback with experienced qualitative researchers able to develop themes from recordings rather than transcripts.

In summary, the future of qualitative research in aphasia must ultimately lead to greater person centredness in aphasia rehabilitation. People with aphasia and their families will use their new-found voice to demand it.

References

Ali, M., Bath, P.M., Lyden, P.D., et al. (2014) Representation of people with aphasia in randomized controlled trials of acute stroke interventions, *International Journal of Stroke*, 9:174–182.

Baker, C., Worrall, L.E., Ryan, B., & Rose, M. (2018) Experiences of mood and depression after post-stroke aphasia, *Aphasiology*, 32(sup1):11–12.

Baker, C., Worrall, L.E., Ryan, B., & Rose, M. (in preparation) Barriers and facilitators to translating stepped psychological care for depression after aphasia: The perspective of stroke health professionals.

Berg, K., Wallace, S., Brandenburg, C., Penn, C., Cruice, M., Isaksen, J., & Worrall, L. (2016) Establishing a consensus on an updated definition of aphasia. *International Aphasia Rehabilitation Conference*; 14–18 December; City University, London.

Bright, F.A.S., Kayes, N.M., Cummins, C., Worrall, L.M., & McPherson, K.M. (2017) Co-constructing engagement in stroke rehabilitation: A qualitative study exploring how practitioner engagement can influence patient engagement. *Clinical Rehabilitation*, 31(10):1396–1405.

Brown, K., Worrall, L., Davidson, B., & Howe, T. (2010) Snapshots of success: An insider perspective on living successfully with aphasia, *Aphasiology*, 24(10):1267–1295, doi:10.1080/02687031003755429.

Brown, K., Worrall, L., Davidson, B., & Howe, T. (2013) Reflection on the benefits and limitations of participant-generated photography as an adjunct to qualitative interviews with participants with aphasia, *Aphasiology*, 27(10):1214–1231, doi:10.1080/02687038.2013.808736.

Cruice, M., Hill, R., Worrall, L., & Hickson, L. (2009) Conceptualising quality of life for older people with aphasia, *Aphasiology*, 24(3):327–347, doi:10.1080/02687030802565849.

Davidson, B., Worrall, L., & Hickson, L. (2008) Exploring the interactional dimension of social communication: A collective case study of older people with aphasia. *Aphasiology*, 22(3):235–257.

Delbecq, A.L., Van de Ven, A.H., & Gustafson, D.H. (1975) *Group Techniques for Program Planning: A Guide to Nominal Group and Delphi Processes*. Glenview, Illinois: Scott, Foresman.

Foster, A.M., Worrall, L.E., Rose, L.E., & O'Halloran, R. (2013) Turning the tide: Putting acute aphasia management back on the agenda through evidence-based practice, *Aphasiology*, 27(4):420–443, doi:10.1080/02687038.2013.770818.

Foster, A., O'Halloran, R., Rose, M., & Worrall, L. (2014) "Communication is taking a back seat": Speech pathologists' perceptions of aphasia management in acute hospital settings, *Aphasiology*, 30(5):585–608, doi:10.1080/02687038.2014.985185.

Foster, A.M., Worrall, L.E., Rose, M.L., & O'Halloran, R. (2015) "I do the best I can": An in-depth exploration of the aphasia management pathway in the acute hospital setting, *Disability and Rehabilitation*, 38(18):1765–1779, doi:10.3109/09638288.2015.1107766.

Grawburg, M., Howe, T., Worrall, L., & Scarinci, N. (2013) A qualitative investigation into third-party functioning and third-party disability in aphasia: Positive and negative experiences of family members of people with aphasia, *Aphasiology*, 27(7):828–848, doi:10.1080/02687038.2013.768330.

Grawburg, M., Howe, T., Worrall, L., & Scarinci, N. (2019) Family-centered care in aphasia: Assessment and rehabilitation of third-party disability in family members. *Topics in Language Disorders*, 39(1):29–54.

Greener, J., Enderby, P., & Whurr, R. (1999) Speech and language therapy for aphasia following stroke, *Cochrane Database of Systematic Reviews*, Issue 2, doi:10.1002/14651858.CD000425.

Grohn, B., Worrall, L., Simmons-Mackie, N., & Hudson, K. (2014) Living successfully with aphasia during the first year post-stroke: A longitudinal qualitative study, *Aphasiology*, 28(12):1405–1425.

Hersh, D., Worrall, L., Howe, T., Sherratt, S. & Davidson, B. (2012) SMARTER goal setting in aphasia rehabilitation. *Aphasiology*, 26(2):220–233, doi:10.1080/02687038.2011.640392.

Hickey, J., Kirstine, S., Linda, W., & Emma, P. (2019) Implementing aphasia recommendations in the acute setting: Speech-language pathologists' perspectives of a behaviour change intervention, *Aphasiology*, doi:10.1080/02687038.2018.1561416.

Howe, T., Davidson, B., Worrall, L., Hersh, D., Ferguson, A., Sherratt, S., & Gilbert, J. (2012) You needed to rehab ... families as well': family members' own goals for aphasia rehabilitation, *International Journal of Language & Communication Disorders*, 47(5):511–521.

Howe, T., Linda, W., & Louise, H. (2007) Interviews with people with aphasia: Environmental factors that influence their community participation, *Aphasiology*, 22(10):1–26, doi:10.1080/02687030701640941.

Howe, T., Worrall, L., & Hickson, L. (2008) Observing people with aphasia: Environmental factors that influence their community participation. *Aphasiology*, 22(6):618–643, doi:10.1080/02687030701536024.

Kagan, A., Black, S., Duchan, J., Simmons-Mackie, N., & Square, P. (2001) Training volunteers as conversation partners using "Supported Conversation for Adults with Aphasia" (SCA): A controlled trial, *Journal of Speech, Language & Hearing Research*, 44(3):624–638.

Lanyon, L., Worrall, L., & Rose, M. (2018a) Combating social isolation for people with severe chronic aphasia through community aphasia groups: Consumer views on getting it right and wrong, *Aphasiology*, 32(5):493–517.

Lanyon, L., Worrall, L., & Rose, M. (2018b) "It's not really worth my while": Understanding contextual factors contributing to decisions to participate in community aphasia groups, *Disability and Rehabilitation*, doi:10.1080/09638288.2017.1419290.

Lanyon, L., Worrall, L., & Rose, M. (2017) Exploring participant perspectives of community aphasia group participation: From "I know where I belong now" to "Some people didn't really fit in," *Aphasiology*, 32(2):139–163, doi:10.1080/02687038.2017.1396574.

Luck, A.M., & Rose, M.L. (2007) Interviewing people with aphasia: Insights into method adjustments from a pilot study, *Aphasiology*, 21(2):208–224.

McCoyd, J., & Kerson, T. (2006) Conducting intensive interviews using email, *Qualitative Social Work*, 5(3):389–406.

McLellan, K.M., McCann, C.M., Worrall, L.E., & Harwood, M.L.N. (2013) "For Māori, language is precious. And without it we are a bit lost": Māori experiences of aphasia, *Aphasiology*, 28:453–470.

O'Halloran, R., Worrall, L., & Hickson, L. (2007) Development of a measure of communication activity for the acute hospital setting: Part I. Rationale and preliminary findings, *Journal of Medical Speech Language Pathology*, 15(1):39–50.

O'Halloran, R., Grohn, B., & Worrall, L. (2012) Environmental factors that influence communication for patients with a communication disability in acute hospital stroke units: A qualitative metasynthesis, *Archives of Physical Medicine and Rehabilitation*, 93(1):S77–S85, doi:10.1016/j.apmr.2011.06.039.

O'Halloran, R., Worrall, L., Toffolo, D., Code, C., & Hickson, L. (2004) *The Inpatient Functional Communication Interview (IFCI)*. Oxon, UK: Speechmark.

O'Halloran, R., Worrall, L., & Hickson, L. (2011) Environmental factors that influence communication between patients and their healthcare providers in acute hospital stroke units: An observational study. *International Journal of Language and Communication Disorders*, 46(1):30–47.

Parr, S., Byng, S., & Gilpin, S. (1997) *Talking about Aphasia: Living with Loss of Language after Stroke*. Buckingham; Bristol, PA: Open University Press.

Rose, T.A., Worrall, L.E., Hickson, L.M., & Hoffmann, T.C. (2010). Do people with aphasia want written stroke and aphasia information? A verbal survey exploring preferences for when and how to provide stroke and aphasia information. *Topics in Stroke Rehabilitation*, 17:79–98, doi:10.1310/tsr1702-79.

Sherratt, S., Worrall, S., Pearson, C., Howe, T., Hersh, D., & Davidson, B. (2011) "Well it has to be language-related": Speech-language pathologists' goals for people with aphasia and their families, *International Journal of Speech-Language Pathology*, 13(4):317–328, doi:10.3109/17549507.2011.584632.

Simmons-Mackie, N., King, J.M., & Beukelman, D.R. (2013) *Supporting Communication for Adults with Acute and Chronic Aphasia (AAC series)*. Baltimore, MD: Paul H. Brookes.

Shrubsole, K., Worrall, L., Power, E., & O'Connor, D.A. (2018a) Barriers and facilitators to meeting aphasia guideline recommendations: What factors influence speech pathologists' practice? *Disability and Rehabilitation*, doi:10.1080/09638288.2018.1432706.

Shrubsole, K., Worrall, L., Power, E., & O'Connor, D.A. (2018b) The Acute Aphasia Implementation Study (AAIMS): A pilot cluster randomised controlled trial. *International Journal of Language & Communication Disorders*, 53(5):1021–1056, doi:10.1111/1460-6984.12419.

Tesak, J., & Code, C. (2008) *Milestones in the History of Aphasia: Theories and Protagonists*, Hove, UK: Psychology Press. 294 pp + XVI.

Tomkins, B., Siyambalapitiya, S., & Worrall, L. (2013) What do people with aphasia think about their health care? Factors influencing satisfaction and dissatisfaction, *Aphasiology*, 27(8):972991, doi:10.1080/02687038.2013.811211.

Wallace, S.J., Worrall, L., Rose, T., & Le Dorze, G. (2016) Core outcomes in aphasia treatment research: An e-Delphi consensus study of international aphasia researchers, *American Journal of Speech-Language Pathology*, 25(4S):S729–S742, doi:10.1044/2016_AJSLP-15-0150.

Wallace, S.J., Worrall, L., Rose, T., & Le Dorze, G. (2017a) Using the international classification of functioning, disability, and health to identify outcome domains for a core outcome set for aphasia: A comparison of stakeholder perspectives. *Disabil Rehabil*, 12:1–10, doi:10.1080/09638288.2017.1400593.

Wallace, S.J., Worrall, L., Rose, T., & Le Dorze, G. (2017b). Which treatment outcomes are most important to aphasia clinicians and managers? An international e-Delphi consensus study, *Aphasiology*, 31(6):643–673, doi:10.1080/02687038.2016.1186265.

Wallace, S.J., Worrall, L., Rose, T., Le Dorze, G., Cruice, M. et al. (2017c) Which outcomes are most important to people with aphasia and their families? An international nominal group technique study framed within the ICF. *Disabil Rehabil*, 39(14):1364–1379, doi:10.1080/09638288.2016.1194899.

Wallace, S.J., Worrall, L., Rose, T., Le Dorze, G., Breitenstein, C., et al. (2018) A core outcome set for aphasia treatment research: The ROMA consensus statement. *International Journal of Stroke*, 174749301880620, doi:10.1177/1747493018806200.

Worrall, L., Hudson, K., Khan, A., Ryan, B., & Simmons-Mackie, N. (2017). Determinants of living well with aphasia in the first year post stroke: A prospective cohort study. *Archives of Physical Medicine and Rehabilitation*, 98(2):235–240.

Worrall, L., Davidson, B., Hersh, D., Howe, T., Sherratt, S., & Ferguson, A. (2010a) The evidence for relationship-centred practice in aphasia rehabilitation, *Journal of Interactional Research in Communication Disorders*, 1(2):277.

Worrall, L., Sherratt, S., Rogers, P., Howe, T., Hersh, D., Ferguson, A., & Davidson, B. (2010b) What people with aphasia want: Their goals according to the ICF, *Aphasiology*, 25(3):309–322, doi:10.1080/02687038.2010.508530.

Worrall, L., Anemaat, L., Bailey, Y., & Puller, A. (2018) Do aphasia clinicians consider mobile technology a supplement to functional communication assessment? Poster presented at the Aphasiology Symposium of Australasia, Sunshine Coast University Hospital, Caloundra, Australia. November, 2018. P15, https://shrs.uq.edu.au/files/5509/Abstract%20booklet%20%28Compressed.pdf.

12

The Impact of Qualitative Research in Rheumatology

Claudia Oppenauer, Erika Mosor, Valentin Ritschl and Tanja Stamm

CONTENTS

Overview about Qualitative Research in Rheumatology, in Contrast and Combination with Qualitative Research Approaches

Whilst quantitative research methods have significantly contributed to the achievements in medical research, collected huge amounts of measurable data, and led to evidence-based diagnosis and therapy in healthcare, the use of qualitative methods has long been neglected in medicine, qualitative publications are still scarce in high-impact journals. Nevertheless, quantitative data tell us only little about attitudes, experiences, behaviour, or perceptions of patients and their daily living, e.g., in patients with a chronic disease. Furthermore, qualitative methods are most suitable to explore experiences, perspectives, and the clinical reasoning process of healthcare professionals. Saketkoo and Pauling showed that the number of qualitative research publications in Medline has more than tripled in rheumatic diseases from 1950 to 2015 [1]. In rheumatoid arthritis (RA), numerous qualitative studies have been done in various areas, such as shared physician/health professional and patient treatment decision making [2–5], interventions for musculoskeletal pain [5], family, social, and intimate relationship level experiences [6–8], physician/health professional patient interaction [9–16], perceived health benefits of interventions [17–19], adherence [19–22], and patient reported outcomes [23–25].

Moreover, for neglected or rare disease manifestations in rheumatology, qualitative research has become a significant method for evaluation due to the small number of patients [1].

Not only in rare conditions, but also to elicit individual meanings of symptoms, qualitative research has added significantly to the scientific knowledge in medicine. As an example, the meaning of pain differs substantially between different people: Ong and Richards [26] refer to the important potential of qualitative research to assess individual patients' pain experiences. They discuss the various cultural and verbal expressions of pain and the relevance of the combination of body, gesture talk, and the spoken word. Since pain is highly linked with other health and disease conditions, complex methods are needed to properly assess how patients experience pain and how this interferes with daily life activities and quality of life [27]. The potential of qualitative research for clinical practice in rheumatology is also highlighted by a study about flare in RA and a related editorial article [28,29].

The combination of quantitative and qualitative research has been more commonly used in healthcare research, and qualitative methods are integrated at different stages of quantitative research in the last years [30]. For the development of patient reported outcomes measures (PROMs), a mixed methods approach including an active involvement of patients as research partners has become state of the art in rheumatic disease research [1,31,32].

Qualitative Research in Studies That Used the International Classification of Functioning, Disability, and Health

Several studies used qualitative methods and the International Classification of Functioning, Disability and Health (ICF) of the World Health Organisation as a framework for functioning categorisation, The aims of these studies were to explore if the problems and issues important to patients with musculoskeletal and rheumatic diseases are adequately covered in the most commonly used outcome measures and which relevant issues might be missing in these instruments [25,33–35]. The Comprehensive ICF Core Set for RA as an application of the ICF was developed in concordance with the patients' perspectives using focus groups in order to explore the aspects of functioning and health important to patients with RA. Thus, results of the focus groups were linked with the ICF categories, and the ICF Core Set for RA was validated by the qualitative data [34,36]. Whenever new patient-reported instruments are developed or existing instruments are adapted, qualitative research builds the basis for this process: The perspectives of patients and health professionals differ substantially and qualitative research allows for systematic exploration and analysis of the problems and needs important to patients from their perspectives [37–40].

Qualitative Research Issues Specific to RA

The following sections highlight major areas in which qualitative research has contributed to the scientific knowledge, but also the clinical care for RA.

Delivery and Procedures of Clinical Care Including Adherence

Qualitative research showed that patients were often worried and concerned when being informed about the stage and severity of their rheumatic disease by clinicians.

Furthermore, these patients were often not adherent to treatment and reported significant anxieties. Although patients could recall most parts of the information provided by the clinicians, the information was not meaningful for them. They remained concerned and anxious because they had already experienced pain and other symptoms which had influenced their daily activities. It is suggested that patients can be reassured more successfully if clinicians reduce the use of clinical relevant terms and focus more on the patients' perspective and subjective perception of the disease and its consequences on daily life [11].

However, clinicians sometimes underestimate patients' willingness to take aggressive treatments and feel inhibited to recommend these therapies although the effectiveness is proven. Focus groups about the COBRA (based on the Dutch acronym Combinatie therapie Bij Rheumatoide Arthritis) therapy revealed that clinicians worried about negative side effects and did not take the time to explain therapy course and possible negative effects. On the other hand, the patients were aware of the negative effects, but were not worried about an aggressive combination therapy and taking multiple pills if this therapy would suppress their illness symptoms and increase disease status and prognosis [41].

The evaluation of flare is an important issue in RA research and qualitative methods or mixed-methods approaches were used to understand this phenomenon from the perspective of patients. Since early diagnosis and intervention for flare episodes are essential for the course of the disease, qualitative methods are particularly suited to gain insight in patients' perspectives. One study revealed that patients consulted physicians as a last strategy when symptoms of flare were no longer bearable, when flare had major consequences on daily life activities, and when self-management strategies such as the use of analgesics or distraction techniques were no longer effective [28]. Flurey and colleagues showed that patients with different characteristics appear to manage RA life in different ways. Male patients were more likely to consult physicians at an early stage of flare because of ineffective self-management techniques compared to women. Yet, education programmes could help to support patients to detect flare symptoms at an early stage and seek medical help before the symptoms affect daily life activities [42].

Qualitative methods also provide deep insights on perceptions of risk and predictive testing held by first degree family members of RA patients with an increased risk of developing RA. Interviews revealed that knowing the actual risk would increase their anxiety and would determine future decision making. The uncertainty of the test results was related to significant worries and was experienced even worse when pain symptoms had already been experienced. Relatives asked for emotional support and specific risk information in order to understand and cope adequately with the risk information provided [43,44].

Qualitative research has been also successfully used in the exploration of the phenomenon of non-adherent behaviour. Non-adherence is defined as the extent to which patients stick to pharmacological and/or non-pharmacological treatment recommendations [45–48]. A wide variety of clinical variables have been identified in statistical analyses that facilitate non-adherence. Yet, these study results were partly inconclusive and contradict each other, e.g., higher numbers of disease-modifying antirheumatic drugs (DMARDs) were described to increase adherence rates [49,50], whilst in another study, higher numbers of previous DMARDs (biologic or other) were a predictor for a reduced DMARD survival [51]. These findings, however, do not give reasons why patients chose to stop the intake of DMARDs. Shorter drug survival may be related to more severe disease and less efficacy, more toxicity, and/or the values, beliefs and experiences of patients. According to the World Health Organisation, the perspective of patients, such as their motivation, values, beliefs, opinions, and needs, are essential factors that need to be considered in non-adherence [47,52]. These values, beliefs, and experiences of patients are the core focus of qualitative research [33].

eHealth

The evaluation of technological innovations, such as electronic recording and monitoring of disease activity and PROMs via apps, is an important target for qualitative research in order to investigate needs and attitudes about electronic data collection and sharing PROM data between different clinical sites and researchers. Results demonstrated that patients accepted electronic data sharing if this improved communication with healthcare providers and the access to relevant RA information [53].

A qualitative focus group study explored the needs of RA patients concerning eHealth technology support for medication use [54]. Results of the focus groups demonstrated that patients especially needed informational, practical, and emotional support concerning medication use. The use of eHealth technologies was considered to be useful for these issues. Although patients addressed concerns regarding personal interaction with health professionals, privacy and data security, and the quality and reliability of the online information. Furthermore, the patients pointed out that eHealth technologies should be used additionally rather than replacing current practices. Despite the patients' perspectives, health professionals' views about the role of eHealth technologies for, e.g., web-based educational resources for diagnostic criteria, clinical therapies, or dosage calculators are also necessary. In a study by MacDonald et al. [55], healthcare professionals discussed the shift of a very paternalistic physician-patient communication to a 'two-way' collaborative conversation enhanced by eHealth technologies. In their opinion, Internet-based patient platforms can support patients to share their disease conditions and provide possibilities for discussing problems, as well as connecting and supporting each other. The health professionals in this study also discussed ethical and practical concerns about the transition of empowered patients, and the challenge to transfer this ideal into practice. The role of false information about disease course or medications on the Internet and its challenging necessity to steer the patients towards the correct path were important issues in the interviews as well.

Outcomes

Patients' experience of disease activity compared to the physicians'/health professionals' perspective was the focus of some recent qualitative studies. A study [56] using focus groups revealed that patients with subjective high disease activity, but with low disease activity estimated by the rheumatologists experienced more stress, difficulties in activities of daily living, and had problems with medication intake. The non-satisfying relationship also had a negative impact on the subjective estimation of the disease activity of the patients. Furthermore, fatigue and pain significantly contributed to a worse disease perception and were also discussed as a main reason for avoiding physical exercises and activity in general.

Qualitative research could also reveal that patients with RA have different sets of beliefs and apprehensions linked with their disease which commonly relate to psychological factors about the development, progression, and manifestation of their disease and which had a major impact on their treatment expectations. These beliefs changed over the course of the disease and were in most cases inappropriate from the medical point of view. Psychological interventions and more in-depth physician explorations with the patients could help to support the patients in reducing inappropriate beliefs and treatment expectations, as well as anxieties and worries about the disease which would enhance treatment adherence and improve long-term outcome [57].

The emphasis on the patients' experience and PROMs have also led to the development of organisations like the independent initiative Outcome Measures in Rheumatology (https://omeract.org/). Outcome Measures in Rheumatology has also contributed to the development and validation of clinical and radiographic outcome measures in RA, osteoarthritis, psoriatic arthritis, fibromyalgia, and other rheumatic diseases. Patient perspectives were considered by Outcome Measures in Rheumatology in various ways, including active participation of patients and patient experts in study groups, as well as by carrying out qualitative studies.

Most Commonly Used Methods in Qualitative Research in RA

For the development of PROMs, a combination of quantitative and qualitative methods is essential to establish psychometric properties. Usually, the first draft of a questionnaire is presented to experts in workshops or panel discussions and to patients in focus groups in order to modify and reduce items before the questionnaire is assessed for reliability and validity in a larger sample [58].

Depending on the research objectives and questions, qualitative methods in RA mainly cover the following approaches: phenomenology, ethnography, and content analysis. Phenomenology and content analysis provide the most commonly used qualitative methods for data acquisition in healthcare research: interviews and focus groups. Both methods give deep insights into patients' and caregivers' attitudes, perceptions, and experiences in a narrative data form. Whilst individual interviews can give very elaborate patients' and caregivers' views on a specific topic, the group dynamics and interactions of a focus group can help to gain data about different perspectives of the focus group members and also reveal controversial topics. Ethnographic approaches commonly use observation(s) of patients in combination with interviews for cultural or social sensitive reasons [1], but also for the identification of patient-physician/health professional communication concerning educational health and therapy information [59]. Another option for analysing qualitative data are historical analyses that use narrative data such as newspapers, journals and digital blogs or forums, and the use of social media as well as non-verbal data such as artistic expressions of patients' hands [1,60].

Quality of Qualitative Research

In all these approaches, stringent quality assurance methods need to be implemented to prove the rigor and accuracy of the qualitative analysis. These might include peer review of a part of the analysis, member checking of the accurateness of the results with the participants, triangulation to a third external resource either literature or data generated by means of a different method, and reflexivity of the researcher.

Discussion

Although qualitative research has started to be used more commonly in healthcare research as well as in medicine and the number of scholars who see its value is constantly increasing, there are still some relevant barriers. First of all, qualitative research employs a different research paradigm in that it celebrates and highlights the meanings of individual concepts, a variability of experiences and demand reflexivity in the process of data generation and analysis. Qualitative research therefore commonly involves small sample sizes with in-depth data gathering and analysis that will lead to a deeper understanding of a certain phenomenon with a variety of experiences, rather than using large sample sizes to quantify a certain phenomenon. For these reasons, qualitative research is essential to explore reasons for behaviour, motivation, possibilities for implementation of lifestyle modifications in patients' lives, as well as views on new technologies including eHealth. Several examples in RA have been described in the previous sections which can hardly be replaced by quantitative study designs. Furthermore, a qualitative study can be a methodologically strong first step in the development or adaptation of PROMs. Likewise, qualitative results can be used for generating hypotheses, in requirements engineering, in systemic modelling approaches, in evaluation studies, and for mixed methods approaches – to complement quantitative data. And vice versa, quantitative data can also be part of qualitative studies, examples are descriptive statistics and statistical models.

Most important in qualitative research is that the authors describe and justify each single step of their research process. Despite the use of rigorous methods to justify and prove accuracy of qualitative data and findings, it is still difficult to publish qualitative studies in high impact journals and receive competitive funding. Unfortunately, qualitative research is often judged against quality criteria for quantitative research, especially regarding sample sizes, generalisability, objectivity, reliability, or validity of the research data. However, qualitative research needs to strictly follow a research paradigm which is different from quantitative research in its epistemological and ontological theories. Qualitative research, thus, has its own reporting criteria, e.g., the consolidated criteria for reporting qualitative research guidelines [61]. These involve a 32 item checklist which can be used before submitting a qualitative research study to a journal in order to face the most commonly used criticisms and providing all the information necessary for the reviewers such as information on the analysis (number of coders, code structure, etc.), providing the interview guide, and argumentation for the use of qualitative research [1].

In conclusion, qualitative research in RA has contributed substantially to a deeper understanding of patient perspectives, their motivations and reasons for behaviour, as well as a comprehensive bio-psycho-social understanding of the living environment of human beings.

References

1. Saketkoo, L.A. and J.D. Pauling, Qualitative methods to advance care, diagnosis, and therapy in rheumatic diseases. *Rheumatic Diseases Clinics of North America*, 2018. 44(2): 267–284.
2. Suter Lisa, G., L. Fraenkel, and S. Holmboe Eric, What factors account for referral delays for patients with suspected rheumatoid arthritis? *Arthritis Care & Research*, 2006. 55(2): 300–305.

3. Ballantyne Peri, J., A.M. Gignac Monique, and A. Hawker Gillian, A patient-centered perspective on surgery avoidance for hip or knee arthritis: Lessons for the future. *Arthritis Care & Research*, 2007. 57(1): 27–34.
4. Kroll, T.L., et al., "Keep on truckin" or "It's got you in this little vacuum": Race-based perceptions in decision-making for total knee arthroplasty. *Journal of Rheumatolgy*, 2007. 34(5): 1069–1075.
5. Klein, D., et al., A qualitative study to identify factors influencing COXIB prescribed by family physicians for musculoskeletal disorders. *Family Practice*, 2006. 23(6): 659–665.
6. Mann, C. and P. Dieppe, Different patterns of illness-related interaction in couples coping with rheumatoid arthritis. *Arthritis Care & Research*, 2006. 55(2): 279–286.
7. Barlow, J.H., et al., Does arthritis influence perceived ability to fulfill a parenting role?: Perceptions of mothers, fathers and grandparents. *Patient Education and Counseling*, 1999. 37(2): 141–151.
8. Backman Catherine, L., et al., Experiences of mothers living with inflammatory arthritis. *Arthritis Care & Research*, 2007. 57(3): 381–388.
9. Sanders, C., J.L. Donovan, and P.A. Dieppe, Unmet need for joint replacement: A qualitative investigation of barriers to treatment among individuals with severe pain and disability of the hip and knee. *Rheumatology (Oxford)*, 2004. 43(3): 353–357.
10. Rhodes, L.A., et al., The power of the visible: The meaning of diagnostic tests in chronic back pain. *Social Science & Medicine*, 1999. 48(9): 1189–1203.
11. Donovan, J.L. and D.R. Blake, Qualitative study of interpretation of reassurance among patients attending rheumatology clinics: "Just a touch of arthritis, doctor?" *BMJ*, 2000. 320(7234): 541.
12. Haugli, L., E. Strand, and A. Finset, How do patients with rheumatic disease experience their relationship with their doctors?: A qualitative study of experiences of stress and support in the doctor–patient relationship. *Patient Education and Counseling*, 2004. 52(2): 169–174.
13. Ward, V., et al., Patient priorities of care in rheumatology outpatient clinics: A qualitative study. *Musculoskeletal Care*, 2007. 5(4): 216–228.
14. Hay, M.C., et al., Prepared patients: Internet information seeking by new rheumatology patients. *Arthritis Care & Research*, 2008. 59(4): 575–582.
15. Arthur, V. and C. Clifford, Rheumatology: The expectations and preferences of patients for their follow-up monitoring care: A qualitative study to determine the dimensions of patient satisfaction. *Journal of Clinical Nursing*, 2004. 13(2): 234–242.
16. Hale, E.D., et al., "Joining the dots" for patients with systemic lupus erythematosus: Personal perspectives of health care from a qualitative study. *Annals of the Rheumatic Diseases*, 2006. 65(5): 585.
17. Marshall, N.J., et al., Patients' perceptions of treatment with anti-TNF therapy for rheumatoid arthritis: A qualitative study. *Rheumatology*, 2004. 43(8): 1034–1038.
18. Woolhead, G.M., J.L. Donovan, and P.A. Dieppe, Outcomes of total knee replacement: A qualitative study. *Rheumatology*, 2005. 44(8): 1032–1037.
19. Thorstensson, C.A., et al., How do middle-aged patients conceive exercise as a form of treatment for knee osteoarthritis? *Disability and Rehabilitation*, 2006. 28(1): 51–59.
20. Campbell, R., et al., Why don't patients do their exercises? Understanding non-compliance with physiotherapy in patients with osteoarthritis of the knee. *Journal of Epidemiology and Community Health*, 2001. 55(2): 132.
21. Veenhof, C., et al., Active involvement and long-term goals influence long-term adherence to behavioural graded activity in patients with osteoarthritis: A qualitative study. *Australian Journal of Physiotherapy*, 2006. 52(4): 273–278.
22. Sale Joanna, E.M., M. Gignac, and G. Hawker, How "bad" does the pain have to be? A qualitative study examining adherence to pain medication in older adults with osteoarthritis. *Arthritis Care & Research*, 2006. 55(2): 272–278.
23. Hewlett, S., Patients and clinicians have different perspectives on outcomes in arthritis. *The Journal of Rheumatology*, 2003. 30(4): 877–879.

24. Kirwan, J., et al., Outcomes from the patient perspective workshop at OMERACT 6. *The Journal of Rheumatology*, 2003. 30(4): 868–876.
25. Stamm, T.A., et al., Validating the international classification of functioning, disability and health comprehensive core set for rheumatoid arthritis from the patient perspective: A qualitative study. *Arthritis Rheumatol*, 2005. 53(3): 431–439.
26. Ong, B.N. and J.C. Richardson, The contribution of qualitative approaches to musculoskeletal research, in *Rheumatology (Oxford)*. 2006. pp. 369–370.
27. Sanders, C., J. Donovan, and P. Dieppe, The significance and consequences of having painful and disabled joints in older age: Co-existing accounts of normal and disrupted biographies. *Sociology of Health & Illness*, 2002. 24(2): 227–253.
28. Hewlett, S., et al., "I'm hurting, I want to kill myself": Rheumatoid arthritis flare is more than a high joint count – An international patient perspective on flare where medical help is sought. *Rheumatology*, 2012. 51(1): 69–76.
29. Paskins, Z. and A.B. Hassell, Qualitative research in RA, in *Rheumatology (Oxford)*. 2012. pp. 3–4.
30. Pope, C. and N. Mays, Critical reflections on the rise of qualitative research. *BMJ*, 2009. 339.
31. Bradley Elizabeth, H., A. Curry Leslie, and J. Devers Kelly, Qualitative data analysis for health services research: Developing taxonomy, themes, and theory. *Health Services Research*, 2007. 42(4): 1758–1772.
32. Adamson, J., et al., "Questerviews": Using questionnaires in qualitative interviews as a method of integrating qualitative and quantitative health services research. *Journal of Health Services Research Policy*, 2004. 9(3): 139–145.
33. Stamm, T.A., et al., Concepts of functioning and health important to people with systemic sclerosis: A qualitative study in four European countries. *Annals of the Rheumatic Diseases*, 2011. 70(6): 1074–1079.
34. Coenen, M., et al., Validation of the international classification of functioning, disability and health (ICF) core set for rheumatoid arthritis from the patient perspective using focus groups. *Arthritis Research & Therapy*, 2006. 8: R84.
35. Coenen, M., et al., Individual interviews and focus groups in patients with rheumatoid arthritis: A comparison of two qualitative methods. *Quality Life Research*, 2012. 21(2): 359–370.
36. Stamm, T.A., et al., Validating the international classification of functioning, disability and health comprehensive core set for rheumatoid arthritis from the patient perspective: A qualitative study. *Arthritis Rheumatol*, 2005. 53(3): 431–439.
37. Carr, A., et al., Rheumatology outcomes: The patient's perspective. *The Journal of Rheumatology*, 2003. 30(4): 880–883.
38. Kirwan, J.R., et al., OMERACT 10 patient perspective virtual campus: Valuing health; measuring outcomes in rheumatoid arthritis fatigue, RA sleep, arthroplasty, and systemic sclerosis; and clinical significance of changes in health. *Journal of Rheumatology*, 2011. 38(8): 1728–1734.
39. Kirwan, J.R., et al., Patient perspective: Choosing or developing instruments. *Journal Rheumatology*, 2011. 38(8): 1716–1719.
40. Stamm, T.A., et al., I have a disease, but I am not ill: A narrative study of occupational balance in people with rheumatoid arthritis. *OTJR: Occupation, Participation and Health*, 2008. 29(1): 32–39.
41. van Tuyl, L.H., et al., Discordant perspectives of rheumatologists and patients on COBRA combination therapy in rheumatoid arthritis. *Rheumatology (Oxford)*, 2008. 47(10): 1571–1576.
42. Flurey, C.A., et al., A Q-methodology study of flare help-seeking behaviours and different experiences of daily life in rheumatoid arthritis. *BMC Musculoskelet Disord*, 2014. 15: 364.
43. Stack, R.J., et al., Perceptions of risk and predictive testing held by the first-degree relatives of patients with rheumatoid arthritis in England, Austria and Germany: A qualitative study. *BMJ Open*, 2016. 6(6): e010555.
44. Mosor, E., et al., SAT0719-HPR "and suddenly you are a person at risk of developing rheumatoid arthritis!" different perspectives of individuals on predictive testing – results of an international qualitative interview study. *Annals of the Rheumatic Diseases*, 2017. 76(Suppl 2): 1511.

45. Haynes, R.B., et al., Interventions for enhancing medication adherence. *The Cochrane Database of Systematic Reviews*, 2005. 2005(4): CD000011.
46. Van Den Bemt, B.J.F., H.E. Zwikker, and C.H.M. Van Den Ende, Medication adherence in patients with rheumatoid arthritis: A critical appraisal of the existing literature. *Expert Review of Clinical Immunology*, 2012. 8(4): 337–351.
47. World Health Organisation, *Adherence to Long-term Therapies: Evidence for action*. 2003, Geneva, Switzerland: World Health Organisation.
48. DiMatteo, M.R., Variations in patients' adherence to medical recommendations: A quantitative review of 50 years of research. *Medical Care*, 2004. 42(3): 200–209.
49. Curkendall, S., et al., Compliance with biologic therapies for rheumatoid arthritis: Do patient out-of-pocket payments matter? *Arthritis Care & Research*, 2008. 59(10): 1519–1526.
50. Borah, B.J., et al., Trends in RA patients' adherence to subcutaneous anti-TNF therapies and costs. *Current Medical Research and Opinion*, 2009. 25(6): 1365–1377.
51. Zink, A., et al., Treatment continuation in patients receiving biological agents or conventional DMARD therapy. *Annals of the Rheumatic Diseases*, 2005. 64(9): 1274–1279.
52. Treharne, G., A. Lyons, and G. Kitas, Medication adherence in rheumatoid arthritis: Effects of psychosocial factors. *Psychology, Health & Medicine*, 2004. 9(3): 337–349.
53. Navarro-Millan, I., et al., Perspectives of rheumatoid arthritis patients on electronic communication and patient reported outcome data collection: A qualitative study. *Arthritis Care Research (Hoboken)*, 2018.
54. Mathijssen, E.G., et al., Support needs for medication use and the suitability of eHealth technologies to address these needs: A focus group study of older patients with rheumatoid arthritis. *Patient Prefer Adherence*, 2018. 12: 349–358.
55. Macdonald, G.G., et al., Ehealth technologies, multimorbidity, and the office visit: Qualitative interview study on the perspectives of physicians and nurses. *Journal of Medical Internet Research*, 2018. 20(1): e31.
56. Walter, M.J.M., et al., Focus group interviews reveal reasons for differences in the perception of disease activity in rheumatoid arthritis. *Quality of Life Research*, 2017. 26(2): 291–298.
57. Berenbaum, F., et al., Fears and beliefs in rheumatoid arthritis and spondyloarthritis: A qualitative study. *PLoS ONE*, 2014. 9(12): e114350.
58. Man, A., et al., Development and validation of a patient-reported outcome instrument for skin involvement in patients with systemic sclerosis. *Annals of the Rheumatic Diseases*, 2017. 76(8): 1374.
59. Kottak, N., et al., An ethnographic observational study of the biologic initiation conversation between rheumatologists and biologic-naive rheumatoid arthritis patients. *Arthritis Care Research (Hoboken)*, 2018.
60. Hinojosa-Azaola, A. and J. Alcocer-Varela, Art and rheumatology: The artist and the rheumatologist's perspective. *Rheumatology (Oxford)*, 2014. 53(10): 1725–1731.
61. Tong, A., P. Sainsbury, and J. Craig, Consolidated criteria for reporting qualitative research (COREQ): A 32-item checklist for interviews and focus groups. *International Journal for Quality in Health Care*, 2007. 19(6): 349–357.

13

Challenging Assumptions about 'Normal' Development in Children's Rehabilitation: The Promise of Critical Qualitative Research

Yani Hamdani and Barbara E. Gibson

CONTENTS

Introduction to Critical Qualitative Research

Critical perspectives draw attention to the sociopolitical dimensions inherent in research and practice and share a key premise of rejecting prevailing notions of science as being 'value-free' (Eakin, Robertson, Poland, Coburn, & Edwards 1996; Green & Thorogood 2018). Rather, critical approaches seek to make social values and assumptions – whether hidden or unacknowledged – visible, particularly in research aimed at understanding and addressing social phenomena (Eakin et al. 1996; Green & Thorogood 2018; Kincheloe, McLaren & Steinberg 2011). By identifying these assumptions, we can examine how they shape the aims of rehabilitation and their effects on young disabled people when they underpin and are enacted in practice. For example, critical disability scholars argue that societies value and are structured around able bodies. Thus, people with physical, cognitive, and other impairments are construed as disabled and experience social disadvantage and marginalisation (Hammell 2006; Hughes 2009). Examining these sorts of assumptions through critical research can open up possibilities for mitigating unintended harms and rethinking the aims of rehabilitation.

Critical research traditions are explicitly political and aimed at emancipating groups by focusing on social change rather than changing individuals (Gibson & Teachman 2012). They aim to unpack the social, political, and historical conditions that contribute to establishing assumptions about 'proper' ways of being and doing for the purpose of revealing how power operates in social relations (Eakin et al. 1996; Foucault 1980; Gibson 2016; Gibson, Nicholls, Setchell & Groven 2018; Kincheloe et al. 2011). In critical research, power is understood to have many dimensions (Eakin et al. 1996; Gibson et al. 2018). For example, Lukes (1974) identifies three dimensions of power. One dimension can be described as overt, in which certain groups have social dominance or privilege over other groups (e.g., non-disabled people over disabled people, adults over children). This dominance or privilege may be inadvertent or go unrecognised. A second, more subtle dimension of power is reflected when inequities amongst groups are recognised, yet remain unresolved or unaddressed (e.g., systemic sexism or racism) (Gibson et al. 2018). A third dimension involves covert forms of power, in which particular ways of thinking about how to be or to act in society become privileged and valued over other ways of thinking. This form of power operates to produce conditions of disadvantage or marginalisation for some groups in society (Bacchi 2009, 2012; Foucault 1980; Njelesani, Teachman, Durocher, Hamdani & Phelan 2015). For example, guided by notions of normal development, rehabilitation practices that promote the transition to adulthood for young disabled people may inadvertently disadvantage some people, such as young people labelled with intellectual and developmental disabilities (IDD), who are unable to or experience challenges in achieving typical adult roles and milestones (e.g., employment, independent living, moving out of the family home).

Critical qualitative research in healthcare and rehabilitation aims to examine taken for granted assumptions, including those related to normalisation and normal development, to reveal how they shape knowledge in particular ways that become taken for granted as 'true' (Gibson 2016; Hammell 2006, 2015). By identifying and unpacking these assumptions, we can examine how they shape the aims of rehabilitation and their effects on young disabled people when enacted in practice. A critical approach proposes that notions of normal development can be questioned to reveal and mitigate any unanticipated harmful effects on young people. The idea is not to 'criticise', as in find fault in a disapproving way, but rather to engage in professional self-scrutiny that 'makes the familiar strange' or imagines possibilities for how 'things could be otherwise' (Gibson et al. 2018). In general, critical research traditions are explicitly political, aimed at emancipation, and focused on mitigating unintended harms. On this note, we now provide an empirical example involving examining assumptions about normal development in transition to adulthood policies to illustrate the contributions that critical qualitative research can make in advancing children's rehabilitation.

Problematising Policies on Transition to Adulthood: A Research Example

This study was led by the first author (Yani Hamdani) as part of her doctoral work and arose from her experiences as an occupational therapist developing and implementing transition to adulthood programs in a children's rehabilitation hospital and questioning their impact on the health and daily life circumstances of young disabled people and their families. The study design included analysis of three documents relevant to public policies on transition to adulthood and qualitative interviews with 13 parents of young people labelled with IDD. Our analysis revealed that taken for granted assumptions about normal ways of being, becoming, and conducting oneself as an adult shaped implicit understandings of the 'disabled child' as problematic and 'in need of' intervention in comparison to the 'non-disabled child'. Embedded in transition policies, these assumptions had multiple effects, both beneficial and harmful on young people labelled with IDD and their parents. The study results have implications for rethinking notions of normal development and traditional indicators of adulthood (e.g., independence, employment) as guiding principles for transition programs and for children's rehabilitation more broadly. We describe the study and provide examples from the documents and interviews to illustrate the critical approach taken in our analysis.

Background

Transition to adulthood for disabled youth has been identified as a public policy problem in many advanced democracies in recent years. In the province of Ontario, Canada, the problem is predominantly framed as a service access issue, particularly when young people 'age out' of paediatric health services by 19 years of age and public education by 21 years of age, and must transfer to adult-oriented programs and services. In response, transition policies and practices have been developed which aim to: (1) prepare youth for leaving public services funded for children, (2) prepare them for roles and activities associated with adult life, and (3) link them to adult-oriented services and supports. These policies and programs are shaped by both explicit and implicit assumptions about disability, normal development, and what constitutes a proper adulthood. Enacted in policies and practices, these assumptions can have implications for how transition to adulthood is understood as a problem and addressed in children's rehabilitation. Thus, they have consequences for young disabled people who are the target of transition interventions, as well as for their parents who provide them with care and support. For this research example, we focus on our examination of normal development in Ontario-based transition policies.

Normal development is a primary organising concept in children's rehabilitation. Based on the attainment of step-wise milestones pegged to pre-existing norms, frameworks of normal physical and cognitive development are generally accepted in public policies and practices designed to serve disabled children (Priestley 2003). For example, the idea of 'developmentally appropriate' care abounds in best practice guidelines in adolescent medicine (American Academy of Pediatrics 1996; Canadian Paediatric Society 2007; Rosen et al. 2003). The variety of checklists, frameworks, and textbooks focused on promoting and supporting normal development attests to its significance in guiding not only rehabilitation practices, but also health and social care, education, and parenting practices more broadly. Normal development is primarily understood as a relatively predictable trajectory of progressively achieved physical, intellectual, emotional, and social milestones from childhood to adulthood (Gibson, Teachman & Hamdani 2015, 2016; Hamdani, Mistry, & Gibson 2015). The goals and expected outcomes of normal development are defined by the perceived norms and competencies for adult life (Priestley 2003). Key indicators of a 'successful' adulthood include independent living, employment, financial self-reliance, and forming intimate relationships. Children are expected to progress along a normal social and developmental trajectory, to the extent possible, on the journey to adulthood. Normal development, as a concept, can be helpful in guiding rehabilitation practices for many children and youth, including children and youth labelled disabled. Yet, as we have discussed previously (Gibson, Teachman, & Hamdani 2015, 2016), when examined from a critical perspective, these practices can have some unintended harmful consequences for young people whose developmental and social trajectories differ from the norm, such as young people labelled with IDD.

Purpose and Study Aims

The purpose of the study described here was to understand how transition is *problematised* in Ontario policies and the implications for the health and daily lives of youth labelled with IDD and their parents (Hamdani 2016). By problematise, we mean examine how the issue of transition is constructed as a particular kind of problem in particular social and political contexts. In our case, the Canadian context is generally referred to as an advanced democracy or Western industrialised society (other examples include Australia, United States, or United Kingdom). The aim of this study was: (1) to identify and examine taken for granted assumptions particularly about childhood disability and normal development embedded in Ontario's transition policies and (2) to explore the effects of policies shaped by these assumptions on the parents of young people labelled with IDD. Parents were the focus of this particular study because they have advocated for and navigated policies and services on behalf of their children labelled with IDD from birth to early adulthood, thus, have first-hand experiences of the effects over the life course. In addition, family caregivers of young people with severe and complex disabilities are often largely responsible for their on-going care and support into adulthood and beyond. Research ethics approval for the study was received from the University of Toronto.

Conceptual Approach

A critical lens guided this study and is reflected in the research aims and methodologies. We also drew on critical scholarship on normal development as a lens for analysis. Critical scholars argue that developmental discourses (patterned ways of thinking) (Lupton 1992) are used to privilege and normalise particular world views about the proper outcome of development and have introduced the idea of 'developmentalism' (Burman 2012; Walkerdine 1993). Riggs (2006) describes developmentalism as the 'particular logic that surrounds dominant accounts of childhood, wherein children are presumed to follow a relatively proscribed pathway to reach maturity' (p. 58). Normal development is assumed to take a specific form, whereby children develop certain skills and attributes that assist them in becoming good, 'contributing' adult citizens (Gibson, Teachman, & Hamdani 2015, 2016). Said differently, a particular kind of adulthood is generally accepted as the right and natural goal of child development – one in which independence, productivity (mainly paid work), and contribution to society are valorised. These ideas are embedded in health, rehabilitation, and social policies focused on developing 'the child'. Whilst well-intended – developmentalism logics will necessarily aim to minimise deficits and maximise functioning in ways that reproduce ableist notions of good and poor life quality. Moreover, critical scholars argue that classic child development theory constructs children as 'incomplete adults' (Priestley 2003) or 'adults-in-the-making' (Burman 2012; Walkerdine 1993). Thus, young people who do not or cannot 'successfully' achieve particular 'adult' skills of independence remain as 'adults-in-the-making', experiencing exclusion from full citizenship and social participation in adulthood. We drew from this scholarship as a critical lens for analysing our data.

Data Sources

Three Ontario-based documents and interviews with 13 parents of young people labelled with IDD were the data sources for analysis. The documents represented policies or proposed courses of action in publicly funded rehabilitation, education, and social services relevant to transitions for young disabled people (see Table 13.1). They were chosen because they were the most influential texts in shaping policies and practices in each of the three public sectors.

Twelve mothers and one father from across the Greater Toronto Area in Ontario participated in semi-structured interviews. Their children had been diagnosed with Down syndrome, autism, intellectual disabilities, and cerebral palsy and were in the age range of 17 years old–27 years old. This was an important step, as the analysis of documents on their own would not reveal the effects of underlying assumptions about disability and transition to adulthood on young disabled people and their families who experience the policies in action. We were interested in how these assumptions were taken up, echoed, or resisted by the people experiencing the enactment of policies in their daily lives, in our case, parents of young people labelled with IDD.

TABLE 13.1

Data Sources: Documents Representing Transition Policy in Three Publicly Funded Sectors

Public Sector	Document
Rehabilitation	*'The Best Journey To Adult Life' for youth with disabilities: An evidenced-based model and best practices guidelines for the transition to adulthood* (Stewart et al. 2009)
Education	*Transition Planning: A Resource Guide* (Ontario Ministry of Education [MEDU], 2002)
Social services (specific to IDD)	*Provincial transition planning framework: Transition planning for young people with developmental disabilities* (Ministries of Community and Social Services [MCSS] and Child and Youth Services [MCYS], 2011)

Analysis Methods

The study drew on a policy analysis approach called 'What's the problem represented to be?', which emphasises problem-questioning, rather than problem-solving associated with conventional policy analysis (Bacchi 2009). It takes the position that policymaking creates particular understandings of what the problem is and what should be done about it. The aim is not to solve the issue per se, but rather to unpack underlying assumptions and consider their potential effects on the target population. In the study, we used this approach to understand how social values and assumptions about disability and child development shaped understandings of the policy issue, what counted as a successful transition to adulthood, and the potential consequences for young disabled people and their families. In doing so, we drew on critical scholarship on normal development to examine how key ideas, such as disability, adulthood, and independence, were represented and applied in the policies.

Our analyses involved interrogating the documents' texts and interview transcripts guided by a series of six interrelated questions from *Analyzing Policy: What's the problem represented to be?* (Bacchi 2009, p. xii).

1. What's the 'problem' represented to be in a specific policy?;
2. What presuppositions or assumptions underlie this representation of the 'problem'?;
3. How has this representation of the 'problem' come about?;
4. What is left unproblematic in this problem representation? Where are the silences? Can the 'problem' be thought about differently?;
5. What effects are produced by this representation of the 'problem'?; and
6. How/where has this representation of the 'problem' been produced, disseminated and defended, and how could it be questioned, disrupted, and replaced?

The analysis involved going back and forth between these questions to dig deeper – that is, to go below the surface of explicitly stated ideas to reveal implicit assumptions about disability, development, and transition to adulthood. We looked for key concepts, binaries (e.g., normality/disability), and categories (e.g., childhood, adulthood) as analytic devices for unpacking both explicit and implicit meanings that shaped how the issue of transition was constituted as a problem. This involved an iterative process of analysis, including writing analytic summaries and reflexive memos, discussing them in PhD committee meetings, iteratively engaging with the data and critical scholarship on disability and development, and documenting decisions in order to support a transparent and rigorous analysis. These methods allowed for an examination of what assumptions about disability and normal development were contained within transition policies and to explore their intended and unintended consequences for young people labelled with IDD and thus their parents.

Results

Documents

'Normal' Ways of Being and Becoming an Adult

Across the documents, the transfer from child- to adult-oriented services was explicitly identified as problematic. Yet, our analysis revealed underlying assumptions about 'normal' ways of being and becoming an adult. These assumptions shaped implicit understandings of what was held problematic, largely focused on social expectations to become as independent and productive as possible in adult life. All of the documents focused specifically on disabled youth, implying that their transitions to adult life were problematic in some way compared to another group – presumably *non-disabled* youth. Disabled youth were targeted for intervention when they reached an arbitrarily determined age when they were no longer eligible for child-mandated (up to 18 years old–21 years old) health, education, and social services. For example, the rehabilitation document stated that it addressed the 'transition to adulthood across the continuum of rehabilitation services' (Stewart et al. 2009 p. 6). Similarly, the social services document addressed the issue of 'lack of planning and inadequate transition support' specifically for young people labelled with IDD and aimed to foster a 'smooth transfer to adult services and a good transition experience' (Ministry of Community and Social Services & Ministry of Child and Youth Services 2011, p. 3). The explicitly stated purpose of the education document was 'to facilitate transition planning from school to work, further education and community living for exceptional students' (Ministry of Education 2002, p. 3), meaning students with disabilities. Interestingly, gifted students also fell under the category of 'exceptional students', but were not required to have a transition plan. On the surface, the problem was construed as a service transfer issue in the documents. However, digging below the surface of these texts revealed implicit assumptions about proper and socially expected ways of being, becoming, and conducting oneself as an adult.

The problem of service transfer rested on an inherently understood problem in which the social and developmental trajectories of young disabled people were judged inadequate or at risk of failure because they deviated from some preconceived norms. For example, the education document stated:

> (A)lmost all students will need or wish to engage in productive employment, supportive employment, or meaningful volunteer work (*MEDU* 2002, p. 20).

Suggested transition goals included:

> (I)ndependent living in the community and daily living skills for independence (*MEDU* 2002, p. 21, 24 & 27).

These statements suggested the relative importance and value placed on particular traits and activities in adulthood, that is, productivity (mainly work) and independence, which all students are expected to achieve or at least approximate. Similarly, the social services document, which focused specifically on young people with IDD, stated that transition planning should:

> ...help the young person prepare for adulthood and to plan for adult services in a manner that promotes social inclusion, greater self-reliance and as independent a life as possible (*MCSS & MCYS* 2011, p. 9).

The terms 'self-reliance' and 'independent' are not explicitly described in the document, rather the importance and value in achieving them were assumed and unquestioned. Thus, taken for granted assumptions about normal indicators of a successful adulthood, largely centred around achieving independence in employment and daily living, were embedded in the documents. An emphasis on achieving independence to the extent possible reflects its high social value as an adult trait, implying that dependence is acceptable in childhood, but less desirable and to be avoided in adulthood. Collectively, assumptions about normal ways of being and becoming an adult in the documents functioned to represent young disabled people as 'in need of intervention' because of their risk of dependency on others in adult life. The rehabilitation document differed somewhat from the other two in that it did not promote the achievement of typical or 'normal' adult roles and activities, but instead worked to reframe notions of 'active citizenship':

> (T)he goal of transition should not be focused on a series of outcomes such as employment, independent living and hobbies; but rather, active citizenship and involvement in meaningful occupations. (Stewart et al. 2009, p. 20)

Active citizenship as a goal is a rather unique idea in healthcare and rehabilitation and is interesting to consider for supporting social participation of young disabled people. However, what is meant by 'active' is not explicitly described in the document, thus is left open to interpretation. The descriptor 'active' suggests that a particular type of citizen is socially valued and preferred compared to, for example, an 'inactive' or 'passive' citizen. Thus, the idea of active citizenship potentially carries with it expectations for participation or contribution in particular ways, but if or how this would differ from more traditional roles of independence and paid work is unclear.

Parent Accounts

Pursuing 'Normal' Adulthood to the Extent Possible

For the most part, parents reproduced ideas reflected in the documents about achieving or approximating as close to a 'normal' developmental trajectory to adulthood as possible for their children. What was interesting was the multiple and creative ways they reformulated the meaning of independence to reflect their child's and family's circumstances. For example, Jane (all names are pseudonyms) stated that:

> 'It's kind of ironic, but for Joy (her 24-year-old daughter labelled with Down syndrome) to become more independent as she gets older, she is also going to have to become more co-dependent with other people.'

Similarly, Daniel discussed how he envisioned a '...supported life independent *of* us. We'd still be part of it...' for his daughter (25 years old, labelled with intellectual disability).

These accounts reflect a view of independence that was not about their daughters doing things for themselves. Rather, it was about shifting their dependence to other people and supports, and in doing so, approximating an imagined 'typical' relationship between parents and their adult children. Yet, the parents still recognised dominant social expectations and value placed on independence in adult life, including approximating independence in daily life management and decision-making. Thus, similar to the documents, the parents' accounts reflected prevailing social values and expectations about an independent adulthood in Western societies.

The parents also reproduced ideas about the ideal outcomes for adult life following high school. For example, Evelyn, a mother, described:

> It's always the same route. You graduate from high school and you continue on with education in school to have some training in order to position yourself in society.

Her comment revealed an inherent assumption that the 'same route' or trajectory from school to further education and eventual employment was expected. Moreover, her comments suggested that it was important to pursue this path to establish oneself financially and socially in adult life. She did not question or consider if another route might be more realistic, feasible, or better for her daughter (who was 27 years old and labelled with intellectual disability). Rather, her account reflected that she had internalised social values and beliefs about a productive, independent adulthood, which shaped her transition planning goals towards these ends.

The parents also shed light on some of the effects of the challenges they experienced in planning for their children's transition to adult life. For example, Linda (whose son was 19 years old and on the autism spectrum) stated:

> We do need transitions [planning & support]... As parents, at the time when you're most tired, everything stops. Special Services at Home[1] gets yanked, if you're lucky enough to get it now at 18, and school stops. You just enter a wasteland, at the time that you need the supports most, psychologically.

In this excerpt, Linda describes the significant fatigue, uncertainty, and distress she experienced even with transition planning and supports, which reflected the parents' accounts as a whole. They also discussed other consequences for their lives, such as deferring their own employment, future retirement, and social time with their own friends in order to support their adult children – consequences that were not accounted for in the transition documents. In addition, both young disabled people and their parents experienced social disadvantages and exclusion from mainstream social life – young disabled people because they failed to achieve developmental markers that afford access to the social roles and activities that signify adult status, and parents because they were expected to fulfil their social responsibilities of providing care and support for children until these markers were achieved, even if their achievement was challenging or not possible.

[1] Special Services at Home is a program publicly funded and managed by MCSS in Ontario, which helps families who provide care for a child identified as having developmental and/or physical disabilities to pay for special services (e.g., skill development programs, respite services) at home or in the community.

Summary

Our analysis revealed that underlying the explicitly identified problem of *transition to adulthood* was an implied problem of *disabled children being at risk of dependency and a non-productive adulthood.* Taken for granted assumptions about normal development – that is, normal or socially preferred ways of being, becoming, and conducting one's self as an adult – shaped an implicitly understood problem represented as the 'disabled child'. Represented in this way, disabled children were identified as being 'in need of' normalisation and intervention compared to non-disabled children because they were at risk of failing to achieve a typical social and developmental trajectory from childhood to adulthood. In other words, they were at risk of being dependent on others for financial and personal care and support in adult life. These outcomes were to be minimised or avoided to the extent possible.

Taken for granted assumptions about normal development functioned to create a social hierarchy in which particular ways of being and doing were privileged and preferred over less desired ways. Embedded in transition policies and reproduced in parent accounts, these assumptions had multiple effects. Some are generally considered beneficial effects for young disabled people, such as feelings of success for working towards or achieving traditional transition goals, even if modified. Yet, they also had unanticipated harmful effects for some people. For example, both young people labelled with IDD and their parents experienced marginalisation and exclusion from mainstream community life (e.g., employment, social opportunities). Parents also experienced stress and fatigue whilst spending countless time and effort to pursue and support transition goals, such as post-secondary education, employment training, or skills for independence, for their children. Shedding light on these types of harms, which were not addressed in the transition policies in any substantial way, offers opportunities to rethink the aims of transition interventions in children's rehabilitation.

Implications for Children's Rehabilitation

Our critical research example highlights several implications for policies and practices related to transition to adulthood, and to children's rehabilitation more broadly. First and foremost, it illuminates the need for a critical rethink of the emphasis on 'normal' – normal bodies, normal development – towards embracing diverse ways of being, becoming, and doing for young disabled people. For example, transition policies may unintentionally de-emphasise other possible, atypical ways of living a good life as an adult that may actually be healthier, or more feasible, desirable, or suited to the life circumstances of young disabled people and their parents. More emphasis can be placed on making and maintaining friendships or engaging in social and recreation activities as valuable goals in their own right, rather than pursuing independence and employment as the main or only goals. Moreover, rehabilitation programs can direct attention to fostering positive disability identities and drawing on strength-based rather than deficit-focused approaches in interventions. Shifts in thinking about 'normality' as the guidepost for disability, development, and transition to adulthood are beginning to emerge, particularly in the field of childhood disability and rehabilitation (Gibson et al. 2016; Gibson & Teachman 2012; Gibson, Teachman & Hamdani 2015, 2016; Gibson et al. 2012; Hamdani, Mistry, & Gibson 2015;

Njelesani et al. 2015; Phelan 2011; Phelan & Ng 2015). Such approaches would support young disabled people to create and lead lives that are relevant to their own desires, goals, and life circumstances.

As a point of clarification, we are not suggesting that conventional rehabilitation approaches focused on addressing impairments and developmental deficits are unimportant or unnecessary or that pursuing traditional indicators of adulthood be abandoned or avoided. Rather, we suggest that a variety of traditional and alternative options for living a good life can be discussed, supported, and given equal attention and consideration in rehabilitation encounters, including sensitive discussions with young disabled people and their families about the potential beneficial and harmful consequences of any option. At a minimum, young disabled people and their families should be exposed to a number of ways for living a good life into adulthood and be given opportunities to evaluate the goals and options that make sense for their life circumstances.

Adopting a life course view in children's rehabilitation can highlight social understandings of what roles and responsibilities are expected at different ages and life stages and how they contribute to shaping understandings of disability (Priestley 2003). As we have shown, adults are expected to develop traits of independence for fulfilling roles and responsibilities associated with employment and daily life management in Western societies. In contrast, it is acceptable for children to be dependent on their parents until they develop skills and competencies to fulfil these roles and responsibilities themselves. Thus, socially accepted roles and responsibilities at different life stages shape how generational categories, such as childhood and adulthood, are characterised and understood in relation to one another (Priestley 2003). Childhood, adolescence, and adulthood are important concepts in themselves and form a social stratification system based on generational relationships, much like gender or class relationships (Priestley 2003). They are imbued with cultural meaning and structure in relation to one another that can be examined and connected to understandings of disability and normal development. Adolescence is considered a critical transitional period between dependency in childhood and independence along the road to adulthood (Holmbeck 2002). Several key developmental tasks are associated with adolescence, including identity formation, emotional development, formation of intimate relationships, cognitive development, and accomplishment of formal education goals, community inclusion, and independent living goals (Wood, Reiss, Ferris, Edwards, & Merrick 2010).

Young disabled people are expected to know about their diagnoses, medical conditions, medications, and equipment; to develop skills to self-manage their health and daily lives; and to become proficient in accessing health and social services. The expectation is that by achieving these 'developmental tasks', young disabled people will be prepared for adult life. 'Successful' childhood is thus understood and promoted as progressive movement from complete physical and social dependence to the highest possible level of independence. It is implicitly understood that dependency in adulthood is to be avoided to the extent possible. This pervasive assumption grounded in notions of normal development shapes the aims of children's rehabilitation, social care, and education, and powerfully influences how disabled young people understand themselves and their place in the world.

Rethinking childhood disability and development in children's rehabilitation can also account more strongly for the entwined life course trajectories of young disabled people and their families. Beyond embracing a variety of trajectories for young people themselves, greater emphasis can be placed on the life course trajectories of their parents, and other important people in their lives (e.g., siblings, extended family members, paid and unpaid caregivers).

Parents are expected to take on extraordinary roles and extended responsibilities to foster as close to a normal life course trajectory as possible for their children, particularly children labelled with IDD, yet their own trajectories are neglected or ignored in public policies and practices. A way forward involves thinking about interconnected life course trajectories of families. Such a perspective would include considering the significant unpaid work conducted daily by parents whose children rely on them for personal care and support into adulthood, and also in creating and implementing transition plans. Moreover, this lens can draw attention to the ways in which the life trajectories of these parents follow different paths than parents of non-disabled children when it comes to providing ongoing and necessary personal and financial support into adulthood and beyond.

Promise of and Future Directions in Critical Qualitative Research

Critical research holds promise for revealing and addressing taken for granted assumptions, logics, and principles that drive practices and structure programs in children's rehabilitation, which other approaches often miss, ignore, or fail to acknowledge. Research in this vein has the potential to disrupt and challenge ingrained ways of understanding and addressing childhood disability and normal development towards creative approaches that acknowledge the diverse needs and circumstances of children and families. Future research can examine what constitutes a successful outcome for young people who do not follow a typical social and developmental trajectory. For example, what would a successful transition to adulthood look like if an array of ways of being, becoming, and doing over the life course were valued, rather than ways associated with the milestones and markers of normal development? This research can explore alternative options for living a good life in adulthood, which can inform changes to the aims of transition policies and practices, whilst also considering parents and families who are often involved in supporting these options beyond the time point in which young disabled people are no longer eligible for children's health, education, and social services.

Further work can be informed by a disabled children's childhood studies approach to inquiry. The main premise of this approach is that disabled children and their childhoods should be valued in their own right – not in comparison to other groups and social categories (Curran & Runswick-Cole 2014). Moreover, this approach explicitly addresses the experiences of disabled children in the contexts of both the Global North and Global South, with the former generally associated with wealthy, Western industrialised societies (Curran & Runswick-Cole 2014). In addition, a disabled children's childhood studies approach begins with the concerns and perspectives of young disabled people, and their families and allies, rather than researchers, policymakers, and service providers. Adopting this approach in future research, coupled with theorising disabled children's life course trajectories in their own right rather than in comparison to normal developmental and social trajectories, can inform new ways of understanding life stages and moving across them as a young disabled person. In addition, further research that compares how life course trajectories of disabled children are thought about in the Global South compared to the Global North can shed new light on the social values and assumptions about childhood, disability, and development embedded in different social, political, and cultural contexts, and open possibilities for rendering them changeable.

Conclusion

In this chapter, we have made a case for the value of critical qualitative rehabilitation research. Using the example of transitions policy for young people with IDD, we have outlined the potential contributions of a critical approach to knowledge generation in children's rehabilitation. Critical approaches identify the taken for granted assumptions that structure and guide actions, including policies, practices, research, and teaching, to reveal unintended and sometimes harmful effects on the groups they aim to serve and help. In children's rehabilitation, the most pervasive and deeply ingrained assumptions are related to how childhood disability and development are understood as problems that need to be fixed and addressed through policies, programs, and practices of normalisation. Understanding rehabilitation as a social process with consequences beyond its intended goals requires different kinds of methodologies that do not assume in advance what counts as a good or poor outcome. The inherent promise of critical qualitative research is to open possibilities for supporting multiple ways for young disabled people and their families to live healthy and well over the life course.

References

American Academy of Pediatrics Committee on Children With Disabilities and Committee on Adolescence. (1996). Transition of care provided for adolescents with special health care needs. *Pediatrics, 98*, 1203–1206.

Bacchi, C. (2009). *Analysing Policy: What's the Problem Represented to Be?* Frenchs Forest, N.S.W: Pearson Education.

Bacchi, C. (2012). Why study problematizations? Making politics visible. *Open Journal of Political Science, 2*(1), 1–8.

Burman, E. (2012). Deconstructing neoliberal childhood: Towards a feminist antipsychological approach. *Childhood, 19*(4), 423–438.

Canadian Paediatric Society. (2007). Care of adolescents with chronic conditions (position statement AH 2007-01). *Paediatric Child Health, 12*(9), 785–788.

Curran, T., & Runswick-Cole, K. (2014). Disabled children's childhood studies: A distinct approach? *Disability and Society, 29*(10), 1617–1630.

Eakin, J., Robertson, A., Poland, B., Coburn, D., & Edwards, R. (1996). Towards a critical social science perspective on health promotion research. *Health Promotion International, 11*(2), 157–165.

Foucault, M. (1980). *Power/knowledge*. New York: Pantheon Books.

Gibson, B. E., & Teachman, G. (2012). Critical approaches in physical therapy research: Investigating the symbolic value of walking. *Physiotherapy Theory and Practice, 28*(6), 474–484.

Gibson, B. E., Teachman, G., & Hamdani, Y. (2015). Rethinking 'normal development' in children's rehabilitation. In K. McPherson, B. E. Gibson & A. Leplège (Eds.), *Rethinking Rehabilitation: Theory and Practice* (pp. 69–79). Boca Raton, FL: Taylor & Francis Group.

Gibson, B. E., Teachman, G., Wright, V., Fehlings, D., Young, N. L., & McKeever, P. (2012). Children's and parents' beliefs regarding the value of walking: Rehabilitation implications for children with cerebral palsy. *Child: Care, Health and Development, 38*, 61–69.

Gibson, B. E., Nicholls, D., Setchell J., & Groven, K. (2018). Introduction. In B. E. Gibson, D. Nicholls, J. Setchell, & K. Groven (Eds.), *Manipulating Practices*. Oslo, Norway: Cappelen Damm Akademisk.

Gibson, BE. (2016) *Rehabilitation: A Post-Critical Approach*. Boca Raton, FL: CRC Press.

Green, J., & Thorogood, N. (2018). *Qualitative Methods for Health Research* (4th ed.). Thousand Oaks, CA: Sage.

Hamdani Y. (2016). "Problematizing transition to adulthood for young disabled people." Doctoral dissertation, University of Toronto. Available from http://hdl.handle.net/1807/76453 (Accessed 6 February 2019).

Hamdani, Y., Mistry, B., & Gibson, B. E. (2015). Transitioning to adulthood with a progressive condition: Best practice assumptions and individual experiences of young men with DMD. *Disability and Rehabilitation, 37*(13), 1144–1151.

Hammell, K. W. (2006). *Perspectives on Disability and Rehabilitation: Contesting Assumptions Challenging Practice*. Philadelphia, PA: Elsevier.

Hammell, K. W. (2015). Rethinking rehabilitation's assumptions: Challenging 'thinking-as-usual' and envisioning a relevant future in children's rehabilitation. In K. McPherson, B. E. Gibson, & A. Leplège (Eds.), *Rethinking Rehabilitation: Theory and Practice* (pp. 45–67). Boca Raton, FL: Taylor & Francis Group.

Holmbeck, G. N. (2002). A developmental perspective on adolescent health and illness: An introduction to the special issues. *Journal of Pediatric Psychology, 27*(5), 409–416.

Hughes, B. (2009). Disability activisms: Social model stalwarts and biological citizens. *Disability & Society, 24*(6), 677–688.

Kincheloe, J. L., McLaren, P., & Steinberg, S. R. (2011). Critical pedagogy and qualitative research. In N. K. Denzin & Y. S. Lincoln (Eds.), *The Sage Handbook of Qualitative Research* (pp. 163–177). Thousand Oaks, CA: Sage.

Lukes, S. (1974) *Power: A Radical View*. London, UK: Macmillan.

Lupton, D. (1992). Discourse analysis – a new methodology for understanding the ideologies of health and illness. *Australian Journal of Public Health, 16*(2), 145–150.

Njelesani, J., Teachman, G., Durocher, E., Hamdani, Y., & Phelan, S. K. (2015). Thinking critically about client-centred practice and occupational possibilities across the life-span. *Scandinavian Journal of Occupational Therapy, 22*(4), 252–259.

Ontario Ministry of Community and Social Services (MCSS) & Ministry of Child and Youth Services (MCYS). (2011). Provincial transition planning framework: Transition planning for young people with developmental disabilities. Retrieved from www.opsba.org (Accessed 22 June 2018).

Ontario Ministry of Education (MEDU). (2002). Transition planning: A resource guide. Retrieved from http://www.edu.gov.on.ca/eng/general/elemsec/speced/guide/specedpartae.pdf (Accessed 22 June 2018).

Phelan, S. K., & Ng, S. N. (2015) A case review: Reframing school-based practices using a critical perspective. *Physical & Occupational Therapy in Pediatrics, 35*:4, 396–411, doi:10.3109/01942638.2014.978933.

Phelan, S. K. (2011). Constructions of disability: A call for critical reflexivity in occupational therapy. *Canadian Journal of Occupational Therapy, 78*(3), 164–172.

Priestley, M. (2003). *Disability: A Life Course Approach*. Malden, MA: Polity.

Riggs, D. W. (2006). Developmentalism and the rhetoric of best interests of the child: Challenging heteronormative constructions of families and parenting in foster care. *Journal of GLBT Family Studies, 2*(2), 57–73.

Rosen, D. S., Blum, R. W., Britto, M., Sawyer, S. M., Siegel, D. M., & Society for Adolescent Medicine. (2003). Transition to adult health care for adolescents and young adults with chronic conditions: Position paper of the society for adolescent medicine. *Journal of Adolescent Health, 33*(4), 309–311.

Stewart, D., Freeman, M., Law, M., Healy, H., Burke-Gaffney, J., Forhan, M., et al. (2009). *'The Best Journey To Adult Life' for Youth with Disabilities: An Evidenced-Based Model and Best Practices Guidelines for the Transition to Adulthood*. Hamilton, ON: CanChild Centre for Childhood Disability Research, McMaster University.

Walkerdine, V. (1993). Beyond developmentalism? *Theory & Psychology, 3*(4), 451–469.

Wood, D., Reiss, J. G., Ferris, M., Edwards, L. R., & Merrick, J. (2010). Transition from pediatric to adult care. *International Journal of Child and Adolescent Health, 3*(4), 445–447.

14

Bringing Qualitative Research into Rehabilitation – A Worked Example of Developing a Rehabilitation Program for Patients with Fibromyalgia

Anne Marit Mengshoel and Merja Sallinen

CONTENTS

Introduction

Fibromyalgia (FM) is a chronic musculoskeletal pain condition with no known cure. Present clinical guidelines are based on effect studies showing limited effects, and the guidelines have not taken into account whether such programmes are found meaningful to patients. Qualitative studies describe how complex and challenging it is for a patient to live with FM, but suggest that patients can overcome it and even become symptom-free again. The gap between quantitative and qualitative evidence was the reason the present authors initiated a project to develop a new rehabilitation programme for patients with FM.

The programme was developed in collaboration with a multidisciplinary team with clinical experiences in delivering group-based educational programmes for patients with inflammatory or degenerative musculoskeletal diseases, as well as FM. In the present chapter, we explore our joint efforts in reading and discussing qualitative studies to develop the new rehabilitation programme. To develop a logical interconnected programme, we had to unpack and reflect on the various knowledges underpinning our understandings. First, we briefly describe some of the discourses embedded in rehabilitation that came into play during our work, followed by a short review of the evidence about the FM condition and patients' experiences. We conclude by describing our working process, dilemmas in clinical practice, and how a logical, interconnected programme was reached.

Discourses Framing the Clinicians' Rehabilitation Context

According to Wade and de Jong (2000), rehabilitation aims to help patients with functional restrictions acquire knowledge and skills to maximise their participation in social settings, minimise pain, and relieve distress experienced by the patient, family, and caregivers. However, rehabilitation is a hybrid discipline with theoretical roots in the disciplines of the various health professionals engaged in the field, as such, it lacks a unique and unified theory detailing the parameters of rehabilitation practice (Siegert et al. 2005). Furthermore, perhaps more than in any other area of medicine and healthcare, rehabilitation practice is highly influenced by societal views on disability and disabled people, as well as people's general expectations regarding getting appropriate and effective help from health services when needed. Rehabilitation practice is also highly framed by health politics and economics, which determine what is possible to deliver. Hence, health professionals have to take into consideration several discourses beyond their professional knowledge. In addition, there are discourses embedded in clinical practice that determine what the best clinical practice is and how it should be delivered. In the process of developing the rehabilitation programme, the clinicians frequently referenced discourses from evidence-based practice (EBP) and patient-centredness.

EBP is broadly embraced by health professionals, also within the field of rehabilitation (Dijkers et al. 2012). The idea behind EBP is that practice should be informed by the best evidence from research (Jacobson et al. 1997). The scientific studies included in the EBP model mainly address issues around a disease or illness condition and how a condition should be treated (Greenhalgh 2014). In other words, EBP relies on condition-oriented evidence. Somatic conditions are often described in terms of typical symptoms, biological dysfunctions or deficits related to cause(s), manifestations of a disease, and typical functional limitations considered to be consequences of a disease (Hofmann 2001; Wulff et al. 1999). Therapies are tailored to these deviations in order to normalise them, and effects of therapies are determined by assessing if the therapies lead to less typical condition-related deficits and consequences (van Riel and Fransen 2005). Evidence from randomised clinical trials is considered to be the most reliable design for determining the most effective and appropriate therapy (Anjum et al. 2015). In order to ensure that the effects are likely to happen across individuals and contexts, personal and contextual factors are controlled for in the design (Kerry 2017). Thus, the assumption underpinning condition-specific knowledge is that people with the same diagnosis – regardless of who they are, the contexts in which they are living, and who is delivering the programme – can successfully be treated by similar therapies.

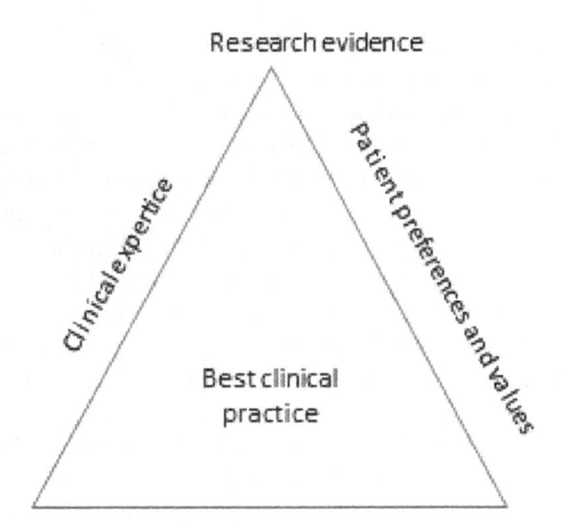

FIGURE 14.1
Evidence-based practice means to integrate a patient's and clinicians' expertise with the best available research evidence.

Another central discourse within rehabilitation referred to by the health professionals who participated in this project was person- or patient-centred practice (Gluyas 2015; Sacristan 2013). Central to patient-centred practice is the idea that patients are regarded as autonomous people who have the right to be heard and actively involved in decisions concerning their life and rehabilitation needs (Gluyas 2015). Further, the patients should be treated with respect by health professionals and a paternalistic attitude should be avoided (Gluyas 2015; Sacristan 2013). In this context, health professionals are expected to clarify a patient's concerns and beliefs, inform them about treatment options, and empower the patient to make decisions, set their own attainable goals, and engage in actions to reach those goals. This approach recommends that clinicians include goal-setting, motivational techniques, and appropriate ways of communicating in their care provision (Gluyas 2015). The person-centred practice focuses on the individual patient's wishes and needs, but is considered to be an integrated part of EBP (Sackett et al. 2007), as illustrated in Figure 14.1.

A Brief Review of Condition-Oriented Evidence on Fibromyalgia

FM is a common disorder with a prevalence estimated to be about 3% to 5% in the general population (Queiroz 2013). FM is a persistent widespread musculoskeletal pain condition accompanied by an array of other symptoms such as fatigue, sleep disturbances, memory problems, irritable bowel, low activity tolerance, and several complaints related to the autonomous system (Choy 2015). Psychological changes are also reported: depression, illness worries, anxiety, inadequate coping skills and psychosocial distress (Anderberg et al. 2000; Ercolani et al. 1994; Gupta et al. 2007; Kurtze et al. 1999; Turk et al. 1996). Typical consequences related to FM are impaired daily functioning and difficulties fulfilling social obligations and continuing to work (Liedberg and Henriksson 2002; Sallinen et al. 2010).

The aetiology of FM is unknown, but stress has been suggested as a plausible triggering factor, as high or longstanding exposure to mental or physical distress has been observed in the period before the onset of FM (Wallace and Wallace 2014). Stress also seems to aggravate symptoms (Yunus 1994). The pathogenesis of FM is explained by hypersensitivity within the central nervous system (Ang and Wilke 1999; McVeigh et al. 2003; Winfield 1999). This means that pain may result from both an amplification of normally pain-free sensory stimuli or the prolongation of normally painful stimuli. An explanation of several other symptoms is related to hyporesponsiveness within the hypothalamic-pituitary-adrenal axis (Crofford et al. 1994; Griep et al. 1993), indicating the existence of inappropriate responses to stressors (Neeck and Riedel 1994). Thus, it has been suggested that biological responses to long-term 'fight and flight' arousal from stress may exhaust systems (Coopens et al. 2018; Van Houdenhove et al. 2005).

Although FM is explained by biological deviations, these cannot be verified by conventional clinical examinations such as blood tests and radiological assessments. Persons with FM do not look sick, and therefore FM is invisible both from 'the inside' and 'the outside'. Health professionals and other people in society may think that patients with FM are malingerers or hypochondriacs, and the symptoms are considered to be imagined or of a psychological nature (Mengshoel et al. 2017). Accordingly, the use of a diagnosis is questioned, and some argue that labelling the suffering with a diagnosis hinders recovery (Hadler 1996).

Systematic reviews of effect studies have been conducted in order to illuminate the best treatment approach for patients with FM. Based on these reviews, evidence-based clinical guidelines for FM have been developed that recommend the use of tricyclic antidepressive drugs, cognitive behavioural therapy, exercise programmes, and patient education (Brosseau et al. 2008a, 2008b; Carville et al. 2008). However, a meta-analysis showed that antidepressant drugs had minor clinical improvement in pain reduction (Üòeyler et al. 2008). The authors expressed concerns as to whether the benefits were big enough, considering the potential side effects from long-term use. Several systematic reviews have concluded that exercise is an important form of therapy for patients with FM (Bidonde et al. 2014; Busch et al. 2002; Jones et al. 2006; Macfarlane et al. 2017; Sim and Adams 2002). Like drugs, strengthening or conditioning exercise programmes lead to some, but not lasting, symptom relief. Exercise leads to improved physical functioning, and an umbrella systematic review noted that physical activity at a moderate intensity level has no adverse effects (Bidonde et al. 2014). However, it should be noted that exercise must be performed on a regular basis to maintain its benefits.

Education programmes have been developed to help patients manage FM symptoms through learning about the condition and practicing appropriate coping skills. The content of these programmes varies, but in general they include lectures on pain mechanisms, encouragement to exercise regularly, and education in pain-management techniques including relaxation and adjusting daily activities to avoid overstrain (Goldenberg 2008; Mannerkorpi and Henriksson 2007; Mengshoel et al. 1995). Attempts may also be made to modify negative feelings, based on the assumption that negative thoughts and certain behaviours can maintain or aggravate suffering (Burchardt 2002). Patient education programmes overlap to some extent with cognitive behavioural therapy (CBT). CBT is a psychological approach based on a theory that a person's beliefs, attitudes, and behaviours play a central role in determining a patient's experience of suffering. The aim is therefore to change cognition and behaviour inspired by classical and operant learning theories (Davidson 2008). Systematic reviews have shown that patient education and CBT lead to clinically relevant improvements in pain, disability, and mood, but the effect sizes are not large, and the effects often do not last (Bernardy et al. 2013; van Koulil et al. 2007). The limited effects of recommended therapies imply a need for developing new rehabilitation programmes.

A Brief Review of Person-Oriented Evidence on Fibromyalgia

Several qualitative studies have been conducted to explore what it is like to live with FM. Bodily sensations of pain and fatigue are experienced as diffuse, with varying degrees of severity (Cunningham and Jillings 2006; Hellström et al. 1999; Råheim and Håland 2006). Many factors can trigger symptoms, but these may vary for no apparent reason (Sim and Madden 2008). This means that patients find their bodies unreliable (Råheim and Håland 2006; Söderberg et al. 2002), and they carefully monitor their activities to avoid 'overdoing it' (Cunningham and Jillings 2006; Mannerkorpi et al. 1999). Accordingly, both the fear of pain and the pain itself may disturb everyday habits and routines (Richardson et al. 2008). Daily life can be perceived as chaotic and beyond a person's own control (Grape et al. 2017), as activities are planned in accordance with day-to-day symptom levels and are halted if these become worse (McMahon et al. 2012; Richardson et al. 2008). In this way, everyday life becomes ruled by incomprehensible bodily sensations (Åsbring and Närvänen 2004; Richardson et al. 2008; Schoofs et al. 2004). This can lead to grief over undone tasks and unfulfilled social obligations, and patients can be forced to delegate responsibilities to other people, as such, a patient's identity, social roles, and relationships are compromised (Richardson 2005). Patients also experience health professionals and others as questioning the 'realness' of their symptoms (Briones-Vozmediano et al. 2013; Dennis et al. 2013; Mengshoel and Heggen 2004), and they sometimes feel that their credibility and dignity are threatened (Åsbring and Närvänen 2002; Sallinen et al. 2011). Thus, patients with FM have to face both the burdens of living with an inexplicable and disruptive illness and being disrespected by other people (Juuso et al. 2014).

It is often years before a diagnosis of FM is arrived at (Choy et al. 2010). During this process, the patients consult various medical specialists in order to rule out serious illnesses (Mengshoel et al. 2017). Immediate relief is experienced by patients when getting a FM diagnosis, as it means they are not suffering from any fatal or crippling disease (Madden and Sim 2006; Mengshoel and Heggen 2004; Undeland and Malterud 2002). However, the relief wanes over time when patients discover that the diagnosis neither validates their sickness nor is accompanied with effective therapy (Madden and Sim 2016). Patients often try several therapies without success, and when they do not become better, they often find that health professionals give up on them, perhaps thinking they are not doing their best to recover (Mengshoel et al. 2017). At this stage, patients are often told that they must accept the situation and learn to live with it, but the diagnosis provides little explanation of how to understand and live with FM (McMahon et al. 2012; Undeland and Malterud 2007). Often, patients are told to 'listen to their body signals' in order to learn what they can and cannot do. However, what is tolerable one day can be impossible the following day (Richardson et al. 2006). Thus, the body does not necessarily provide any definitive answer about how to adjust a life to an illness.

In acute pain conditions, pain is often related to injurious bodily incidents. This interpretation could also apply to incidents of pain aggravation in chronic pain conditions. In contrast, patients who have recovered from FM understand symptom aggravation as the body's way of warning them about too much mental and physical strain over time (Mengshoel and Heggen 2004). This meaning was used by the patients as a guide to figure out what had to be done to achieve a less stressful life. New episodes of pain, after a patient had become healthy again, were even reversed by a temporary down-regulation of daily life (Mengshoel and Heggen 2004). Other researchers who have interviewed patients who have recovered from FM also find that symptoms are used as a resource for remaking a daily life they can tolerate (Grape et al. 2015; Sallinen et al. 2012; Wentz et al. 2012). In this process, symptoms gradually disappear (Grape et al. 2017). This suggests that life stress can be heightened by uncertainty related to the diagnostic process, the ambiguous meaning of the diagnosis, the lack of efficient therapies, and degrading attitudes from health professionals and other people. Of course, it is also stressful to live with an unmanageable illness that disrupts daily life, social identity, and roles. Accordingly, making sense of the illness situation and adjusting one's life situation accordingly can be important ingredients for modulating stress.

Summing up the evidence, low effects of pharmacological and non-pharmacological therapies for FM have been demonstrated by the condition-oriented evidence, implying that the development of new rehabilitation programmes for these patients is needed. Both quantitative and qualitative studies show, in various ways, the complexity of symptoms and their personal and social consequences – life stress, too, may play a role, for example, in perpetuating symptoms. Few studies address patients' recovery experiences, but evidence from qualitative studies brings hope that patients can overcome FM. We therefore wanted to incorporate this knowledge into the process of developing a new rehabilitation programme. In the following section, we describe our working process.

The Working Process of Developing a New Rehabilitation Programme

The Context and Participants

The project was undertaken at the Lillehammer Hospital of Rheumatic Diseases in Norway. This is a specialised hospital delivering medical diagnostics and therapies to patients with chronic musculoskeletal disorders, as well as multidisciplinary rehabilitation programmes for in- and outpatients. Over the years, the staff has been involved in several research projects, and the hospital has a culture that encourages continuous debates amongst the staff aimed at improving practice. Their rehabilitation programme for patients with FM followed the clinical evidence-based guidelines and included a combination of patient education, CBT, and conditioning exercise. A multidisciplinary team of 12 health professionals to 14 health professionals participated in the present project. The team was comprised of nurses, occupational therapists, physicians, physiotherapists, social workers, a psychologist, and a dietician. Most of the team members had worked for many years in rehabilitation for patients with musculoskeletal disorders. Several had further education, e.g., in counselling, and all were recognised within their professions for their competency. The head of the unit – an occupational therapist – strongly supported the developmental process and attended all of the workshops. The clinicians' reasons for participating were varied from professional curiosity and a wish to do better, to become stronger to resist external threats of future official limitations in funding the programme.

The developmental process was led by researchers (the authors) from the University of Oslo. We had prior clinical experiences in delivering rehabilitation within mental health, primary healthcare, and rheumatology as physiotherapists, and we had participated in research projects that lay broadly within the field of rehabilitation, but with a special focus on FM. The development of the rehabilitation programme was funded by the Norwegian Foundation for Health and Rehabilitation (no. 2017/HE2-184218) and approved by the Norwegian Data Inspectorate for Research (no. 2018/57956/3/EPA).

The Researchers' Pre-understandings

The project leader (AMM) holds a part-time position at the hospital and knew the context and the health professionals, to a certain extent, she occupied an insider position on the project. Nevertheless, her knowledge about the clinicians' rehabilitation practice for patients with FM was fragmented. The other researcher (MS) had an outsider position, she did not know the participants beforehand, was unfamiliar with ongoing discussions, and, being Finnish, was unfamiliar with the Norwegian rehabilitation context. The researchers' diverse positions nurtured the process, helping to develop a good atmosphere for sharing and discussing experiences and asking about issues that, from an insider position, were likely taken for granted and thus not detected.

The researchers had the shared experience of clinicians often being up-to-date in quantitative, condition-oriented research, as clinicians learn to read and critically appraise quantitative studies through their professional education and courses in EBP. But reading and evaluating qualitative studies do not seem to be included in such curricula. Clinicians may feel that qualitative studies report about experiences that are too individual to be transferable to their patients. This raises a timely question about the validity and transferability of research in a clinical context. Quantitative studies illuminate trends and inform about 'mean' patients that do not necessarily exist in the real world (Anjum et al. 2015). This means that it is challenging to translate evidence from quantitative effect studies to provide valid information about an intervention's potential significance to an individual patient in a clinical setting (Haynes et al. 2002). Qualitative studies, in turn, are highly situational and nested in the culture and contexts in which the informants live their lives (Green and Thorogood 2014). Accordingly, informants' experiences do not necessarily match a specific patient in another clinical context. Nevertheless, in our opinion, both qualitative and quantitative studies can inform and enhance clinical reflexivity and reasoning, but neither can dictate what clinicians should do in practice. We therefore acknowledge that there is a gap between research and practice. Because the clinicians claimed to practice patient-centred care and to take a patient's perspective into account in their practice, we found it relevant to bridge this gap by bringing in patient-oriented evidence, discussing it in light of clinicians' own experiences.

We had no given 'formula' to implement, but we envisioned that, together with the clinicians, we could co-develop a programme tailored to patients' personal recovery processes. By talking across clinical experiences, scientific, and professional knowledges, we assumed that everyone's reflexivity would be encouraged, including our own. It is a common opinion that knowledge from evidence should be transferred to clinicians in a kind of 'one-way road' (Lockwood et al. 2004; Manns and Darrah 2006) – however, this contrasted with our goal of establishing a 'bidirectional road'. In retrospect, we discovered that the process can even be described as a 'multidirectional web of roads'.

Workshops and Participants' Roles

In agreement with the head of the rehabilitation unit, we planned to arrange three full-day workshops within a one-month interval. The workshops served as an arena for expressing ideas, sharing experiences, and searching for new understandings in accordance with a participatory, action research method. After the third workshop, the content of the programme had not yet been clarified, so a two-day workshop was arranged to concretise the content and procedures of the programme.

Before each of the first three workshops, the researchers distributed two or three qualitative papers, which were then read by the clinicians. The head of the rehabilitation unit encouraged the professionals to present these papers and discuss them in regular literature meetings at the hospital. She also raised questions for the researchers about what needed to be clarified and further elaborated upon. In addition, between the workshops, she had informal meetings with the professionals in which they continued their reflections and eventually agreed to try out new practical solutions in their clinical practice. The researchers moderated or observed the group discussions, made notes, analysed and summarised discussions orally and in writing, thereby also linking the process to evidential and theoretical understandings of patients' illness and recovery experiences.

Bringing Qualitative Studies and Inquiry into the Process

Reflecting Across Qualitative Studies and Clinical Experiences

During open plenary discussions, qualitative studies were used to facilitate discussions to explore how the health professionals understood and found meaning in the literature and whether the studies resonated with what their patients had told them. For the first meeting, participants read systematic reviews of qualitative interviews of patients with FM that addressed inexplicable, unpredictable pain and fatigue, diagnostics, activity and identity constraints, and explanations of suffering (Mengshoel et al. 2017; Sim and Madden 2008; Toye et al. 2013). This raised reflections in the meeting about uncertainties regarding the meaning and managing of such a complex illness. To further enhance these reflections, two additional texts were selected for reading before the second workshop: a paper discussing the importance of making sense of bodily sensations from a patient perspective (Corbin 2003) and a narrative review of recovery interpreted as a personal learning process (Mengshoel and Grape 2017). The importance of making sense of an unfamiliar body and its relationship to daily life were discussed further in the third workshop, inspired by papers addressing two topics: what it is like for patients to live with and be in treatment for FM (Ashe et al. 2017), and the importance for patients with chronic illnesses to take action to create order in their life situation (Kralik et al. 2004). Regarding the latter, the authors discussed professional-driven vs patient-driven approaches, which inspired a lively discussion amongst participants about the professionals' roles. The clinicians discovered that what they had read in the papers corresponded and gave meaning to what they had heard from their patients. Even more importantly, these papers also facilitated reflections about situations from their own clinical practice and their relationships with their patients. Whilst the discussions were not always centred on the papers' main topic, they all related to concepts or details in the papers that helped the clinicians articulate their own thoughts. Hence, the papers were helpful in bringing otherwise private reflections into the 'public' sphere.

Thematically Focused Explorative Reflections

The open cross-talks could often seem fragmented and difficult to follow. Therefore, we decided to arrange group discussions about the themes that we identified when we created the summaries from the prior meeting, such as the meaning of the diagnosis to patients and to professionals. These discussions were initially performed in a large group, but when we realised that some participants appeared less comfortable voicing their thoughts in a big group, the group was divided in two. In small groups of six or seven, everyone had more space and opportunity to express themselves, and the reflections became more focused and went deeper into the given topic. Here, too, the researchers' role was to facilitate reflections amongst the clinicians, but this time their role also entailed keeping the reflections focused so in-depth information about a topic could emerge. As both Bringing Qualitative Studies researchers were engaged in moderating these discussions, the discussions were audio-recorded.

Importance of Writing up Summaries

After each workshop, the researchers developed written reports summing up what was said in the open and thematically focused discussions. We discussed our own experiences, notes and audio-recordings, and developed themes that were then presented at the next workshop. These presentations served to validate our interpretations, to keep the process on track, and promote further progress. For the final workshop, the researchers drafted a document in which the various themes developed in the process were pulled together and given meaning with the help of theoretical models. This draft was sent to the clinicians before the workshop and helped both the researchers and the clinicians see how various knowledges were connected and formed a logical whole. After more clarifying discussions, the draft was used to translate the programme into clinical procedures and actions. At this point, the clinical team leader took charge of the process to concretise a timetable for the rehabilitation intervention, including what would be done and by whom.

Dilemmas Experienced in Clinical Practice

During the developmental process, several dilemmas in clinical practice became apparent that were not explicitly addressed in the scientific literature. For illustration, we provide some examples below. These dilemmas could not be solved through procedures, but a shared awareness about these issues was found to be valuable. It made us realise that dilemmas can appear when different logics and meanings are set in motion.

A Diagnosis with Various Meanings in Clinical Practice

The papers synthesising qualitative studies about patients' experiences of FM diagnosis (Mengshoel et al. 2017; Sim and Madden 2008) led to lengthy discussions. One discussion addressed the various attitudes towards the FM diagnosis amongst Norwegian rheumatologists that either accepted the reality of symptoms or considered them an exaggeration of trivial complaints. This discussion also linked to an ongoing debate in Norway about whether hospitals specialising in rheumatology should deliver services to these patients. To some extent, the clinicians felt they had to defend their practice against external forces. These controversies are attached to an ontological question as to whether subjective illness experiences are reliable without any objective verification of biological malfunction. Nevertheless, the team was ambivalent about whether the diagnosis was good or bad for the patient. On the one hand, getting a 'proper' diagnosis halted the patients' cycle of seeing new physicians. On the other hand, it was questioned whether the FM diagnosis could attach a patient to a sick role and thus strengthen sickness behaviour and hamper the recovery process. This ambivalence can be interpreted as rooted in various discourses: fear of medicalisation, for example, or health professionals' imperative to help ill people. The team also expressed different views about the clinical relevance of the diagnosis. The medical doctors used the diagnosis as a tool for validating FM from a medical perspective and explaining the patient the biological background of FM and the medical treatment approach they eventually chose. The allied health professionals valued the diagnosis for more instrumental reasons, as it helped them stop the patients from searching for new interpretations. For them, the diagnosis could also mean a fundamental change in a patient's focus from spending energy to convince health professionals about the reality of their suffering into starting their recovery work. This reflects the health professionals' various knowledges and interests within their work.

Ambiguous Understandings of Acceptance and Normality

The professionals acknowledged that their patients with FM were going through at least two processes simultaneously: namely, a process of losing or giving up something that was taken for granted earlier and a process of reaching for recovery. The constant yearning for life as it used to be, often expressed by the patients, seemed to reflect an ambivalent attitude towards starting a recovery process. The professionals pointed out that they felt it is important to explore this ambivalence with the patient in order to enable positive development and acceptance: for example, asking, 'What can you do to make your situation better, and what is holding you back?' The patient must accept the situation as it is in that moment, but at the same time not resign themselves to the idea that it will be the same in the future. Acceptance and normality were closely connected concepts, both relating to a personal process of recovery. Patients' grief over the normal life they had lost and uncertainty about their symptoms could be relieved when patients realised that their experiences were shared by other patients with FM – i.e., these experiences were normal for FM. However, in a process of recovery, a new meaningful normality had to be created. This means that patients had to accept that they would not necessarily return to life as it used to be, but accept that another normal life could be rebuilt that could be as good as the previous one. Acknowledging the patients' processes meant that the health professionals recognised the personal processes that patients were undergoing, but they considered these processes barriers to their own work rather than something to be directly acted upon. Acceptance and normality can thus have both positive and negative connotations in a person's recovery process.

Ambivalences in Interpreting Outcomes

The different meanings of the concept of normality were also discussed in relation to how and by whom progress in the patient's process can be measured or evaluated. It was acknowledged that sometimes the measurement tools that the professionals considered reliable might not detect small changes that were nonetheless perceived as meaningful by the patients. Alternatively, there could be times when there was a clinically significant improvement in objective measurements, but the patient did not see the benefit. It was also stated that encouraging the patient to pay attention to even a small improvement was important to keep up motivation and to prevent dropouts. The need for developing follow-up strategies after the rehabilitation programme was perceived as important because as one of the health professional said: 'recovery does not happen in the blink of an eye – rather than that, it takes time and effort'. These reflections demonstrate that two different interpretations of recovery are operating simultaneously: recovery linked to improved outcomes (i.e., reduction in disease/illness symptoms) caused by time-limited and effective interventions and recovery linked to patients' perceptions of wellness and satisfaction as time-consuming processes.

Uncertainties Related to Own Professional Role

The professionals emphasised that the rehabilitation process is in fact the patient's process and that the pace of the patient should be respected. However, they found it problematic if the patient either 'rushed forward too quickly and crashed' or 'parked here and did not want to move forward'. From the professionals' vantage point, the clinicians were put in an uncertain position: to interfere or not to interfere? They also discussed whether it is ethically acceptable to give up trying to motivate and guide the patient if the patient was not ready or willing to take action her/himself. It was seen to be against the idea of person-centred care if the professionals made a decision to halt the rehabilitation, but it was also their clinical experience that there was no point to continue if the patient was reluctant. Whether or not to interfere was also discussed with regards to patients who repeatedly told the same story about suffering. They felt it was important to listen to a patient's stories, but at the same time this recurrent narrative hindered the patient from starting to search for possibilities to do something about their situation. In this case, a dilemma arose, weighing opposing aims: respect a patient's autonomy or the professionals' obligation to be effective.

The syntheses also brought the issue of tolerating professional uncertainty into the discussion (Mengshoel et al. 2017; Sim and Madden 2008). Uncertainty was reflected upon regarding how to respond to certain questions from their patients, i.e., what is wrong, why this pain, and how can I understand and manage unpredictable variations in symptoms? The professionals felt they lacked good answers to these questions and were therefore uncertain about their own professional expertise. Although work experience, further education, and reading research reports had increased their competence and knowledge over the years, there was still no consensus in the literature that helped them give an explicit answer to the patients' questions. Sometimes the clinicians also felt frustrated with these patients when nothing seemed to help. They pointed out that their uncertainty was easily transferred onto the patients, and, in such a situation, it could be difficult to convince the patient about the benefits of the rehabilitation programme or to motivate the patient to take an active role in their rehabilitation. In turn, patients' earlier negative experiences of encounters with health professionals were sometimes reflected in their relationship to their new providers. The professionals therefore had to actively work to build a good relationship with patients with FM – more so than with other patients they met through their work. Their statements suggested that their relationships with patients with FM were fragile, and the professionals 'watched their steps' carefully. This reflects the fact that, although health professionals feel they should be personal, they also has to behave as experts in their practice, these two aims are not always in harmony.

The Bricolage of Knowledges Underpinning the New Programme

The Programme's 'Why'

A biopsychosocial model helped us display the condition-oriented evidence about FM to help our interpretations by demonstrating how complex FM actually is, as well as how biological, psychological, and social factors may interact with each other. This made it easier for us to understand how life stress can perpetuate symptoms and deficits of FM and, accordingly, why tailoring a rehabilitation programme to modify life stress may be appropriate (Figure 14.2). Moreover, the biopsychosocial model makes it plausible that changes in, for example, how a patient perceives a situation or how their life is lived can influence

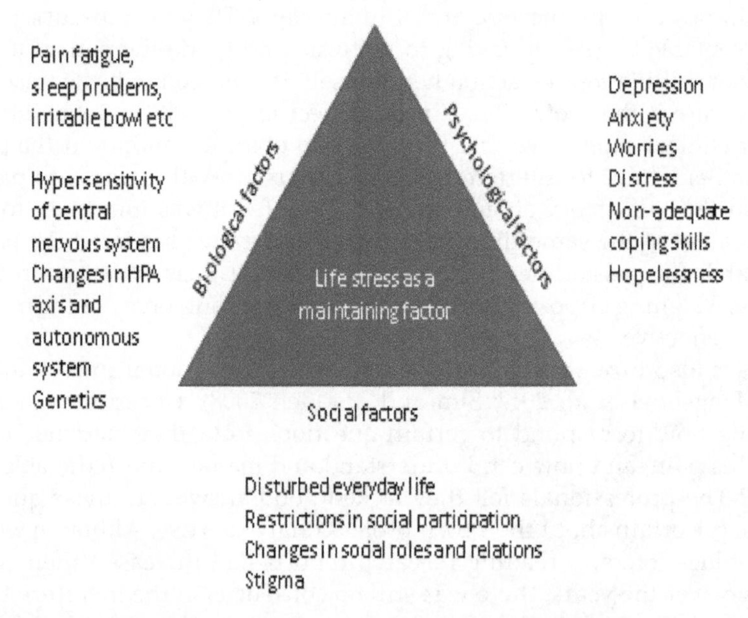

FIGURE 14.2
Complexity of FM and rationale for addressing life stress in a rehabilitation program.

biological, psychological, and social factors. In this way, the programme's purpose and rationale could be explained by condition-oriented evidence.

The biopsychosocial model was already a pillar for the clinicians' work, and, accordingly, the modelling of the programme's 'why' was easily adopted. However, it was difficult to see how the programme's content could be modelled using a biopsychosocial model. In support of this notion, Epstein and Borrell-Carrio (2005) conclude that a biopsychosocial model cannot guide a practice in chosing an explicit or implicit therapeutic methodology, rather, it serves more as a vision for practice, such as in the present case.

The Programme's 'What'

Both the researchers and the clinicians held the opinion that a rehabilitation programme for patients with FM could not be delivered in a 'one-size-fits-all' fashion, but had to be tailored to the needs of each patient, in accordance with the ideals of patient-centredness. For the clinicians, this meant that the patient must determine what they need and what the right solution is for them to reach their life goals. However, patient-oriented evidence shows that patients struggle to understand how symptoms relate to what they are doing in daily life. It is therefore not a given that patients with FM know what they need. They need hints about what to look for, and they must explore and discover what brings stress into their lives and find out how to modify, for example, social obligations, and their own and others' expectations and priorities. One premise underpinning this view is that a patient will be willing to take actions if they find them meaningful and realistic.

The next question to consider for clinical work is: how can health professionals help a patient develop insights into how symptoms relate to what they do in daily life? The literature on patient-centredness does not focus on the importance of a patient's meaning-making process, but according to person-oriented evidence about FM, this is important. A personalised resource-oriented recovery model highlights the patient's strengths and resources for exploring and discovering how illness relates to their own life project in order to get their lives back on track (Egnew 2009; Le Boutillier et al. 2011; Priebe et al. 2014). Each patient has to discover what their body can tolerate in daily life in order to trust their body again; find out what must be prioritised in their lives; and take actions to adjust their lives to their capabilities. For the patient, this may involve finding out what kind of life is possible to live within the boundaries set by an illness, restructuring patterns of living, getting used to new habits and routines, and redefining social roles and obligations (Kearney 1999). As in patient-centred practice, this process must be guided by the patient's priorities, values, abilities, and competences (Priebe et al. 2014). A person's recovery process is powered by their hope, engagement, and strength, and by support and engagement from others. The endpoint of this recovery process cannot be predetermined, but is part of the patient's explorative learning process. The path to recovery may take different turns over time, and a relapse does not necessarily have to be interpreted as a failure, but rather as something that gives new insights. Thus, a personal recovery process, as illustrated by the person-oriented evidence from interviews of patients with FM, communicates well with a resource-oriented recovery model and the clinicians' efforts to engage in delivering patient-centred practice.

Underpinning the new rehabilitation programme is an assumption that although wellness can be over-shadowed by illness, it is not inevitably lost because of it. A patient therefore is believed to have the capacity to reshape their future and bring wellness back to the fore (Lucey 2017). Learning that FM is a chronic illness that one has to learn to accept and live with can deprive a patient of hope and motivation to overcome FM. However, knowing that someone has recovered can provide hope and empower a patient to take action. But if a patient should fail at their recovery, our discussions highlight the fact that health professionals must be aware that the patient should not be blamed.

Final Reflections about What We Learnt

By bringing person-oriented evidence from qualitative studies into the process of developing the rehabilitation programme, we created an opportunity for health professionals to express otherwise personal clinical experiences and discuss them with others. The reflections were facilitated by discussions across qualitative studies and clinical experiences, as well as the researchers' explorative approach in accordance with qualitative research. We actively used theories about personal suffering and healing to interpret the group's reflections, thereby introducing new interpretations to the group. This ended up becoming a fruitful discovery process for us all. Moreover, the gap between clinical experiences, evidence, and patient-centredness was bridged with the help of biopsychosocial and personal resource-oriented models. Thus, we argue that by taking a 'bottom-up' approach, we were able to develop a theory-driven and patient-centred rehabilitation programme that also includes clinical experiences and preferences.

The prior rehabilitation programme aimed to promote a healthy lifestyle amongst patients to improve health. The new programme is more focused, as it targets life stress modifications which is linked to an understanding of the FM condition. Certainly, healthy lifestyles can impact life stress, and it may still be relevant to bring in elements from exercise, pain modulating techniques, and diets. But the difference here is that the purpose of the programme has changed, and this may in turn change the ways strategies are applied. For example, physical activity can serve as a strategy to modulate stress instead of previously to improve physical fitness. Instead of choosing strategies from a 'tool-box' of health strategies, the new programme has no tool-box, rather each patient has to find what is right for them to do to modify their life stress and overcome problems of FM.

In patient-centred practice, it is important to acknowledge the patient's experiences, and we argue that it is also important to understand the meaning of what patients say by taking into account patients' experiences during the programme. Patient-oriented evidence can enable clinicians to make sense of and respond to patients' stories. For years, this has been emphasised by physicians practicing narrative medicine, for example, Clark and Mishler (1992) and Kleinman (1988). Despite the fact that patient-centredness is included in the EBP model, qualitative studies have not been suggested for the sake of understanding experiences. However, we learnt that qualitative studies are important for interpreting both patients' and professionals' experiences. Thus, we suggest that qualitative studies should be brought into the field of rehabilitation to support patient-centred practice.

In summary, with the help of theoretical models and interpretations, qualitative studies, and qualitative explorative interviews and analysis, the content of a theory-driven, patient-centred rehabilitation programme was developed. As the health professionals were actively engaged in the development process, they created an ownership of the programme. Thereby, the programme was directly implementable to practice. New concepts and ways of talking about a patient's recovery process are now being used by the health professionals: for example, they refer to turning points, small and big steps towards change, patients' discoveries, and healing work in context of everyday work, biographical, and identity work. This does not mean that all clinical uncertainties and dilemmas are answered, but they can be articulated and discussed by the team in light of theoretical knowledge about FM, illness, and the patients' personal recovery processes.

References

Anderberg, U.M., Marteinsdottir, I., Theorell, T., & von Knorring, L. 2000. The impact of life events in female patients with fibromyalgia and in female healthy controls. *European Psychiatry*, 15(5), 295–301.

Ang, D. & Wilke, W.S. 1999. Diagnosis, etiology, and therapy of fibromyalgia. *Comprehensive Therapy*, 24(4), 221–227.

Anjum, R.L., Kerry, R., & Mumford, S.D. 2015. Evidence based on what? *Journal of Evaluation in Clinical Practice*, 21(6), E11–E12.

Åsbring, P. & Närvänen, A.L. 2002. Women's experiences of stigma in relationship to chronic fatigue syndrome and fibromyalgia. *Qualitative Health Research*, 12, 148–160.

Åsbring, P. & Närvänen, A.L. 2004. Patient power and control: A study of women with uncertain illness trajectories. *Qualitative Health Research*, 14(2), 226–240.

Ashe, S.C., Furness, P.J., Haywood-Small, S., & Larsen, K. 2017. A qualitative exploration of the experiences of living with and being treated for fibromyalgia. *Health Psychology Open* (July–December) 1–12.

Bernardy, K., Klose, P., Busch, A.J., Choy, E.H., & Häuser, W. 2013. Cognitive behavioural therapies for fibromyalgia. *Cochrane Database of Systematic Reviews*, (9), CD009796.

Bidonde, J., Busch, A.J., Bath, B., & Milosavljevic, S. 2014. Exercise for adults with fibromyalgia: An umbrella systematic review with synthesis of best evidence. *Current Rheumatology Reviews*, 10, 45–79.

Briones-Vozmediano, E., Vives-Cases, C., Ronda-Pérez, E., & Gil-González, D. 2013. Patients' and professionals' views on managing fibromyalgia. *Pain Research & Management*, 18(1), 19–24.

Brosseau, L., Wells, G.A., Tugwell, P., Egan, M., Wilson, K.G., Dubouloz, C.J., Casimiro, L. et al. 2008a. Ottawa panel evidence-based clinical practice guidelines for aerobic fitness exercises in the management of fibromyalgia: Part 1. *Physical Therapy*, 88(7), 857–871.

Brosseau, L., Wells, G.A., Tugwell, P., Egan, M., Wilson, K.G., Dubouloz, C.J., Casimiro, L. et al. 2008b. Ottawa panel evidence-based clinical practice guidelines for strengthening exercises in the management of fibromyalgia: Part 2. *Physical Therapy*, 88(7), 873–886.

Burchardt, C.S. 2002. Non-pharmacological management strategies in fibromyalgia. *Rheumatic Diseases Clinics of North America*, 28, 291–304.

Busch, A.J., Schachter, C.L., & Peloso, P.M. 2002. Fibromyalgia and exercise training: A systematic review of randomized clinical trials. *Physical Therapy Reviews*, 6, 287–306.

Carville, S.F., Arendt-Nielsen, S., Bliddal, H., Blotman, F., Branco, J.C., Buskila, D., da Silva, J.A.P. et al. 2008. EULAR evidence-based recommendations for the management of fibromyalgia syndrome. *Annals of the Rheumatic Diseases*, 67(4), 536–541.

Choy, E. 2015. *Fibromyalgia Syndrome*, 2 ed. Oxford: Oxford University Press.

Choy, E., Perrot, S., Leon, T., Kaplan, J., Petersel, D., Ginovker, A., & Kramer, E. 2010. A patient survey of the impact of fibromyalgia and the journey to diagnosis. *BMC Health Services Research*, 10, 102.

Clark, J.A. & Mishler, E.G. 1992. Attending to patients' stories: Reframing the clinical task. *Sociology of Health & Illness*, 14(3), 344–371.

Coopens, E., Kempke, S., Van Wambeke, P., Claes, S., Morlion, B., Luyten, P., & Van Oudenhove, L. 2018. Cortisol and subjective stress responses to acute psychosocial stress in fibromyalgia patients and control participants. *Psychosomatic Medicine*, 80, 317–326.

Corbin, J.M. 2003. The body in health and illness. *Qualitative Health Research*, 13(2), 256–267.

Crofford, L.J., Pillemer, S.R., Kalogeras, K.T., Cash, J.M., Michelson, D., Kling, M.A., Sternberg, E.M., Gold, P.W., Chrousos, G.P., & Wilder, R.L. 1994. Hypothalamic-pituitary-adrenal axis perturbations in patients with fibromyalgia. *Arthritis & Rheumatism*, 37, 1583–1592.

Cunningham, M.M. & Jillings, C. 2006. Individuals' descriptions of living with fibromyalgia. *Clinical Nursing Research*, 15(4), 258–273.

Davidson, K. 2008. Cognitive-behavioural therapy: Origins and developments. In *Cognitive-Behavioural Interventions in Physiotherapy and Occupational Therapy*, 1 ed. M. Donaghy, M. Nicol, & K. Davidson, Eds., Edinburgh, Scotland: Butterworth Heinemann, pp. 3–17.

Dennis, N.L., Larkin, M., & Derbyshire, S.W.G. 2013. 'A giant mess' – Making sense of complexity in the accounts of people with fibromyalgia. *British Journal of Health Psychology*, 18, 763–781.

Dijkers, M.P., Murphy, S.L., & Krellman, J. 2012. Evidence-based practice for rehabilitation professionals: Concepts and controversies. *Archives of Physical Medicine and Rehabilitation*, 93 (suppl 2), S164–S176.

Egnew, T. 2009. Suffering, meaning, and healing: Challenges of contemporary medicine. *Annals of Family Medicine*, 7(2), 170–175.

Epstein, R.M. & Borell-Carrio, F. 2005. The biopsychosocial model: Exploring six possible things. *Families, Systems and Health*, 23(4), 426–431.

Ercolani, M., Trombini, G., Chattat, R., Cervini, C., Pergiacomi, G., Salaffi, F., Zeni, S., & Marcolango, R. 1994. Fibromyalgic syndrome: Depression and abnormal behavior. *Psychotherapy and Psychosomatics*, 61, 178–186.

Gluyas, H. 2015. Patient-centred care: Improving healthcare outcomes. *Nursing Standard*, 30(4), 50–57.

Goldenberg, D.L. 2008. Multidisciplinary modalities in the treatment of fibromyalgia. *Journal of Clinical Psychiatry*, 69(Suppl. 2), 30–34.

Grape, H.E., Solbrække, K.N., Kirkevold, M., & Mengshoel, A.M. 2015. Staying healthy from fibromyalgia is ongoing hard work. *Qualitative Health Research*, 25(5), 679–688.

Grape, H.E., Solbrække, K.N., Kirkevold, M., & Mengshoel, A.M. 2017. Tiredness and fatigue during processes of illness and recovery: A qualitative study of women recovered from fibromyalgia syndrome. *Physiotherapy Theory & Practice*, 33(1), 31–40.

Green, J. & Thorogood, N. 2014. Qualitative methodology and health research. In *Qualitative Methods for Health Research*, 3 ed. J. Green & N. Thorogood, Eds. London, UK: SAGE Publications, pp. 3–34.

Greenhalgh, T. 2014. Evidence based medicine: A movement in crisis? *British Medical Journal*, 348.

Griep, E.N., Boersma, J.W., & de Kloet, E.R. 1993. Altered reactivity of hypothalamic-pituitary-adrenal axis in the primary fibromyalgia syndrome. *Journal of Rheumatology*, 20, 469–474.

Gupta, A., Silman, A.J., Ray, D., Morriss, R., Dickens, C., Macfarlane, G.J., Chiu, Y.H., Nicholl, B., & McBeth, J. 2007. The role of psychosocial factors in predicting the onset of chronic widespread pain: Results from a prospective population-based study. *Rheumatology*, 46, (4) 666–671.

Hadler, N.M. 1996. If you have to prove you are ill, you can't get well. The object lesson of fibromyalgia. *Spine*, 21(20), 2397–2400.

Haynes, R.B., Devereaux, P.J., & Guyatt, G.H. 2002. Physicians' and patients' choices in evidence based practice. Evidence does not make decisions, people do. *British Medical Journal*, 324, 1350.

Hellström, O., Bullington, J., Karlsson, G., Lindqvist, P., & Mattson, B. 1999. A phenomenological study of fibromyalgia. Patient perspectives. *Scandinavian Journal of Primary Health Care*, 17, 11–16.

Hofmann, B. 2001. Complexity of the concept of disease as shown through theoretical frameworks. *Theoretical Medicine*, 22, 211–236.

Jacobson, L.D., Edwards, A.G.K., Granier, S.K., & Butler, C.C. 1997. Evidence-based medicine and general practice. *British Journal of General Practice*, 47, 449–452.

Jones, K.D., Adams, D., Winters-Stone, K., & Burchardt, C.S. 2006. A comprehensive review of 46 exercise treatment studies in fibromyalgia (1988–2005). *Health Quality Life Outcomes*, 4(1), 67.

Juuso, P., Skär, L., Olsson, M., & Söderberg, S. 2014. Meanings of being received and met by others as experienced by women with fibromyalgia. *Qualitative Health Research*, 24(10), 1381–1390.

Kearney, M.H. 1999. *Understanding Women's Recovery from Illness and Trauma*. Thousand Oaks, CA: Sage Publications.

Kerry, R. 2017. Expanding our perspective on research in musculoskeletal science and practice. *Musculoskeletal Science and Practice*, 32, 114–119.

Kleinman, A. 1988. *The Illness Narratives*. Cambridge, MA: Basic Books.

Kralik, D., Koch, T., Price, K., & Howard, N. 2004. Chronic illness self-management: Taking action to create order. *Journal of Clinical Nursing*, 13(2), 259–267.

Kurtze, N., Gundersen, K.T., & Svebak, S. 1999. Quality of life, functional disability and lifestyle among subgroups of fibromyalgia patients: The significance of anxiety and depression. *British Journal of Medical Psychology*, 72, 471–484.

Le Boutillier, C., Leamy, M., Bird, V.J., Davidson, L., Williams, J., & Slade, M. 2011. What does recovery mean in practice? A qualitative analysis of international recovery-oriented practice guidance. *Psychiatric Services*, 62(12), 1470–1476.

Liedberg, G.M. & Henriksson, C.M. 2002. Factors of importance for work disability in women with fibromyalgia: An interview study. *Arthritis Care & Research*, 47(3), 266–274.

Lockwood, D., Armstrong, M., & Grant, A. 2004. Integrating evidence based medicine into routine clinical practice: Seven years' experience at the Hospital for Tropical Diseases, London. *British Medical Journal*, 329(7473), 1020–1023.

Lucey, J. 2017. *The Life Well Lived: The Therapeutic Journey to Recovery and Wellbeing*. 1 ed. Dublin, Ireland: Transworld Ireland Publishers.

Macfarlane, G.J., Kronisch, C., Dean, L.E., Atzeni, F., Hauser, W., Fluss, E., Choy, E.H. et al. 2017. EULAR revised recommendations for the management of fibromyalgia. *Annals of the Rheumatic Diseases*, 76, 318–328.

Madden, S. & Sim, J. 2006. Creating meaning in fibromyalgia syndrome. *Social Science & Medicine*, 2962–2973.

Madden, S. & Sim, J. 2016. Acquiring a diagnosis of fibromyalgia syndrome: The sociology of diagnosis. *Social Theory & Health*, 14(1), 88–108.

Mannerkorpi, K., Kroksmark, T., & Ekdahl, C. 1999. How patients with fibromyalgia experience their symptoms in everyday life. *Physiotherapy Research International*, 4(2), 110–122.

Mannerkorpi, K. & Henriksson, C. 2007. Non-pharmacological treatment of chronic widespread musculoskeletal pain. *Best Practice & Research Clinical Rheumatology*, 21(3), 513–534.

Manns, P. & Darrah, J. Linking research and clinical practice in physical therapy: Strategies for integration. 2006. *Journal of Physiotherapy*, 92(2), 88–94.

McMahon, L., Murray C, Sanderson S., & Daiches A. 2012. 'Governed by the pain': Narratives of fibromyalgia. *Disability and Rehabilitation*, 34(16), 1358–1366.

McVeigh, J.G., Hurley, D.A., Basford, J.R., Sim, J., & Finch, M.B. 2003. The pathogenesis of fibromyalgia syndrome: An update. *Physical Therapy Reviews*, 8, 211–216.

Mengshoel, A.M., Forseth, K.Ø., Haugen, M.A., Walle-Hansen, R., & Førre, Ø. 1995. Multidisciplinary approach to fibromyalgia – A pilot study. *Clinical Rheumatology*, 14(2), 165–170.

Mengshoel, A.M. & Grape, H.E. 2017. Rethinking physiotherapy for patients with fibromyalgia – Lessons learnt from qualitative studies. *Physical Therapy Reviews*, 22(5–6), 254–259.

Mengshoel, A.M. & Heggen, K. 2004. Recovery from fibromyalgia – Patients' own experiences. *Disability and Rehabilitation*, 26(1), 46–53.

Mengshoel, A.M., Sim, J., Ahlsen, B., & Madden, S. 2017. Diagnostic experiences of patients with fibromyalgia – A meta-ethnography. *Chronic Illness*. doi:10.1177/1742395317718035.

Neeck, G. & Riedel, W. 1994. Neuromediator and hormonal perturbations in fibromyalgia syndrome: Results of chronic stress? In *Fibromyalgia and Myofascial Pain Syndrome*, vol. 8. A. Masi, ed., Kent: Baillière Tindall, pp. 763–776.

Priebe, S., Omer, S., Giacco, D., & Slade, M. 2014. Resource-oriented therapeutic models in psychiatry: Conceptual review. *British Journal of Psychiatry*, 204, 256–261.
Queiroz, L.P. 2013. The world-wide epidemiology of fibromyalgia. *Current Pain and Headaches Report*, 17, 356.
Råheim, M. & Håland, W. 2006. Lived experience of chronic pain and fibromyalgia: Women's stories from daily life. *Qualitative Health Research*, 16(6), 741–761.
Richardson, J.C. 2005. Establishing the (extra)ordinary in chronic widespread pain. *Interdisciplinary Journal for the Social Study of Health, Illness and Medicine*, 9(1), 31–48.
Richardson, J.C., Ong, B.N., & Sim, J. 2006. Remaking the future: Contemplating a life with chronic widespread pain. *Chronic Illness*, 2, 209–218.
Richardson, J.C., Ong, B.N., & Sim, J. 2008. Experiencing and controlling time in everyday life with chronic widespread pain: A qualitative study. *BMC Musculoskeletal Disorders*, 9, 3.
Sackett, D.L., Rosenberg, W.M.C., Gray, J.A.M., Haynes, R.B., & Richardson, W.S. 2007. Evidence based medicine: What it is and what it isn't. *Clinical Orthopaedics and Related Research*, 455, 3–5.
Sacristan, J.A. 2013. Patient-centred medicine and patient-oriented research: Improving health outcomes for individual patients. *BMC Medical Informatics and Decision Making*, 13, 6.
Sallinen, M., Kukkurainen, M.L., & Peltokallio, L. 2011. Finally heard, believed and accepted – Peer support in the narratives of women with fibromyalgia. *Patient Education and Counseling*, 85(2), 126–130.
Sallinen, M., Kukkurainen, M.L., Peltokallio, L., & Mikkelson, M. 2010. Women's narratives on experiences of work ability and functioning in fibromyalgia. *Musculoskeletal Care*, 8(1), 18–26.
Sallinen, M., Kukkurainen, M.L., Peltokallio, L., Mikkelsson, M., & Anderberg, U.M. 2012. Fatigue, worry, and fear – Life events in the narratives of women with fibromyalgia. *Health Care for Women International*, 33, 473–494.
Schoofs, N., Bambini, D., Ronning, P., Bielak, E., & Woehl, J. 2004. Death of a lifestyle: The effects of social support and healthcare support on the quality of life of persons with fibromyalgia and/or chronic fatigue syndrome. *Orthopaedic Nursing*, 23(6), 364–374.
Siegert, R.J., McPherson, K.M., & Dean, S.G. 2005. Theory development and a science of rehabilitation. *Disability and Rehabilitation*, 27(24), 1493–1501.
Sim, J. & Adams, N. 2002. Systematic review of randomized controlled trials of nonpharmacological interventions for fibromyalgia. *Clinical Journal of Pain*, 118, 324–336.
Sim, J. & Madden, S. 2008. Illness experience in fibromyalgia syndrome: A metasynthesis of qualitative studies. *Social Science & Medicine*, 67(1), 57–67.
Söderberg, S., Lundman, B., & Norberg, A. 2002. The meaning of fatigue and tiredness as narrated by women with fibromyalgia and healthy women. *Journal of Clinical Nursing*, 11(2), 247–255.
Toye, F., Seers, K., Allcock, N., Briggs, M., Carr, E., Andrews, J., & Barker, K. 2013. Patients' experiences of chronic non-malignant musculoskeletal pain: A qualitative systematic review. *British Journal of General Practice*, 63(617), 829–841.
Turk, D.C., Okifuij, A., Sinclair, J.D., & Starz, T.W. 1996. Pain, disability, and physical functioning in subgroups of patients with fibromyalgia. *Journal of Rheumatology*, 23, 1255–1262.
Undeland, M. & Malterud, K. 2002. Diagnostic work in general practice: More than naming a disease. *Scandinavian Journal of Primary Health Care*, 20, 145–150.
Undeland, M. & Malterud, K. 2007. The fibromyalgia diagnosis – Hardly helpful for the patients? *Scandinavian Journal of Primary Health Care*, 225, 250–255.
Üòeyler, N., Häuser, W., & Sommer, C. 2008. A systematic review on the effectiveness of treatment with antidepressants in fibromyalgia syndrome. *Arthritis & Rheumatism (Arthritis Care & Research)*, 59(9), 1279–1298.
Van Houdenhove, B., Egle, U., & Luyten, P. 2005. The role of life stress in fibromyalgia. *Current Rheumatology Reports*, 7, 365–370.
van Koulil, S., Effting, M., Kraaimaat, F.W., van Lankveld, W., van Helmond, T., Cats, H., van Riel, P.L.C.M., de Jong, A.J.L., Haverman, J.F., & Evers, A.W.M. 2007. Cognitive-behavioural therapies and exercise programmes for patients with fibromyalgia: State of the art and future directions. *Annals of the Rheumatic Diseases*, 66(5), 571–581.

van Riel, P.L.C.M. & Fransen, J. 2005. To be in remission or not: Is that the question? *Annals of the Rheumatic Diseases*, 64(10), 1389–1390.

Wade, D.T. & de Jong, B.A. 2000. Recent advances in rehabilitation. *British Medical Journal*, 320, 1385–1388.

Wallace, D.J. & Wallace, J.B. 2014. *Making Sense of Fibromyalgia*. 3 edn. Oxford, UK: Oxford University Press.

Wentz, K.A.H., Lindberg, C., & Hallberg, L.R.M. 2012. On parole: The natural history of recovery from fibromyalgia in women: A grounded theory study. *Journal of Pain Management*, 5(2), 177–194.

Winfield, J.B. 1999. Pain in fibromyalgia. *Rheumatic Diseases Clinics of North America*, 25(1), 55–79.

Wulff, H.R., Pedersen, S.A., & Rosenberg, R. 1999. *Medicinsk filosofi (Philosophy of Medicine)*. 5 ed. Copenhagen: Munksgaard.

Yunus, M.B. 1994. Fibromyalgia syndrome: Clinical features and spectrum. *Journal of Musculoskeletal Pain*, 2(3), 5–21.

15

Concept Development through Qualitative Research: The Case of Social Support Networks for People with Intellectual Disability

Anne E. Roll and Barbara J. Bowers

CONTENTS

Text and Concepts in Qualitative Research

Most qualitative research is based on some form of textual analysis. Researchers use documents, observation protocols, and interview transcripts to conduct analysis. In this chapter, we focus on one of the earliest systematic approaches to analysing qualitative data, the grounded theory approach. Originally developed by Glaser and Strauss (1965), the approach has since been revised and interpreted differently by several authors (Glaser 1978; Strauss 1987; Strauss & Corbin 1990; Corbin & Strauss 2008; Bowers & Schatzmann 2009; Bryant & Charmaz 2011; Charmaz 2014, 2016). However, as one of the most commonly used qualitative methodologies, some of its key elements have remained constant. They include the concurrency of data collection and data analysis, early initiation of interview transcript or field note coding, theoretical sampling to support ongoing analysis, and the constant comparison of the emerging concepts with existing and new data. The aim is to arrive at a theory or conceptual model that is grounded in the data. It typically includes identifying a central category or core category which refers to a basic social phenomenon or process and that accounts for most of the observed behaviour (Strauss & Corbin 1998).

In the grounded theory methodology, coding involves labelling concepts, the dimensions of those concepts (often as social processes), and the conditions associated with variations in those processes as described by participants. It is in their talking about a phenomenon that concepts, dimensions, and conditions are discovered. Thus, the conceptual model generated at the conclusion of the study is 'grounded' in the data rather than being guided by received theory. Whilst different approaches for coding and analysing have been suggested (Strauss & Corbin 1990; Glaser 1992; Charmaz 2014, 2016; Bowers & Schatzman 2009), the general idea of analytically breaking the data into core components to build a conceptual model and ultimately a theory has remained consistent. Since these codes are intended to capture what is analytically meaningful in the text, as expressed by the participants, these are analytical concepts. Eventually, according to Strauss (1987) and Strauss and Corbin (1990), the most analytically important concept to which most codes can be related becomes the central concept.

In their well-known study *Awareness of Dying* (1965), for example, in which Glaser and Strauss initially described the grounded theory methodology, the central concept was 'awareness context'. Studying the interaction of staff and relatives with dying people in a hospital, they argued that what the patient knew about his or her state and what others assumed the patient knew was crucial for how they interacted with each other. Glaser and Strauss (1965) identified the following four types of awareness: 'closed awareness' (patients do not suspect their death), 'suspicion awareness' (patients have a suspicion regarding their death), 'awareness of mutual pretense' (nothing is said, but everybody knows), and 'open awareness' (the patient knows it and speaks openly about it).

This foray into grounded theory methodology shows how concepts are used for analytical purposes in one particular qualitative research approach. The conceptual innovations that these studies produce increase scientific knowledge. By doing so, they can also have an impact on how professionals understand and act in certain situations. In Glaser and Strauss' *Awareness of Dying* (1965), the distinction between the different awareness types that the authors developed shaped how health professionals thought about and interacted with people they believed were dying.

This research demonstrates how qualitative research broadens understanding and goes beyond medical knowledge. By developing concepts based on qualitative data collection, it can inform people, researcher, and clinicians about processes that are important for health and healthcare. New concepts and conceptual distinctions that qualitative studies produce therefore can lead to real-world changes that impact the health and well-being of patients.

Professional and Policy Implications of Concepts

The British sociologist Anthony Giddens argued that one difference between the natural sciences and the social sciences is in how concepts are used and how they travel (1986). He argued that in the natural sciences, scientists develop concepts to describe and understand the natural world, but that this natural world does not use these concepts ('single hermeneutic'). However, the social sciences operate with a 'double hermeneutic' because 'the concepts of the social sciences are not produced about an independently constituted subject-matter, which continues regardless of what these concepts are. The "findings" of the social sciences very often enter constitutively into the world they describe' (Giddens 1986: 20). The concepts that are developed to describe social life become an important element of social life itself and thereby change it. Concepts that biologists develop, on the other hand, do not change the material reality these concepts refer to, for example, an atom. Concepts that are developed in the social sciences not only often enter the non-academic world, but by doing so, shape our understanding of this social reality. There are many examples, including concepts such as social class or habitus. The same is also true for new concepts developed in research on health and healthcare. When these concepts move beyond the academic field, they begin to shape how we think about and act in the world. These effects may be particularly strong in certain professional and policy fields, but also with broader audiences.

By exploring lifeworlds that we know very little about and by trying to understand why people act the way they do and the meaning it has for them, qualitative research can develop new concepts that both reflect and shape our understanding of the world beyond academic circles. This is one of the strongest potential contributions qualitative research can make to improving health and well-being, particularly for groups we know relatively little about, allowing us to gain insights into their health-related practices or interactions with the health system. One such group, people with intellectual disability (ID) and their families, will be used to demonstrate how powerful and transformative concept development through qualitative research can be.

Examples from Qualitative Research on Health and Healthcare

Apart from the classic example from Glaser and Strauss (1965) presented above, many other qualitative studies in nursing and health research have developed new concepts that have subsequently shaped healthcare. We will now briefly introduce some studies on diverse subjects such as caregiving, chronic illness, and in somewhat greater detail, how family members of people with ID build social support networks for people with ID. These studies demonstrate the potential of qualitative research to make important contributions to healthcare and rehabilitation by developing new concepts based on experiential data from the perspective of people participating in research studies.

Kathy Charmaz (1983) studied the experience of being chronically ill. With her category 'loss of self', she describes how people lead more restricted lives, experience social isolation, are discredited, and how they experience being a burden to others because of their chronic illness. She describes this as an experience of suffering that goes beyond physical suffering related to direct effects of the illness. This more complex understanding of how patients experience their illness, within their social context, gives healthcare providers a more comprehensive understanding of the patient's needs than would be possible if only considering effects directly related to the illness. This revelation has strong implications for healthcare delivery strategies.

A second example is Barbara Bowers' (1987) study of intergenerational caregiving. She found that caregiving usually involves much more than the traditional definition of hands-on caregiving that healthcare provider and researcher alike had previously focused on. Bowers (1987) described the following five categories of caregiving: anticipatory, preventive, supervisory, instrumental, and protective caregiving. 'Anticipatory caregiving' is caregiving that considers the possible future and prepares for it. 'Preventive caregiving' includes activities that family caregivers carry out to prevent their relatives' conditions from getting worse. Bowers refers to the active involvement of caregivers in the caregiving process by doing things like arranging doctor's appointments, for example, as 'supervisory caregiving' and traditional hands-on caregiving as 'instrumental caregiving'. The last category, 'protective caregiving' involves care designed to protect the self-image of the person they are caring for, a type of caregiving that is most actively engaged in when the person they are caring for has mild cognitive impairment. Caregivers do so, for example, by not confronting the person with their deficits to protect both the person's identity and, in the case of adult children, the parent-child relationship. Giving these different dimensions of caregiving separate names and therefore distinguishing them enables nurses and other health professionals to see how complex caregiving can be and to respond in a way that aligns with the experience of the caregiver. It also helps healthcare providers to better understand and assess family caregiving contributions for older people, which in turn makes it possible to better support them.

A third example is Anne Roll's and Barbara Bowers' (2019) study entitled 'Building and Connecting: Family Strategies for Developing Social Support Networks for Adults with Down Syndrome'. This study is introduced in somewhat more detail in the following section to demonstrate the potential of qualitative research and concept development for improving healthcare and rehabilitation.

The Case of Social Support Networks for People with ID

Whilst it is well known that social networks and social support networks in particular are important for a person's health and well-being, (House, Landis, & Umberson 1988; Valente 2010), little is known about the social support networks of people with ID and – as one of the largest groups of people with ID – people with Down Syndrome (DS) in particular. In recent decades, the life expectancy of people with DS has increased dramatically and has reached an age of approximately 60 years in most developed countries (Bittles 2007). Nevertheless, people with DS are still often dependent on others throughout the life course. The dependency is due to the significant limitations in both intellectual functioning and limitation in adaptive behaviour of people with DS. For example, not many people with DS are able to drive and therefore rely on others for transport, especially if there are no public transport options available. Finding and maintaining work or moving into an apartment and living independently are other important challenges. Whilst it is well known that family members play an important role in supporting their children with DS throughout their lives (Petner-Arrey, Howell-Moneta & Lysaght 2015; Hillman et al., 2013), very little is known about what family members actually do to develop and maintain the social support networks for their sons and daughters with DS. However, because of the critical role that social support networks play in health and well-being more generally, this knowledge would enable healthcare providers to better tailor their support to actual needs and address existing bottlenecks. More broadly, if the generally extensive work of family members was better understood by health and social care providers as well as policy makers, the potential for more effective programming would be enhanced, quality of life for family members and adults with DS would likely be improved, and all too common institutionalisation could be delayed. Understanding how family members develop and maintain social support networks of people with DS was the goal of this study.

Research Process

During her time as a staff nurse in long-term care settings, the first author of this chapter noticed that people with ID who were aging in the community were losing support from their family. This was mostly the case because of their increasing life expectancy and their family members' own aging process. These people with ID in the community were then often admitted to long-term care facilities despite being much younger than most long-term care residents. The importance of social support networks therefore increased and became vital for older people with DS for remaining in the community. Because the goal of this study was to understand the participants' perspectives of the situation as well as how their perspectives resulted in specific actions (social processes), this study adopted a grounded theory approach.

Developing Concepts

Based on the researchers' prior experiences, we assumed that awareness of increasing life expectancy of people with DS would lead to family members engaging in future planning for the person with DS. Initially, the research focused on how family members were planning for the future. In the first interviews, participants were asked how they experienced the social support network of their relatives with DS, what kind of support was provided by others, and how they felt about and planned for the future of their relatives with DS. Consistent with grounded theory, our analysis remained grounded in the descriptions of the participants. To our surprise, planning for the future was rarely mentioned. Family members' accounts primarily focused on the present. Whilst future planning was sometimes mentioned, it was never prominent or central. The following quote from an early interview with a father in his 1980s and a daughter with DS in her late 40s shows this:

'You're asking a serious question, "How are we planning for it?" We're not. We're just going to make it, like I said, as best as we can for her until that day comes.'

Based on our expectations about the importance of planning for the future, we asked ourselves briefly if this father was not caring. How could he not think and plan for the future given his situation and age? However, during the interview, he talked about so many other things he had done and is doing to support his daughter. A more detailed, grounded theory-based analysis of the interview transcripts with the first few family members revealed that the family members of people with DS were also thinking about the future, but were much more focused on the present and about what they have already done, and continue to do, to support the person with DS. Following this insight, new interview questions were developed to reflect this insight and to ask for what family caregivers do to support their relatives with DS and to what end. These data were analysed again and additional data were collected and, over time, through the constant comparison of data and emerging categories two approaches (social processes) for developing and supporting the social support networks of people with DS were identified: the 'building' and the 'connecting' approaches. Based on this analysis, we eventually developed what we call the building and connecting framework (Roll & Bowers 2019). This framework encompasses the two approaches we identified and the associated strategies for helping people with DS develop and maintain social support networks throughout their lives.

The building approach includes strategies that family members use to build a support network around the person with DS, mostly relying on family members and friends. The connecting approach, on the other hand, is characterised by connecting the person with DS to already existing, external, and often professional, actors and organisations. Both approaches and the associated strategies are described in more detail in Roll & Bowers (2019).

Member Checking

This section describes a member checking exercise in which the preliminary concepts are introduced to some research participants and experts in the field of people with DS – in this case, family members of people with DS – to get their feedback. Member checking is a technique used in qualitative research to help improve the accuracy, credibility, validity, and transferability of findings by sharing preliminary or final results with participants to find ask them whether the developing framework reflects their experience, to add dimensions that they don't see, and to add variations in experience and the conditions that seem to account for those variations. In the study by Roll & Bowers (2019), the first member checking exercise was carried out after slightly more than two thirds of all interviews (20 out of a total of 29). The data were continuously being analysed and the preliminary findings could therefore be presented to family members of people with DS to see if they could see their own experiences being reflected in the developing framework. An early version of the figure that presents the building and connecting approaches and their respective strategies was shown and explained to participants. Two general kinds of reactions of participants could be distinguished, although some participants combined both reactions: using the concepts and their adaptation.

Everyday Use

After the building and connecting approaches and the respective strategies had been presented, some family members immediately categorised themselves as either using building or connecting strategies. From that point onwards, almost all participants used the concepts to refer to these two approaches and the associated strategies and to describe what they and others were doing, demonstrating how useful the concepts were in allowing them to express their experiences. None had used this language (or concepts) in the past to think about or describe their situations and had therefore not previously been able to express these components of their experience. This is illustrated by the way this sister of a person with DS responded, referring to her and her mother's behaviour:

> 'Clearly the builders, clearly the builder. Just it always worked, that [person with DS] was always at home. And there was a lot of planning that goes along with making [person with DS] life enriched in work, in recreation. Mother always thought she could handle that, and she did. And she did it really well, and she kept him super, super involved from work, activities, recreation. They did things together. We did things together. It worked'. [127 sister]

Another mother also expressed excitement about the usefulness of these concepts, stating that finally someone gave her the language to explain what she had been doing all these years for her son with DS. By moving him out at an early stage and sharing responsibilities and decisions with professionals, she tried to enable him to have the most independent life possible:

> 'Definitely I am a connector. Now I can finally explain to other moms what I am doing and I feel not guilty about it'. [134 mother]

People who were not family members, but experts in the field of providing care and support for people with DS also used the approaches, primarily for describing changes in the lives of people with DS:

> 'I think there is this transition [relating to a family situation] you just talked about with the building approach towards the connecting approach. He was in the building approach, but his guardians passed away. So now he needs – and she [mother of the person with DS] wants him to have more support with that outside'. [140 caregivers]

In the next case, a mother justified why one approach alone is not working.

> 'I will use a building approach to build skills so that he can better work using a connecting approach and everything. But as a family, like you said, the siblings come in and everything, and they mess it up and everything because they want to protect them and keep them in a building approach'. [mother of a person with DS]

Some participants gave positive feedback and asked where this framework and these concepts came from. We explained that they were developed based on the analysis of the interviews. One mother then exclaimed:

> 'And I had not heard 'building approach' and 'connecting approach' before, so that is something that I will sell. That was good'. [Mother 123]

Potential Contributions of Concepts

Whilst these concepts have only been developed recently, it is possible to speculate about their potential future contributions to illustrate how qualitative research can contribute to healthcare and rehabilitation through concept development.

First, and beginning at the macro level, this framework and the two central concepts could help policymakers understand that two different approaches exist for family members for supporting their relatives with DS. Therefore, variation in the structures and components of support programs might be necessary to accommodate both groups and to support them in ways that are consistent with, and build on, the support provided by families.

These concepts could also be helpful for professional healthcare agencies and could prevent family members from being misjudged or labelled in ways that are not helpful. For example, some family members shared that they were often seen as overprotective if their adult child with DS still lived with them. Other family members reported being seen as uncaring if they chose to share responsibilities with professionals and promoted their adult child's independence. Using this framework could facilitate a more appropriate characterisation of the work that families do and could serve as a basis for developing new, more supportive professional strategies.

And as the member checking exercise has already indicated, these concepts can help family members of people with DS and people with DS themselves to explicitly talk about their preferred approaches and strategies. Volunteer groups and self-help organisations could use these concepts in marketing materials, information sessions, and discussions with clients and families. The framework might also be useful in guiding families as they begin to make decisions about how to care for a child with DS, giving them the opportunity to think about and consciously decide which approach might suit their circumstances and how or when to combine the two approaches.

Like in the cases of the other qualitative studies on nursing and healthcare introduced above, the concepts developed in this study may travel beyond academia to shape policy, healthcare practice, and the everyday lives of the people with DS.

Conclusions

One of the ways qualitative research can contribute to healthcare and rehabilitation is by developing new concepts and making conceptual distinctions. This chapter has focused on the grounded theory research approach which is one of the best-known and most frequently used approaches. It can be distinguished from other qualitative approaches in its insistence on building frameworks, and ultimately theory, grounded in empirical data and taking the perspectives of research participants seriously. Most importantly, this requires the researcher to hear what participants are saying, to render their experiences conceptually, and to avoid imposing preconceived understandings of these experiences.

Naming something is a precondition for talking about it, reflecting on it, considering alternatives, and making conscious decisions for or against something. Developing concepts for what people do – especially when this tends to be invisible to professional observers – therefore is an important first step. And as soon as these concepts leave the academic realm, they can begin to shape social reality. Because they can do so both in positive and in negative ways and the researcher has little to no control over this, it is very important that the underlying research process is rigorous and credible.

Whilst the actual usefulness and impact of the study on the social support networks of people with DS and the role of family members introduced here remains to be seen, other studies have already shown that qualitative researchers can make an important contribution to improving healthcare and rehabilitation through concept development. And as our social worlds are getting more diverse and more complex in many regards, more qualitative concept development is necessary to improve healthcare and rehabilitation in the future.

References

Bittles, A. H., Bower, C., Hussain, R., & Glasson, E. J. (2007). The four ages of Down syndrome. *European Journal of Public Health*, 17(2), 221–225. doi:10.1093/eurpub/ckl103.

Bowers, B. J. (1987). Intergenerational caregiving: adult caregivers and their aging parents. *ANS. Advances in nursing science*, 9(2), 20–31. doi:10.1097/00012272-198701000-00006.

Bowers, B., & Schatzman, L. (2009). Dimensional analysis. In Morse, J., Stern, P., Corbin, J., Bowers, B., Charmaz, K., Clarke, A. (Eds.), *Developing Grounded Theory. The Second Generation* (pp. 86–126). New York: Routledge.

Bryant, A. & Charmaz, K. (2011). Grounded theory. In Williams, M., & Vogt, W. P. *The SAGE Handbook of Innovation in Social Research Methods* (pp. 205–227). London, UK: SAGE Publications. doi:10.4135/9781446268261.

Charmaz, K. (1983). Loss of self: A fundamental form of suffering in the chronically ill. *Sociology of Health & Illness*, 5: 168–195. doi:10.1111/1467-9566.ep10491512.

Charmaz, K. (2014). *Constructing Grounded Theory* (2nd ed.). Thousand Oaks, CA: Sage.

Charmaz, K. (2016). The power of constructivist grounded theory for critical inquiry. *Qualitative Inquiry*, *23*(1), 34–45. doi:10.1177/1077800416657105.

Corbin, J., & Strauss, A. (2008). *Basics of Qualitative Research* (3rd ed.)*: Techniques and Procedures for Developing Grounded Theory* Thousand Oaks, CA: Sage. doi:10.4135/9781452230153.

Giddens, A. (1986). *The Constitution of Society: Outline of the Theory of Structuration*. Cambridge, UK: Polity.

Glaser, B. G. (1978). *Theoretical Sensitivity: Advances in the Methodology of Grounded Theory*. Mill Valley, CA: Sociology Press.

Glaser, B. G. (1992). *Emergence Versus Forcing: Basics of Grounded Theory Analysis*. Mill Valley, CA: Sociology Press.

Glaser, B. G., & Strauss, A. L. (1965). *Awareness of Dying*. New Brunswick, NJ: Aldine.

Hillman, A., Donelly, M., Dew, A., Stancliffe, R. J., Whitaker, L., Knox, M., Shelley, K., & Parmenter, T. R. (2013). The dynamics of support over time in the intentional support networks of nine people with intellectual disability. *Disability & Society*, *28*(7), 922–936. doi:10.1080/09687599.2012.741515.

House, J. S., Landis, K. R., & Umberson, D. (1988). Social relationships and health. *Science (New York, N.Y.)*, *241*(4865), 540–545.

Petner-Arrey, J., Howell-Moneta, A., & Lysaght, R. (2015). Facilitating employment opportunities for adults with intellectual and developmental disability through parents and social networks. *Disability and Rehabilitation*, 1–7. doi:10.3109/09638288.2015.1061605.

Roll, A. E., & Bowers, B. J. (2019). Building and connecting: Family strategies for developing social support networks for adults with down syndrome. *Journal of Family Nursing*. doi:10.1177/1074840718823578.

Strauss, A. L. (1987). *Qualitative Analysis for Social Scientists*. New York: Cambridge University Press. doi:10.1017/CBO9780511557842.

Strauss, A. L., & Corbin, J. M. (1998). *Basics of Qualitative Research: Techniques and Procedures for Developing Grounded Theory*. Thousand Oaks: Sage Publications.

Strauss, A., & Corbin, J. M. (1990). *Basics of Qualitative Research: Grounded Theory Procedures and Techniques*. Thousand Oaks, CA: Sage Publications.

Valente, T. W. (2010). *Social Networks and Health. Models, Methods and Application*. Oxford, UK: Oxford University Press.

16

The Importance of Social Support in the Rehabilitation of Female Bariatric Surgery Patients: Lessons Learned from Qualitative Inquiry

Jennifer Paff Ogle, Juyeon Park and Mary Lynn Damhorst

CONTENTS

Selected excerpts from this book chapter were previously published in the following work:
Ogle, J. P., Park, J., Damhorst, M.L. and Bradley, L. A. (2016). Social Support for Women Who have Undergone Bariatric Surgery. Qualitative Health Research, 26(2), pp. 176–193.

Introduction

Bariatric surgery represents a major medical procedure that requires a significant rehabilitation process, including considerable post-surgery lifestyle modifications. This rehabilitation process includes adhering to a strict dietary regimen (van Hout et al. 2006) and learning to manage new interpersonal situations (Sogg and Gorman 2008) whilst adjusting to dramatic weight loss. The experience of bariatric surgery also is often characterised by stress and anxiety (Shiri et al. 2007). As bariatric patients navigate the surgery and rehabilitation process, they may experience stresses such as physiological problems, psychological challenges (e.g., fear of dying, depression), difficulties maintaining post-surgery diet and physical activity routines, interpersonal challenges (e.g., social isolation, divorce, shifts in social circles, jealousy over weight loss), and body image concerns (Ogden et al. 2006; van Hout et al. 2006).

In this chapter, we examine the value of qualitative inquiry in lending understanding about the role of *social support* in helping women to negotiate the stresses encountered along the bariatric surgery journey, including the rehabilitation process. To this end, we explore stories shared and lessons learned from our own in-depth interviews with 13 women who had undergone bariatric surgery (Ogle et al. 2016). To set a context for this discussion, we first consider the concept of social support and the ways in which qualitative research can be employed to '[reach] the parts other methods cannot reach' (Pope and Mays 1995, p. 42).

Setting the Context

Social Support for Bariatric Surgery Patients

Social support refers to the activities and behaviours that people undertake to help others facing demanding circumstances to reach personal goals and/or to navigate stressful situations (Tolsdorf 1976). Social support fosters self-acceptance and self-esteem and fulfils needs for warmth, intimacy, and interpersonal communication (Albrecht and Adelman 1987). Four forms of social support are commonly discussed within the literature: emotional/affective, informational, instrumental, and companionship (Bambina 2007). *Emotional/affective* support includes demonstrations of care, concern, love, reassurance, sympathy, and empathy. *Informational* support entails disseminating facts or direction/counsel that may assist someone to address a circumstance or problem by enriching his/her understanding of the circumstance or problem and/or by suggesting resolutions to the problem (Bambina 2007; Thoits 2011). *Instrumental* support comprises offering behavioural or material aid with everyday tasks or problems, thus providing individuals more time and resources to release themselves from everyday responsibilities when they are facing a distressing situation in their lives (Bambina 2007; Thoits 2011). Lastly, *companionship* support involves participating in or sharing of daily activities and thoughts with others.

Thoits (2011) has suggested that, in health contexts, social support is offered to distressed individuals by two categories of persons: primary group members and secondary group members. Primary group members are significant others who lack first-hand experience with the stressor that is provoking anxiety in a distraught individual. Secondary group members are individuals in a distressed person's social network who share first-hand experience with the stressor at hand. According to Thoits, different group members are poised to provide differing forms of support to distressed individuals. Primary group members are best positioned to offer demonstrations of care and to provide practical aid, whereas secondary group members are best suited to offer empathic understanding, to provide information/guidance, and to serve as role models. Support persons who concurrently occupy primary and secondary roles – that is, significant others who are similar experientially to the distressed individual relative to the given stressor – are particularly well-positioned to offer effective support to a distressed individual.

Findings from existing work suggest that social support can promote positive surgery experiences and outcomes amongst individuals who undergo bariatric surgery. For example, Vishne et al. (2004) identified a correlation between perceptions of social support and satisfaction with bariatric surgery outcomes (Vishne et al. 2004). Several other studies provide support for a positive correlation between support group participation and post-operative weight loss (Elakkary et al. 2006; Orth et al. 2008; Song et al. 2008). Further, in response to open-ended questionnaire items, bariatric patients have emphasised the value of support group involvement in assisting them to cope with the difficulty of adjusting to a new dietary routine post-surgery (Hafner et al. 1991). Prior to our qualitative inquiry (Ogle et al. 2016), however, understanding about *how* social support operates in the lives of bariatric patients to promote well-being and positive rehabilitation outcomes was limited.

Qualitative Methods as Means to Uncover the 'Parts Other Methods Cannot Reach'

Qualitative research is grounded in interpretive philosophical traditions that insist on the importance of understanding the perspectives of the people involved and the meanings that individuals ascribe to lived experiences and to human or social problems (Creswell 2013; Pope et al. 2002; Pope and Mays 2006). Generally speaking, qualitative research seeks *understanding* rather than *quantification*[1] of social phenomena, adopting analytical categories to characterise such phenomena (Pope et al. 2006). Because qualitative research brings to the fore the viewpoints of people with healthcare concerns, it is especially valuable for gaining understanding about support-related care and interactions, including what support and interactions mean to patients, what patients gain from them, and what patients find frustrating about them (Grypdonck 2005).

In-depth interviews – the data collection approach we adopted in our study of female bariatric patients (Ogle et al. 2016) – can be particularly useful in exploring experiences of care and support because they allow researchers to gain richness of understanding about issues and experiences. Because in-depth interviews emphasise people's 'own words' rather than researcher-generated categories and terms, interviews 'give voice' to people under study and can reveal issues unanticipated by the researchers (Pope et al. 2002; Sofaer 1999, p. 1105). In-depth interviews also are especially apt for highlighting the perspectives of those whose voices are rarely heard (Sofaer 1999), including marginalised populations such as individuals who are overweight or obese and who seek bariatric surgery.

[1] Because sampling strategies used with qualitative approaches do not seek to identify a statistically representative group of participants, even expressing findings in terms of relative frequencies may be misleading. In some instances, however, simple counts may be reported (Pope, Ziebland, and Mays 2006).

Although qualitative methods often are associated with the development of new theory or models, they also can be particularly valuable in the refinement of existing theory in that they may move inquiry beyond description towards meaningful explanation that is not wedded to *a priori* understanding (Anderson-Hudson and Ozanne 1988; Creswell 2013; Pope et al. 2002; Sofaer 1999). With our qualitative approach, we were able to expand existing theoretical understanding of social support for bariatric patients by generating detailed descriptions of the interactions amongst patients and supporters as reported by patients. The 'stories and details of people's lives' are an avenue to understanding (Seidman 2006, p. 1).

Social Support and the Rehabilitation of Female Bariatric Patients

Themes and Theoretical Insights from Participant Accounts

We recruited our 13 participants from a bariatric surgery support group. The support group was sponsored by a university hospital system located in a mid-sized city in the western United States. Each support group session was facilitated by a certified bariatric nurse. We limited participation in the study to women who had undergone surgery within the past 36 months. This ensured that participants' recollections of the surgery experience would be readily accessible. We opted to focus upon women's experiences of bariatric surgery because more than 80% of those who seek bariatric surgery procedures are female (Farinholt et al. 2013).

Participants in the study ranged in age from 26 years to 66 years, but most were middle-aged (mean = 53 years). One participant identified as 'Hispanic', the remaining participants described themselves as 'white' or 'Caucasian'. Nine participants were married, the others were not romantically involved at the time of the research. Three participants noted that their close family members had undergone bariatric surgery before their own procedures; many others were acquainted with people who had undergone bariatric surgery prior to their own procedures.

We adopted an in-depth, semi-structured approach for the interviewing process (Merriam and Tisdell 2015), with each interview lasting between 1 hour and 3 hours. We drew from the grounded theory tradition, shifting back and forth between data collection and analysis in a non-linear, iterative process of constant comparison (Corbin and Strauss 2008; Creswell 2013). Emergent design is a common feature of this iterative process, making the conduct of interviews a fluid process. Although research and interview questions were carefully pre-planned and strongly grounded in previous literature, interaction with the first few participants alerted the researchers to new issues and ideas that were then incorporated in the remaining interviews. Thus, analysis began early in the data collection process and expanded throughout the remainder of the study.

In addition, analytic categories and themes were allowed to emerge from the data rather than being determined only through *a priori* theory and research findings. Thus, analyses were used to confirm or support previous research and theory as well as to move understanding forward with new understandings (Merriam and Tisdell 2015). To this end, the interviews and analyses were undertaken in an inductive, reflexive process in which we continually worked to avoid clinging blindly to previous work whilst also building on an array of previous work to deepen understanding and to formulate a comprehensible accounting of the data (Hibbert et al. 2014; Merriam and Tisdell 2015).

We organised the following discussion around key themes/findings that emerged from our analyses. Throughout the discussion, we use pseudonyms to refer to participants and incorporate references to prior work that illuminate or support our interpretations of the data.

The Importance of Support and the Varied Others Who Provided It

Analyses revealed that participants' experiences of bariatric surgery were marked by both triumphs and trials. In confronting the challenges encountered throughout the bariatric journey, participants regarded social support as essential:

> '[Social support] is important; I mean you've got to have that support. I couldn't imagine going through this by myself. And there's times...that you want to beat your head up against the wall, you want to fall down and stop and cry. And I've done all that stuff. Um, but I've always had someone there to help pick me back up' (Marilyn). (Ogle et al. 2016, p. 179)

Analyses also elucidated the kinds of interactions that participants experienced as supportive as well as 'the who' of those interactions (Ogle et al. 2016, p. 179). All participants noted that they gained support from an assemblage of people in their lives. Although, in some cases, there was overlap in the forms of support offered by various supporters, most frequently, the forms of support provided to participants differed across supporters' social locations. This finding confirmed Thoits's (2011) proposition that different groups of supporters specialise in providing various forms of support to distraught individuals. Consistent with Thoits's conceptualisation, participants received support from 'close others' (i.e., primary group members such as spouses, family members, and friends) as well as 'like others' (i.e., secondary group members such as other bariatric patients). Social support provided by close others reflected the 'emotional intimacy and physical proximity' that these individuals shared with participants (Ogle et al. 2016, p. 184), whereas support provided by like others often was provided within the context of the support group and revealed empathic understanding of participants' lived experiences of the bariatric journey. Additionally, our work expands Thoits' conceptualisation by recognising a third group of supporters – health professionals – who cannot readily be categorised as 'primary' or 'secondary' group members. Absent 'the emotional and proximal bonds' of primary group members and the first-hand experiences of secondary group members (Ogle et al. 2016, p. 179; Thoits 2011), the social support provided to participants by health professionals was informed primarily by their professional experiences, including the competence and sensitivities they had developed over the years.

Types of Support Provided

A chief contribution of our findings is data that allow deeper understanding of *how* supporters provided support, as seen through the eyes of participants. Supporters were described as:

1. Assuaging participants' uncertainty and anxiety,
2. Serving as role models and companions for participants,

3. Nurturing participants' sense of mattering, and
4. Relieving participants of everyday responsibilities during a stressful stage in their lives.

Assuaging Uncertainty and Anxiety

Throughout their narratives, participants expressed uncertainty and anxiety they had experienced during the bariatric journey. Prior work has established that social support may temper uncertainty about health conditions (Albrecht and Adelman 1987; Thoits 1983), and this was clearly borne out within our sample. Participants articulated how varied others in their lives – including health professionals, like others, and close others – offered emotional/affective and informational support that appeased their uncertainty and anxiety about the surgery.

Several participants shared that health professionals offered support that helped them to navigate doubt and hesitation about the decision to undergo bariatric surgery. Health professionals did not indiscriminately endorse bariatric surgery over other means of weight loss, but empowered participants to make decisions about the surgery by providing them information about the health and quality of life benefits of bariatric surgery. Health professionals also offered guidance to participants about which bariatric procedure might be most well-suited for them. Additionally, surgeons granted tentative participants 'permission' to move forward with bariatric surgery as an alternative over more conventional weight loss/management strategies, which had previously been sources of frustration for participants:

> 'I was a little uncertain... My newest doctor, he's like, "You know the definition of insanity, right? Doing the same thing over and over again and expecting a different result". I'm like, "I've tried Jenny Craig, Weight Watchers... all sorts of different things". And, he's like, "You need, you need to look at this [surgery], and you need to accept it for what it is, and if you want to live you know past 45, then this is what you're going to need to do"' (Marilyn). (Ogle et al. 2016, p. 180)

Exchanges with like others within the context of the support group also worked to alleviate participants' insecurities and concerns as they made various deliberations about the surgery. Like others dispensed advice to participants about different surgeons and medical facilities, advantages and disadvantages of various bariatric procedures, and insurance/Medicare coverage of bariatric surgery. This guidance was valued because it represented first-hand perspectives from individuals who had recently navigated the bariatric journey and gave participants increased confidence in their decision-making processes.

Even after committing to the surgery, participants harboured varied concerns and anxieties about the surgery, itself, and the lifestyle changes that would necessarily follow. As the surgery approached, participants sought and received social support from like others, close others, and health professionals that served to soothe this distress. Both like others and close others offered expressions of care and reassurance, frequently providing prayers and/or a charitable listening ear. Whereas like others were well-positioned to offer empathic understanding that resonated with participants facing concerns, the support offered by close others was especially valued because of the strong (relational) ties they shared with participants:

> 'I started going to support group eight months before the surgery and those women and men are absolutely incredible. I got three emails the night before I went into surgery... Two days before [the surgery], I ran into one of the girls at [the grocery store], and she asked if she could pray with me and gave me a little pep talk....They have been incredible, so that took my nerves totally down to a manageable level, I felt like I was going in [to the surgery] with an armful of people who had already been there' (Aurora). (Ogle et al. 2016, p. 182)

> '[My husband] and I, we're just really close, so just every day, we talked about [the surgery]...We'd be like, "Now what are we going to do when I have this surgery?"...I was hooked on Diet Pepsi. [After the surgery], there's absolutely no carbonated drinks, ever...I'd sit there and say, "I don't think I can do it". And, he'd be like, "Yeah, but is it worth not having a Diet Pepsi?"...So, it did take me several months working with [my husband], mostly' (Betty). (Ogle et al. 2016, p. 185)

Health professionals allayed participants' pre-surgery apprehensions by listening closely to participants, recognising the legitimacy of their concerns, and providing reassurances and explanations:

> 'They calmed [my concerns]...The anaesthesiologist listened, and I told him how...I've had problems with the anaesthesia before, and they listened, and they wrote it down, and they took good care of me, and they really did a great job...They didn't put me under as far... I think talking to them ahead of time and letting them tell me that they were going to pay attention and stuff was good' (Connie). (Ogle et al. 2016, p. 181)

Finally, health professionals and like others provided informational support that helped to quell participants' uncertainty about physiological and psychological issues encountered post-surgery. In this vein, health professionals shared scientifically grounded knowledge with participants during support group meetings and follow-up medical appointments. Participants regarded knowledge claims dispensed by health professionals to be highly trustworthy and reliable, perceiving health professionals to be 'expert' and 'authoritative'. Much of the guidance provided by health professionals addressed how to manage the physiological problems encountered post-surgery (e.g., dumping syndrome[2]) and/or how to successfully enact the post-surgery lifestyle regimen. Additionally, psychologists helped participants anticipate potential personal and interpersonal challenges they might encounter post-surgery (e.g., addiction transference, social isolation, interpersonal difficulties), raising their awareness, and, hence, their preparedness for confronting these trials.

A wide range of knowledge also was exchanged amongst participants and like others within the support group, including what to eat at various phases of the rehabilitation process, how to navigate eating at restaurants, where to purchase reasonably priced clothing as one's body quickly changed sizes, how to surmount weight plateaus, which resources to use/consult, and how the surgery impacted others in one's life. Beyond assisting participants to manage some of the 'concrete' challenges of bariatric surgery, listening to like

[2] Dumping syndrome is frequently experienced by individuals after gastric bypass surgery and refers to the quick 'dumping' of food from the stomach pouch into the small intestine. Symptoms include abdominal cramping, fast heartbeat, lightheadedness, and diarrhea. Dumping syndrome can be prevented by avoiding the consumption of certain foods (WebMD, 2017).

others share their lived experiences with bariatric surgery helped to normalise the triumphs and trials of the surgery experience for participants:

> 'I love the support group... it's been awesome just to hear everyone's stories and talk about what their struggles are and be like, "Hey I'm like that too!" Afterward we get together and talk about it like, "How did you get through it?" "What did you do to make that stop happening?"' (Barb). (Ogle et al. 2016, p. 183)

In turn, appreciating that their lived experiences were shared by other, similarly situated individuals provided comfort and consolation to participants as they sought to cope with sometimes unfamiliar terrain of the bariatric journey.

Serving as Role Models and Companions

For participants, one of the most important functions that like others played was that of 'role models'. Observing and modelling others who have effectively negotiated a stressful situation has the capacity to positively shape the coping efforts of distressed individuals, to increase their sense of control, to foster hope within them, and to help them imagine themselves as similarly successful in the future (i.e., to assist them in striving towards a goal) (Markus and Nurius 1986; Thoits 2011). In this respect, participants frequently turned to like others as 'aspirational models' of bariatric 'success stories', invoking these stories and the experiences of like others as motivation to help move them along towards similar forms of success for themselves. For participants, 'success' was characterised in terms of evidencing weight loss or weight loss maintenance that had not been possible prior to surgery and/or witnessing post-surgery improvements in health, mobility, and/or appearance:

> 'My [close relatives, who also underwent bariatric surgery] are doing absolutely amazing, as far as what they're supposed to do. The younger one, who had diabetes, she went to her doctor a few weeks ago, and her A1C was normal, her blood pressure was normal, and she hadn't been on her meds since she had the surgery... And, they've both lost weight. They're just doing so well. That is an incentive for me to continue. I'm not losing weight as fast as they are...They're really working hard at it. Well, I am, too... they are sort of an inspiration to me because they're doing so well' (Rachel). (Ogle et al. 2016, p. 183)

Of particular interest is that Rachel turned to her family members as a source of inspiration in her bariatric journey, confirming Thoits's (2011) argument that significant others who also are positioned as like others may be especially effective in providing social support.

Participants also looked to some like others as negative role models, or 'cautionary tales' of what represents a bariatric 'misstep' or 'defeat' and what outcomes that they wished to sidestep for themselves. In this way, findings expand Thoits's (2011) framework of social support by proposing that role models are not just aspirational, but may be admonitory, as well. Thus, within our sample, participants observed how other bariatric patients had encountered various challenges – most frequently, with gaining back weight lost through surgery – and invoked the experiences of these like others to consider how they might avoid a similar fate for themselves:

> '[Bariatric surgery] is not the end all or be all of weight loss or weight gain. It's something that you use to achieve what you want to achieve. Like I said, [my relative's cousin] had

> the surgery, but she's gained almost all of her weight back because she didn't continue to use it for what it was meant to be. You have to always be aware of what you're eating, because otherwise, you will gain your weight back' (Rachel). (Ogle et al. 2016, p. 183)

Researchers have proposed that significant others may take on a companionate presence in the everyday lives of distressed individuals, providing emotional sustenance and companionship support to them (Bambina 2007; Thoits 2011). This was observed within our sample, with close others serving as 'joint collaborators' in the participants' bariatric journeys and rehabilitation processes (Ogle et al. 2016, p. 186). In the role of 'joint collaborator', close others teamed with participants in differing surgery routines to encourage, motivate, or otherwise provide support to them. For example, close others joined participants in their post-surgery diet and physical activity regimens, helped participants to navigate purchases of food and clothing, joined participants at support group meetings, and, in a few cases, even underwent surgery with participants. Owing to their intimate engagement in participants' bariatric experiences, close others shared in participants' 'journeys of progress' (see Ogle et al. 2016, p. 186):

> 'My husband would take me for walks in the park... and we increased tree by tree by tree... I had a hard time getting into walking with this...[but], he's really encouraged me... I weighed 238 pounds, I could hardly walk from one tree to the next, and we just kept increasing. About six months in, he said, and this is when I started enjoying it, he says, "I bet you can't run up that hill." And, I thought, well, I ran up the hill, and that just had such an empowering, I could run! And, I started that day, I would run from tree to tree, and walk farther, and walk and run and walk. But, he really did encourage me. That is something I will never forget' (Wanda). (Ogle et al. 2016, p. 186)

Participants were keenly appreciative of the role that close others assumed in inspiring them in their march of progress towards improved health and fitness and expanded empowerment, frequently reading close others' companionship and collaboration as testimony of their care and concern. Additionally, during her interview, Wanda suggested that her husband's involvement in her post-surgery routine expanded her sense of accountability to the routine, noting that his engagement and presence made her sense that she was part of something 'bigger than' herself (cf. Bambina 2007, p. 11).

Nurturing a Sense of Mattering

A sense of mattering, or the inclination to regard the self as important, arises from interpersonal interactions and has been associated with psychosocial well-being (Schieman and Taylor 2001). Accordingly, Thoits (2011) recognises lived interactions that foster perceptions of mattering as a mechanism of social support that promotes well-being and health. Throughout their narratives, participants expressed how interactions with health professionals, like others, and close others nurtured a sense of mattering within them, which in turn, served as a source of affective/emotional social support at various junctures in their bariatric journeys.

In a pre-surgery context, interactions with health professionals sometimes addressed a sense of lack within participants and reassured them that they 'mattered enough' to choose bariatric surgery. For instance, Wanda's husband was reluctant to support his wife's decision to have the surgery, owing to the cost of the procedure. The bariatric navigator at the surgery centre encouraged Wanda to continue negotiations with her husband, reminding her, 'Where there's a will, there's a way, and you are worth it'. Reflecting on this encouragement, Wanda remarked, 'And, that just really…I thought, "I am worth it"', reflecting in her the perception that she *did* matter (Ogle et al. 2016, p. 180).

As they contemplated the surgery decision, participants also received support from close others suggesting that they mattered enough to their loved ones that these significant others would embrace them, regardless of whether or not they committed to the surgery procedure:

> 'My husband was extremely supportive. He was supportive if I decided not to, and he said, "I'll be your biggest supporter if you decide to do it". …That was everything…I felt complete acceptance from him, whether or not I did the surgery…I felt like whatever choice I made, I was acceptable' (Frances). (Ogle et al. 2016, p. 184)

Frances's remark that she felt 'complete acceptance' from her husband 'whether or not' she chose to pursue the surgery reflects the protective function that a sense of mattering can serve in potentially stressful situations (Cobb 1976; Thoits 2011). Other participants, too, recalled interactions with close others that conveyed to them that they mattered, reminding these participants that their significant others were invested in them and their successes (cf. Rosenberg and McCullough 1981). For example, when her grandmother encouraged her to pursue bariatric surgery, this reinforced for Marilyn her worth as a person who deserved to engage in a behaviour that would enhance the quality of her life. And, after surgery, when close others asked how participants were 'getting along' or whether they could 'lend [them] a hand', this, too, underscored for participants that others were interested in their welfare and progress (Ogle et al. 2016, p. 184).

Exchanges with like others, particularly within the context of the support group, communicated to participants that they mattered enough to be celebrated for their accomplishments and successes (e.g., weight loss or maintenance):

> 'And in my experience, it's not common for women to celebrate each other's successes – it's almost like it's a bigger deal to discuss a person's failures or their downfall, and [the support group] is a whole group of people, and that's their whole basis of existing... is to celebrate each other's successes' (Aurora). (Ogle et al. 2016, p. 182)

Several participants shared that, prior to surgery, they had accrued relatively limited experience with being celebrated. Rather, they had frequently been targets of weight-based discrimination. As such, being applauded for their successes – especially for successes that 'rested on the surface of their bodies' – was especially significant for them (Ogle et al. 2016, p. 182).

Assisting with Practical Needs

Within our sample, participants frequently received instrumental support from close others. This is perhaps not surprising, as the provision of such aid is an expectation of those with whom we share strong relational ties (cf. Messeri et al. 1993). Instrumental support was most frequently offered to participants by spouses and family members, but when they could not assist, friends filled in as their proxies.

Participants identified two forms of instrumental support that helped them to navigate the bariatric rehabilitation process. First, close others provided help with executing the tasks of daily life during and after the surgery (e.g., food shopping and preparation, transportation to and from medical appointments, pet care), relieving the participants from everyday responsibilities throughout this stressful period in their lives (cf. Bambina 2007; Thoits 2011). Second, close others promoted positive surgery outcomes for participants by issuing gentle reminders to participants to observe their post-surgery dietary regimens. Because these reminders signified 'behavioural assistance with practical accountabilities', they constituted a form of instrumental support (Ogle et al. 2016, p. 186):

> 'I have to walk around with snacks...[Friends] have asked me, "Did you remember to, do you need to have your snack?", you know, just to remind me...You know, people have said, "Okay, you need to take a break and eat a string cheese".... So, they've been flexible...[and] understanding' (Helen). (Ogle et al. 2016, p. 186)

Participants' Desire for More or 'Better' Support

All participants in the sample shared that they received social support from a constellation of others in their lives, noting that this support promoted positive functioning for them. At the same time, however, several participants acknowledged a desire for more or perhaps 'better' support at different junctures in their bariatric journeys, reminding us that, at times, relationships constitute sources of strain or stress rather than support (Rook 1990). For example, some participants experienced opposition from others about the decision to undergo bariatric surgery. Securing support from individuals staging resistance often required negotiations, with the participants steering these interactions:

> '[My adult daughters]... weren't all on board until I kind of had a meltdown and said, "I'm not asking permission, I'm asking you to support me...This is something I have to do", and then, it turned them around... [They] started being real supportive of it' (Betty). (Ogle et al. 2016, p. 186)

Other participants experienced feelings of ambivalence and concern when they recognised that their family members' support for their decision to undergo bariatric surgery was premised upon their family members' desires for them to render their bodies more 'socially acceptable' through dramatic weight loss made possible through the surgery.

At times, participants met with opposition from close others at later points in their bariatric journeys. For example, Connie's foster children posed resistance to modifying their diets to accommodate her post-surgery regimen, which confirms prior findings that after bariatric surgery, family members sometimes struggle to adapt to lifestyle changes necessitated by the surgery (Bylund et al. 2013).

However, most frequently, participants desiring more or 'better' support voiced concerns about being misunderstood and/or being targets of misperceptions about the lived reality of bariatric surgery. For example, many participants noted that others in their lives falsely perceived that, after surgery, participants would not enjoy eating or could not go out to eat. Participants also shared that people frequently assumed that they had taken the 'easy way out' to losing weight – an assumption that participants found to be very hurtful. They also found that others did not understand their post-surgery dietary regimen, frequently proposing that participants consume foods or beverages that were not within the confines of their eating plans or harassing them for eating too little or too much. To cope with these misperceptions, participants often sought to redress confusion through edification:

> '[I have] a friend... who expressed some concerns... many of them irrational... "Oh my God, you're never going to be able to eat again!" "You're never going to be able to enjoy food again!"... I tried to explain where she had misconceptions... but... it hasn't sunk in... [I: "So, what did you do when she expressed those concerns?"] Well, I tried to educate her, but she's not, she doesn't always... listen carefully' (Helen). (Ogle et al. 2016, p. 187)

Finally, a handful of participants shared a desire for more enthusiastic or keen responses from their family members in recognition of their post-surgery triumphs (e.g., weight losses). Connie attempted to rationalise her daughter's lack of zeal or interest for her bariatric successes by positioning this reaction within the context of her daughter's personal circumstances:

> 'My one daughter has been a little more standoffish; she doesn't offer compliments unless I seek them out... it would be nice if she was a little more excited, you know. But again, I think that's more about what she's kind of going through in her personal self; she doesn't want her mom to be smaller than her, and... I totally get that' (Connie). (Ogle et al. 2016, p. 187)

Lessons Learned from Our Qualitative Inquiry and Implications for Moving Forward

Our qualitative inquiry illuminated the perspectives of largely middle-aged women who had undergone bariatric surgery within the past 36 months, with an emphasis upon the role of social support in helping them to cope with the stresses of the surgery experience and the ensuing rehabilitation process. In reflecting upon our findings – and the interpretive processes used to generate them – we evidenced several worthwhile 'lessons learned' about the value of adopting a qualitative approach to gain insights into people's healthcare concerns and to develop recommendations for patient care. It is these lessons to which we now turn our attention.

Lesson #1: Harness the Potential of Qualitative Methods to Do What They 'Do Best' in a Healthcare Context – to Identify 'What Really Matters' to Patients and to Unpack Complex Issues and Processes Related to Healthcare

Although prior work had produced limited understanding of *how* social support operates in the lives of bariatric patients to promote positive psychological and health outcomes, our findings richly characterised the forms of social support at work in participants' lives and highlighted the roles that this support played in buffering the demands of undergoing and rehabilitating from bariatric surgery. In particular, through inductive analysis of participants' narratives, we discovered that supporters: (a) assuaged participants' uncertainty and anxiety by providing information and understanding/expressions of care, (b) served as role models and companions for participants, inspiring them to forge ahead in their journeys towards improved health and fitness, (c) nurtured participants' sense of mattering through demonstrations of value and concern, and (d) relieved participants of everyday responsibilities during a stressful stage in their lives by providing instrumental aid. Thus, our work was the first to offer deep insights into the *lived* interactions that support rehabilitation from bariatric surgery. Importantly, our qualitative approach also allowed us to identify what participants found frustrating during their bariatric experience, in that many of them expressed a desire for more or better support (cf, Grypdonck 2005). Thus, findings 'fleshed out' the process of social support and the meaning of this support in participants' lives and in their rehabilitation journeys, from the perspectives of the participants, themselves.

Lesson #2: Recognise the Value of Qualitative Methods in Verifying and Complementing Existing Theory

Although qualitative methods are often associated with the development of new theory, they also present a valuable way to confirm and complement existing theory, especially when the existing theory aligns closely with patterns observed within a given qualitative data set (Corbin and Strauss 2008). Thus, although the inductively generated themes we discussed within this chapter represent the particulars of how social support unfolded in our participants' bariatric journeys, findings also indicate that types of social support identified in prior research – namely, informational, emotional/affective, instrumental, and companionship support (Bambina 2007) – functioned in participants' lives, working in diverse ways to promote their well-being. For example, informational support helped participants to proactively confront specific, potentially stress-inducing decisions and situations (e.g., the decision to pursue bariatric surgery, which bariatric procedure to choose, how to troubleshoot various post-surgery challenges). Instrumental support helped participants to complete practical, daily tasks when they were unable to do so independently. Emotional and companionship support assisted participants as they sought to address affective concerns such as anxiety about the surgery or the surgery decision and/or when others in their lives perceived that they needed encouragement, reassurance, or motivation. Thus, the talk of the participants highlighted the ways in which the support extended to them varied across the surgery experience depending on their situational support needs and confirming existing work. Overall, our findings highlighted the contextual grounding of support or the idea that, to be helpful, support provided should align with the needs triggered by the particular situation (cf, Bianco 2001).

Lesson #3: Acknowledge the Value of Qualitative Findings in Extending (or Refuting) Existing Ways of Knowing, Remain Open to New Interpretations That Do Not Strictly Cohere to *A Priori* Theory

Throughout the research process, scholars who conduct qualitative/interpretive work remain open to new information, grounding their interpretations in the data, and allowing their study to 'unfold' cooperatively with the assistance of the participants and the insights gained from the data. This is consistent with the interpretivists' assumption that one cannot possess *a priori* knowledge of participants' diverse, lived realities (Anderson-Hudson and Ozanne 1988, p. 513). Thus, although participants' accounts verified Thoits's (2011) suppositions about the support behaviours provided by close others and like others (i.e., primary and secondary others, respectively), a key contribution of our qualitative inquiry was to recognise a third group of supporters – health professionals – not included within Thoits's typology, underscoring the value of not limiting interpretations to *a priori* theoretical understandings (Pope and Mays 1995; Sofaer 1999). Although health professionals maintained weak ties with participants (Adelman et al. 1987), they nonetheless provided valuable forms of emotional/affective and informational support to them. Certainly, in some cases, support provided by like others helped participants to achieve goals similar to the support provided by health professionals (e.g., to feel encouraged, to address problems). From participants' perspectives, however, like others and health professionals brought differing forms of credibility to bear upon the support provided. In the case of the like other, credibility was built based upon experiences shared between the supporter and the participant. For the health professional, credibility was rooted in professional expertise, which produced a sense of authority and trustworthiness. Both types of credibility were valued by participants.

Our qualitative inquiry expands Thoits's framework in other ways as well. As noted, findings extend Thoits's (2011) ideas by suggesting that even role models who are not aspirational may function as social support resources, inviting productive and enriching developments in the self. Again, this finding was not anticipated, but instead, emerged unexpectedly from participants' narratives, amplifying our understanding of the ways in which role models may be invoked in the social support process.

Lesson #4: Value Qualitative Approaches for Their Capacity to Reveal Issues of Hegemony and Power and to 'Give Voice' to Those Whose Voices Have Been Marginalised in Other Contexts

As Sofaer (1999) reminds us, qualitative/interpretive methods – and in particular, in-depth interviews – are ideally suited to clarifying values/power relations and to amplifying the perspectives of the disempowered. Indeed, in their accounts, participants highlighted the ways in which issues of power operated within their social networks and were negotiated within the context of the social support provided, influencing their bariatric journeys in both positive and negative ways. Key here were issues of power that shape sociocultural understandings of what represents an acceptable body. Although Thoits (2011) acknowledges that social support may foster perceptions of mattering, our work illuminates the significance of social support in promoting a sense of mattering amongst a marginalised population such as our participants – a group of women whose bodies had at one time disrupted cultural ideals of thinness and who had therefore been targets of obesity bias and discrimination. Specifically, participants' narratives bring to the fore the way in which interactions with health professionals, like others, and close others prompted participants to feel like they *mattered*, which may have been particularly salient for participants because, as larger persons, they had frequently been recipients of the message that they *did not matter*. Thus, to be valued by others represented a departure in participants' experience and allowed them to find value in themselves and to build confidence and self-respect. Conversely, recognising that others supported participants' decision to move forward with surgery only because their bodies transgressed norms of social acceptability was associated with negative feelings about the self, leaving participants frustrated and ambivalent.

Lesson #5: Consider the Implications of Qualitative Research Findings for Evidence-Based Practice

Because qualitative methods are grounded in personalised knowledge, researchers have argued that findings from interpretive work should figure centrally in evidence-based practice, which has emerged as the standard of care within the health profession. Evidence-based practice is associated with the 'thoughtful...and judicious use of the best evidence available to develop the best [health care] practices for individual patients' (Sandelowski 2004, p. 1369). Accordingly, findings from our work may suggest practical implications for the care of bariatric patients. For instance, that so many of our participants benefitted from support received from like others and health professionals within the context of their support group prompts us to recommend that a support group model be adopted at all healthcare facilities performing bariatric procedures; prior work, as well, points to the value of the support received from such groups (Elakkary et al. 2006; Hafner et al. 1991; Orth et al. 2008; Song et al. 2008). If a given facility does not have the resources to offer a support group independently, perhaps it could join together with another facility in the area to provide such a service. Online, interactive support groups, which require further study for their impacts and effectiveness, also could enhance support systems, particularly for patients who live far distances from group facilitators/one another or who have demanding work and family schedules.

A second – and clear – implication for practice stems from our finding that some participants experienced a desire for more or 'better' support. That several of our participants felt inadequately supported implies, perhaps, that supporters of individuals seeking bariatric surgery may need direction or guidance in how they can best provide support, an observation that Linda shared within her narrative:

> 'What would be nice would be some kind of a hand-out or little booklet for your family members to read so they can say, "Well [they're] not always going to feel [their] best. There might be times they don't feel good. But be nice to them because they're in pain. Don't try to get them to eat or drink something that they're not supposed to"' (Linda). (Ogle et al. 2016, p. 189)

As Linda suggests, guidance to supporters could include distributing educational materials such as hand-outs or brochures to supporters. Alternatively, such guidance also could take shape in the form of an online resource or app, which would be broadly available to a variety of potential supporters. Ideally, the development of such resources would be informed by input from varied stakeholders – including bariatric patients, health professionals, and supporters – and could be employed as tools in diverse settings (e.g., individual or group counselling/support sessions, appointments with health professionals).

Additionally, some participants encouraged their supporters to join them at doctor's appointments and/or to attend support group meetings with them. In such contexts, accurate information was shared and supporters' misperceptions were resolved. In the following comment, Betty explains how she sought to leverage the support of health professionals to normalise her experiences of bariatric surgery for her husband, so that the couple could arrive at a mutual understanding or definition of the situation (Ball 1972), thereby relieving some of the anxiety prompted by her husband's previous misunderstandings about her surgery:

> '[My husband] has been to all of [the support group meetings]...Sometimes...he thinks I should do something better than I am...He gets on me, like, "that looks like an awful lot of pasta. Are you supposed to have that much pasta?"...But, in these meetings, he'll hear other people say things...And, I'll just kind of look like at him like.... "See? That's just how it is!"...So, when he comes with me to doctor's appointments...and to the support group, he hears. And, he hears [the doctor] say, "She's doing great. Whatever she's doing right now, let her do it how she's doing it. She's doing great". So, I think that helps [him] understand more.' (Betty)

Accordingly, when possible, support group facilitators may wish to engage members of participants' social support networks in the group's activities. In some cases, it may even be appropriate to design events or activities exclusively for members of bariatric patients' social support networks. Helping supporters to better understand the lived experiences and support needs of bariatric patients ultimately will enhance the quality of patients' rehabilitation journeys.

In conclusion, our qualitative approach to studying the role of social support in the bariatric patient experience: (a) provided nuanced and complex understanding of the effects of and needs for social support, (b) facilitated relating the data to varied theories and past work that together deepened understanding, (c) uncovered some supports not clearly identified in prior work, and (d) suggested potential ways to enhance supportive experiences for bariatric patients. As such, the accounts we collected from female bariatric patients offer an important window on the perspectives, subjective constructions, and meaning-making of these patients as they recall their lived experiences during the bariatric process.

References

Adelman, M. B., Parks, M. R. and Albrecht, T. L. (1987). Beyond close relationships: Support in weak ties. In: T. L. Albrecht and M. B. Adelman, eds., *Communicating Social Support*. Newbury Park, CA: Sage Publications, pp. 126–147.

Albrecht, T. L. and Adelman, M. B. (1987). Communicating social support: A theoretical perspective. In: T. L. Albrecht and M. B. Adelman, eds., *Communicating Social Support*. Newbury Park, CA: Sage Publications, pp. 18–39.

Anderson-Hudson, L. A. and Ozanne, J. L. (1988). Alternative ways of seeking knowledge in consumer research. *Journal of Consumer Research, 14*(4), pp. 508–521.

Ball, D. W. (1972). The definition of the situation: Some theoretical and methodological consequences of taking W.I. Thomas seriously. *Journal for Theory of Social Behaviour, 2*(1), pp. 61–82.

Bambina, A. (2007). *Online Social Support*. Youngstown, OH: Cambria Press.

Bianco, T. (2001). Social support and recovery from sport injury: Elite skiers share their experiences. *Research Quarterly for Exercise and Sports, 72*(4), pp. 376–388.

Bylund, A., Benzein, E. and Persson, C. (2013). Creating a new sense of we-ness: Family functioning in relation to gastric bypass surgery. *Bariatric Surgical Practice and Patient Care, 8*(4), pp. 152–160.

Cobb, S. (1976). Social support as a moderator of life stress. *Psychosomatic Medicine, 38*(5), pp. 300–314.

Corbin, J. and Strauss, A. (2008). *Basics of Qualitative Research*. 3rd ed. Thousand Oaks, CA: Sage.

Creswell, J.W. (2013). *Qualitative Research and Research Design: Choosing Among Five Approaches*. 3rd ed. Thousand Oaks, CA: Sage.

Elakkary, E., Elhorr, A., Aziz, F., Gazayerli, M. M. and Silva, Y. J. (2006). Do support groups play a role in weight loss after laparoscopic adjustable gastric banding? *Obesity Surgery*, 16(3), pp. 331–334.

Farinholt, G. N., Carr, A. D., Chang, E. J. and Ali, M. R. (2013). A call to arms: Obese men with more severe comorbid disease and underutilization of bariatric operations. *Surgical Endoscopy, 27*(12), pp. 4556–4563.

Grypdonck, M. H. F. (2005). Qualitative health research in the era of evidence-based practice. *Qualitative Health Research, 16*(10), pp. 1371–1385.

Hafner, R. J., Watts, J. M. and Rogers, J. (1991). Quality of life after gastric bypass for morbid obesity. *International Journal of Obesity, 15*(8), pp. 555–560.

Hibbert, P., Sillince, J., Diefencbach, T. and Cunliffe, A. (2014). relationally reflexive practice: A generative approach to theory development in qualitative research. *Organizational Research Methods, 17*(3), pp. 278–298.

Markus, H. and Nurius, P. (1986). Possible selves. *American Psychologist, 41*(9), pp. 954–969.

Merriam, S. B. and Tisdell, E. J. (2015). *Qualitative Research: A Guide to Design and Implementation.* 4th ed. San Francisco, CA: Jossey-Bass.

Messeri, P., Silverstein, M. and Litwak, E. (1993). Choosing optimal support groups: A review and formulation. *Journal of Health and Social Behavior, 34*(2), pp. 122–137.

Ogden, J., Clementi, C. and Aylwin, S. (2006). The impact of obesity surgery and the paradox of control: A qualitative study. *Psychology & Health, 21*(2), pp. 273–293.

Ogle, J. P., Park, J., Damhorst, M. L. and Bradley, L. A. (2016). Social support for women who have undergone bariatric surgery. *Qualitative Health Research, 26*(2), pp. 176–193.

Orth, W. S., Madan, A. K., Taddeucci, R. J., Coday, M. and Tichansky, D. S. (2008). Support group meeting attendance is associated with better weight loss. *Obesity Surgery, 18*(4), pp. 391–394.

Pope, C. and Mays, N. (1995). Reaching the parts other methods cannot reach: An introduction to qualitative methods in health and health services research. *British Medical Journal, 311*(6996), pp. 42–45.

Pope, C. and Mays, N. (2006). Qualitative methods in health research. In: C. Pope and N. Mays, eds., *Qualitative Research in Health Care,* 3rd ed. Malden, MA: Blackwell, pp. 1–11.

Pope, C., van Royen, P. and Baker, R., (2002). Qualitative methods in research on healthcare quality. *Quality and Safety in Health Care, 11*(2), pp.148–152.

Pope, C., Ziebland, S. and Mays, N., (2006). Analysing qualitative data. In: C. Pope and N. Mays, eds., *Qualitative Research in Health Care,* 3rd ed. Malden, MA: Blackwell, pp. 63–82.

Rook, K. (1990). Parallels in the study of social support and social strain. *Journal of Social & Clinical Psychology, 9*(1), pp. 118–132.

Rosenberg, M. and McCullough, C. B. (1981). Mattering: Inferred significance and mental health among adolescents. *Research in Community & Mental Health, 2,* 163–182.

Sandelowski, M. (2004). Using qualitative research. *Qualitative Health Research, 14*(10), pp. 1366–1386.

Schieman, S. and Taylor, J. (2001). Statuses, roles, and the sense of mattering. *Sociological Perspectives, 44*(4), pp. 469–484.

Seidman, L. (2006). *Interviewing as qualitative research: A guide for research in education and the social sciences.* New York: Teachers College Press.

Shiri, S., Gurevich, T., Feintuch, U. and Beglaibter, N. (2007). Positive psychological impact of bariatric surgery. *Obesity Surgery, 17*(5), pp. 663–668.

Sofaer, S. (1999). Qualitative methods: What are they and why use them? *Health Services Research, 34*(5, Pt. 2), pp. 1101–1118.

Sogg, S. and Gorman, M. J. (2008). Interpersonal changes and challenges after weight-loss surgery. *Primary Psychiatry, 15*(8), pp. 61–66.

Song, Z., Reinhardt, K., Buzdon, M. and Liao, P. (2008). Association between support group attendance and weight loss after Roux-en-Y gastric bypass. *Surgery for Obesity and Related Diseases, 4*(2), pp. 100–103.

Thoits, P. A. (1983). Main and interactive effects of social support: Response to LaRocco. *Journal of Health and Social Behavior, 24*(1), pp. 92–95.

Thoits, P. A. (2011). Mechanisms linking social ties and support to physical and mental health. *Journal of Health and Social Behavior, 52*(2), pp. 145–161.

Tolsdorf, C. C. (1976). Social networks, support, and coping: Exploratory study. *Family Process, 15*(4), pp. 407–417.

van Hout, G. C. M., Boekestein, P., Fortuin, F. A. M., Pelle, A. J. M. and van Heck, G. L. (2006). Psychosocial functioning following bariatric surgery. *Obesity Surgery, 16*(6), pp. 787–794.

Vishne, T. H., Ramadan, E., Alper, D., Avraham, Z., Seror, D. and Dreznik, Z. (2004). Long-term follow-up and factors influencing success of Silastic vertical gastroplasty. *Digestive Surgery, 21*(2), pp. 134–141.

WebMD. (2017). Dumping Syndrome. Available at: https://www.webmd.com/digestive-disorders/dumping-syndrome-causes-foods-treatments#1 (Accessed 20 December 2017).

17

Qualitative Research on Caregiving Outcomes

Shilpa Krishnan, Monique R. Pappadis and Timothy A. Reistetter

CONTENTS

Introduction

Each year, around 44 million Americans provide 37 billion hours of unpaid informal care for adults or children with chronic conditions (National Alliance for Caregiving and American Association of Retired Persons [AARP] Public Policy Institute 2015). Caring for a loved one can be a deeply rewarding experience, as individuals come closer to each other at a time of adversity. However, caregiving is also physically and emotionally demanding (Krishnan et al. 2017b). It is not a surprise that caregiving is an international need. Informal caregivers play a very important role in managing the health of individual who needs assistance. An informal caregiver is usually a spouse, partner, family member, neighbour, or friend. Informal caregivers usually are not paid for the services they provide to their loved one needing assistance. Informal caregiving involves a range of services such as assistance with activities of daily living and instrumental activities of daily living. In contrast, formal caregivers are those who are paid for their services (e.g., nurse practitioner). In this chapter we use the terminology 'caregivers' to describe informal caregivers.

Qualitative research provides us with rich narrative data on an individual's behaviour, experiences, perspectives, beliefs, values, or motivation in a given situation. The first section of this chapter focuses on the role of caregivers in patient-centred care. The second section describes the methods, data collection processes, and analyses used in qualitative and mixed methods research to explore caregiver outcomes.

Role of Caregivers in Patient-Centred Care

Patient-centered care is a multistage process, and incorporating the caregiver's needs and perspectives is part of this process (Gillick 2013). Including caregivers in the patient's continuum of care will strengthen the relationship of the patient and the caregiver and also empower caregivers to continue with their caregiving duties. A qualitative study exploring mobility outcome preferences of stroke survivors from the caregiver's perspectives revealed that stroke survivors and their caregivers differ in their outcome preferences (Krishnan et al. 2018). Caregivers were more often concerned for the stroke survivor's safety, wanted to prevent falls, and have appropriate home modifications. Caregivers provide the first source of information on the patient's health history, abilities, and needs. In spite of this, informal caregivers are usually marginalised by the healthcare system.

Caring for a Seriously Ill Patient

Critically ill individuals may not be able to make their own healthcare decisions. In such instances, their caregivers take on an additional role as a substitute decision maker. The frequency, intensity, and duration of caregiving increases whilst caring for a seriously ill patient, e.g., multiple chronic conditions, end of life, dementia, or Alzheimer's disease (Schulz et al. 2018). These caregivers may also have the power of attorney that gives them legal power to make healthcare decisions for their loved one. The interactions and communications between family and heath care providers, also known as *therapeutic alliance*, must begin before formal end-of-life conversations. Qualitative methods have been utilised to strengthen the therapeutic alliance and identify the facilitators and barriers to establishing such alliance early on, with family members caring for critically ill individuals (Kalocsai et al. 2018).

Qualitative research can also be utilised to perform a program evaluation, e.g., test the feasibility and effectiveness of a program from the caregivers' perspectives. Healthcare professionals and policymakers will routinely want information on the sustainability, feasibility, and utility of an intervention or program to understand whether it ultimately benefits patients. Engaging caregivers in the program evaluation process provides a unique perspective for clinicians to assess the healthcare service delivery. For instance, Boucher (2018) engaged caregivers through focus group interviews and face-to-face semi-structured interviews to understand the acceptability of a community-based palliative program (Boucher et al. 2018). Boucher's study noted that some informal caregivers expressed positive feelings related to acceptability of the new community-based palliative care service. A wife of a 72-year-old male patient mentioned,

> I don't feel embarrassed to share feelings with them, because they understand it, and they're very good listeners and that's very important. I think that's lacking in our medical delivery system and it's not lacking here.

However, some informal caregivers were fearful to accept the community-based palliative care service, as they perceived that this service would inhibit their loved one's access to necessary medical services.

Collective Caregiving in Hospice Setting

Hospice care provides supportive and palliative care during the end of life for patients with terminal illness or injury. Use of hospice care is associated with better pain control, improved patient satisfaction, and decreased hospital and ICU mortality (Kleinpell et al. 2016). Family members of patients receiving hospice care report greater satisfaction and improved caregiver outcomes compared to other settings of care (Teno et al. 2004). There has been an increase in the number of studies using qualitative approaches to explore the perceptions and experiences of patients of hospice and their caregivers. A qualitative study explored the knowledge and perception of hospice care, barriers to hospice enrolment, and the preferences to improve access and knowledge amongst patients with metastatic cancer and their caregivers (El-Jawahri et al. 2017). Using semi-structured interviews provided an in-depth look at the perceived barriers of caregivers to using hospice care, e.g., fear of outcomes (*Maybe there is a false sense of security that everything is okay as long as they stay out of hospice*), dealing with the guilt of perceived abandonment (*I think every family strives to provide the services the patient needs because they feel a sense of abandoning the patient if they dole that off on someone else*), and lack of understanding the role of hospice care.

Caregiving Preparedness

The process of caregiving usually involves a steep learning curve. Informal caregivers are not usually prepared to provide caregiving services. The role of informal caregivers is not static, but continually changes depending upon the need of the patient. Sometimes a caregiver is a 'tech support', 'friend', 'chef', 'house cleaner', 'advocate', or 'healthcare provider'. Given the multifaceted process of caregiving, it is important to provide education and training to caregivers based on their current needs. Qualitative methods can be used to assess the knowledge of caregivers to carry out complex caregiving activities such as medical procedures, personal care, medication management, or care coordination tasks. For instance, an exploratory qualitative study sought to understand the support needs of 15 caregivers for home mechanical ventilation safety from the healthcare team (Schaepe and Ewers 2018). This study revealed that the caregivers anticipated knowledge and skills from healthcare professionals for various strategies, especially when the providers were not available (e.g., changing a tracheostomy tube). Caregivers mostly felt unprepared and did not know what to do during emergency.

Caregivers' Relationships

Caregivers caring for their loved one may have complicated relationships. Separately considering the views of individuals and their caregivers who experience a change together may not provide a holistic view of the disease and rehabilitation process. A narrative approach where the patient and caregiver provide the shared life story will help address the ambiguity, especially amongst spousal caregivers (Riekkola Carabante et al. 2017). Spousal caregivers often feel lonely and often experience a reduced connection with their existing social networks. The complexity of social interactions increases because of the their loved one's changed behaviour. The information from qualitative studies will help rehabilitation professionals develop programs for caregivers as they incorporate support from their social network.

Developing, evaluating, and providing accessibility to dyadic interventions that incorporates both the individuals' relationship and their shared identity will promote a healthy relationship amongst caregivers and those they care for (Kitwood and Bredin 1992). A qualitative study assessed the feasibility of a therapeutic community-based group intervention using semi-structured interviews by incorporating the perspectives of 12 dyads (Clark et al. 2018). The dyadic intervention helped caregivers develop empathetic relationships and enhanced the personal relationships with their loved ones. In addition, the caregivers also developed new social networks and friendships with other caregivers in their community group.

Cultural Differences in Caregiving

Racial and ethnic minority caregivers provide more care to their loved ones compared to non-Hispanic whites. This is partly because minority caregivers are less likely to use formal services. Caregiving needs and experiences significantly differ among various ethnic backgrounds. A qualitative study explored the experiences amongst caregivers from different ethnic groups based on their cultural values and beliefs (Pharr et al. 2014). Pharr's study included 35 caregivers from various ethinicities including European Americans, Asian Americans, Hispanic Americans, and African Americans. The results of their study revealed that caregiving was considered very natural amongst some cultural groups, where carers assumed caregiving to be their responsibility. Pharr's study also revealed that women and younger adults usually adopt the responsibility of caregiving among some ethnic groups. Another qualitative study revealed that Korean caregivers do not have adequate knowledge and understanding of the disease process (e.g., demetia), which restricts them from seeking out supportive services (Richardson et al. 2017).

Culture not only includes race/ethnicity, but also sexual or gender orientation, rurality, religion, language, and other characteristics and norms of a particular group of individuals. Qualitative studies have identified sexual and gender minority caregivers experiencing sexual and gender prejudice, have valued friends or community members as their families choice for support. This cohort's needs often go unrecognised, and they value the importance of acknowledging the diversity within their cultural group (Washington et al. 2015). Rurality could also affect patients' access to services and caregivers' need for support services. Caregivers of stroke survivors living in rural areas described less family support across the care continuum (Cameron et al. 2013). Several studies have used qualitative methods to develop, culturally adapt, or improve health programs to reach caregivers and patients living in rural areas (Danzl et al. 2013, Cherry et al. 2017, Dionne-Odom et al. 2018). Spendelow et al. (2017) identified several coping strategies exhibited by male carers that ranged from 'finding meaning and purpose' in life to exhibiting a masculine gender role identity by 'promoting the association of traditional masculinity' with caring (Spendelow et al. 2017).

Caregivers Caring for Multiple Individuals, 'Sandwich Generation'

A significant proportion of caregivers care for multiple individuals. The 'sandwich generation' refers to those middle-aged caregivers who care for their parents whilst raising a child below 18 years old or supporting an adult child (Parker and Patten 2013). Adults younger than 40 years and Hispanics are more likely to be included in this cohort. Sandwich generation caregivers are more likely than other caregivers to be stressed, be pressed for time, and face economic and financial burden.

Around 60 percent of informal caregivers hold either full- or part-time jobs (Family Caregiver Alliance 2016). The burden of caregiving usually strains the informal caregiver's work environment. A qualitative study exploring the impact of caregiving on 'sandwich generation' caring for older adults with osteoarthritis revealed that these caregivers often find it challenging to balance their work duties and dual caregiving responsibilities (Barker et al. 2017). These caregivers are more likely to have missed time from work and have inadequate productivity. Paid leave is short, usually less than 1 month, and caregivers find it challenging to balance their responsibilities at work with their caregiving duties.

Caregiving Burden

Caregivers are at an increased risk for behavioural health and other health-related problems (Haines et al. 2015). In addition to providing patient care, informal caregivers need support themselves. Caregiving can be time consuming, physically demanding, and emotionally stressful (Krishnan et al. 2017b). Although caregivers face a huge economic and financial burden (Ferrell and Kravitz 2017), their needs are not fully assessed. Qualitative research methodology provides a way to capture and assess the burden and needs of caregivers. It is important to effectively screen caregivers to ensure that they do not harm the patient for whom they provide care.

Respite services provide caregivers a temporary break in their caregiving activities, which can significantly reduce their physical and emotional burden. To understand the feasibility of respite care, a qualitative study interviewed 24 Scottish caregivers' on their communication experiences with respite care staff. Researchers were interested in the caregivers' perceptions of barriers with the facilitators whilst sharing information about the older adult they care for and the most effective modes of sharing relevant information (McSwiggan et al. 2017). McSwiggan's study revealed a delay in receiving information on respite care services and eligibility to receive these services.

Qualitative and Mixed Methods to Explore Caregiver Outcomes

Guidelines for Reporting Qualitative Research

The consolidated guidelines for reporting qualitative studies guideline includes a 32-item checklist designed to promote transparent reporting of qualitative studies (Tong et al. 2007). A qualitative study sought to understand the interactions of informal caregivers with primary care healthcare providers in the decision-making process within the primary care team caring for chronically ill elderly patients (Doekhie et al. 2018). Doekhie in her study presented a table describing the processes the study adhered to each of the 32 items. For example, whilst describing the researcher's relationship with the participants, Doekhie states,

> There was no relationship between the researcher/interviewer with the patients, informal caregivers, and 32 of the professionals. There was a relationship with six of the professionals. The researcher met these professionals during academic conferences or they were introduced to the primary researcher by colleagues of the research department for the purpose of this research project.

Data Collection Methods

Qualitative research methods include collecting, analysing, interpreting, and presenting results from a narrative. Watching what people do (participant observation) provides more in-depth information compared to listening to what they do (Bernard et al. 1984). To explore the distribution of responses across a group, one-on-one interviews should be utilised (Bernard et al. 2016). Focus groups allow the researcher to explore complex constructs and quickly gain information from multiple participants in a relatively short time (Krueger and Casey 2014). Responses in a focus group interview will not be independent, as people will feed off one another. To complement all data collection methods, field notes provide an additional rich source of data. Qualitative studies can utilise a combination of multiple data collection approaches to discover an underlying phenomenon or build a theory. Barker and Womack's studies incorporated caregivers' perspectives using multiple data collection approaches (Barker et al. 2017, Womack et al. 2018).

In qualitative research, data collection and analysis should be closely connected (Walker 2014). The researchers should have a general sense of how the data will be analysed to design a semi-structured questionnaire. Structuring the semi-structured questions and data collection methods depend upon our assumption and what we may want to acquire from the data. Let us look at an example. Informal women caregivers tend to have higher levels of depression and psychological distress compared to their male counterparts (Schoenmakers et al. 2010). To understand the differences in characteristics amongst a cohort of individuals (in this case, higher emotional distress amongst informal women caregivers), the data were collected using focus groups that included informal women caregivers.

Methodological Approach

It is important to recognise the qualitative methodological approach before deciding to conduct qualitative research. For instance, the sampling, data collection, and analysis for a study utilising a grounded theory framework will be inherently different from a study employing a discourse analysis framework.

Grounded Theory

Grounded theory is a widely used qualitative methodology that relies on the lived experiences of individuals and the social constructs that build upon these experiences (Glaser and Strauss 2017). Grounded theory is primarily inductive in nature, which means the research study is exploratory and is conducted to acquire information to build a theory. The research questions using grounded theory help explain 'how' and 'why' individuals behave a certain way in similar or different contexts. The data for grounded theory can be ethnographic (participant observation), focus group discussions, or in-depth interviews.

Womack (2018) adopted the principles of a constructivist grounded theory framework in her study of 11 occupational therapists who were routinely involved in training informal caregivers to manage the health of older adults. The constructivist grounded theory relies on making meaning of the data from the participant's experiences to generate a theoretical interpretation (Charmaz 2000). Compared to healthcare providers who follow the biomedical paradigm, rehabilitation professionals, including occupational therapists, position caregivers to play a greater role in the rehabilitation of the individual. Womack's goal was to understand the complexity of interactions of occupational therapists with informal caregivers (Womack et al. 2018). The participants recruited in this study were targeted purposefully through a LISTSERV of occupational therapists caring for older adults. The data for Womack's study were collected through two open-ended focus group interviews over 2 days and were supplemented by handwritten observation notes by the researchers and reflective memos from each participant. Grounded theory relies on multiple data collection sources for rich, empirical, and trustworthy data.

The first stages of coding in grounded theory begins with line-by-line coding (open-coding), to identify useful concepts and develop low-level categories. Womack's study utilised open-ended codes such as *caregiver caught in potentially unsafe situation* (Womack et al. 2018). Using constant comparative analysis, the data for the rest of the interviews are coded by comparing the similarities and differences between the emerging concepts. The constant comparative approach, as the name implies, involves comparing similarities and differences to trace out emerging codes and develop a theory (Hallberg 2006). Higher-level analytical categories (axial or selective coding/focused codes) are developed at later stages of the analysis by linking and associating the codes to one another. One of Womack's focused codes was *therapist is expert responsible for ensuring safety of the situation* (Womack et al. 2018). The researchers should develop and maintain a codebook of memos describing the definitions and rationale for each of the categories coded (Strauss 1987). A theoretical model is generated beginning with the analysis of the first interview and refined as emerging concepts arise from additional interviews. The model is refined using constant comparative analysis. Womack's study hypothesised a theoretical model in which occupational therapists perceive themselves as trainers of caregivers, where the occupational therapists expertise is prioritised to make healthcare and treatment decisions for older adults (Womack et al. 2018).

Content Analysis

Qualitative content analysis has several different techniques: conventional, directed, or summative (Hsieh and Shannon 2005). Conventional content analysis is a technique used to describe a phenomenon. Codes are developed from the actual text or words, and the names of categories are derived from the data. This technique is often used when there is not an *a priori* theory driving the study. Directed content analysis involves using a prior theory or hypothesis and analysing data to confirm or validate the theory or framework (Bernard et al. 2016). It is common practice to rank order the frequency of codes and use exemplars to provide a description of the codes or themes identified. Often called 'quantitative content analysis' or 'text data mining', this method can be performed using popular qualitative data analysis software, such as *NVivo, MaxDictio of MAXQDA Plus* or *Analytics*

Pro, or *ATLAS.ti*. Summative content analysis is often performed by identifying certain words or concepts, quantifying their frequency of occurrence, and then interpreting the context or meaning of the words used. Hence, content analysis is considered quantitative in nature compared to grounded theory, which is purely qualitative. Data collection in content analysis is similar to other qualitative approaches in the use of interviews, focus groups, or observations. Caregiver qualitative studies using content analysis have also included unique media forms, such as mobile apps (Grossman et al. 2018), diaries (Egerod et al. 2017), or social media (Gage-Bouchard et al. 2017).

Phenomenology

Phenomenology, based on the European philosophy, utilises personal narratives to describe the lived experience of an individual of a phenomenon, (Sokolowski 2000). This process includes using open-ended questions and avoiding the interviewers' and researchers' biases, also known as 'bracketing'. The concept of bracketing must be initiated whilst forming the research questions of the study (Bernard et al. 2016) and followed through the data collection, analysis, and interpretation stages (Chan et al. 2013). A qualitative study using the phenomenological approach adopted the principle of 'bracketing' by consciously putting aside the research team's professional background and experience in nursing and psychology, whilst probing young adults with parental multiple sclerosis on the impact of caregiving in their daily lives (Moberg et al. 2017).

Open-ended questions allow the researcher to capture individuals' ideas in their own words compared to close-ended questions (yes/no) (Cannell and Kahn 1968). A qualitative study explored the perspectives of adult children on the impact of caregiving for an individual with osteoarthritis, utilising an interpretive phenomenological approach (Barker et al. 2017). Unlike grounded theorists, phenomenologists include only data sources that might explain the phenomenon or experience (e.g., individuals who have lived through an experience). To completely describe the phenomenon, Barker's study recruited only adult children caring for parents with 'severe' osteoarthritis that caused significant levels of pain and mobility limitations. The data analysis for a study using the phenomenological approach is similar to the grounded theory (as described above), except that the researchers do not build a theoretical model (Starks and Trinidad 2007).

Framework Analysis

Framework analysis consists of five key stages: (1) familiarisation – immersing oneself in the data by listening to audio recordings, reading transcripts, studying fieldnotes, and then listing key ideas and recurrent themes; (2) identifying a thematic framework – based on the identified concepts and themes that may be applied to transcripts and refined as needed; (3) indexing – all data are read and coded according to the thematic framework, either numerically or descriptively; (4) charting – thematic references are rearranged by core themes, which may be developed by *thematic* analysis by themes across all respondents or by case for each respondent across themes; and (5) mapping and interpretation – analysing key characteristics that may be used to create a schematic diagram of the phenomenon studied (Ritchie et al. 1994). Cameron et al. (2013) used framework analysis to identify the changes in support needs of stroke family caregivers across the care continuum. Specifically, they used the "Timing it Right" framework to inform their analysis, a conceptual framework to address the need of caregivers of stroke survivors across five phases of recovery: (1) admission to acute care; (2) medical stabilisation; (3) preparing for discharge home; (4) initial adjustment to living at home; and (5) adaptation to community living (Cameron and Gignac 2008).

Framework analysis may also be used to create typologies, detect associations between concepts, and explain how, when, and why a phenomenon occurs. For example, in one study, caregiver perceptions during the end-of-life period were characterised along two axes, one which identified four caregiver-cancer patient relationships, and one involving subjective caregiving experiences made up of distinct concepts: care spontaneity, death, sympathy for patient emotions, impressions on witnessing death, and introspective reflections in bereavement (Mori et al. 2012).

Photovoice

Photovoice is a community-based participatory action research methodology that relies on the concept that the participants (e.g., caregivers) are experts on their own life (Wang et al. 1996). Participants are provided cameras to photograph events in their life related to a specific research question. Participants also provide reflections on each photograph and are asked to comment on 'why a particular situation exists', and 'what can be done to bring about a change, if needed'. This methodology incorporates a participant driven process, in which participants meet in a group to identify relevant themes depicted through the photographs and reflections. Faucher (2015) used this methodology to understand the supports and challenges perceived by caregivers caring for older adults (Faucher and Garner 2015). The results of the study (photographs) were presented in an art exhibit which was attended by stakeholders and policymakers. This is a powerful method to bring about a desirable change on a grass-roots level. Photovoice is a powerful visual methodology that can be used as a supplemental qualitative methodology. It can also be used to explore contextual factors that may serve as facilitators or barriers to an individual's or community's health.

Qualitative Analysis Software

Software applications such as *Atlas.ti* (Friese 2014), *NVivo* (Castleberry 2014), or *MAXQDA* (Saillard 2011) can be used to code qualitative data. A scoping review exploring the needs of stroke survivors from the perspectives of caregivers utilised *NVivo 10* to analyse, code, and manage the qualitative data (Krishnan et al. 2017a). Doekhie's study utilised *Atlas.ti* to analyse the qualitative interview transcripts to understand the involvement of informal caregivers with primary care providers (Doekhie et al. 2018). Schaepe's study utilised *MAXQDA 11* to explore the support needed by caregivers caring for individuals on home mechanical ventilation (Schaepe and Ewers 2018).

Meta-ethnography Aka Qualitative Meta-synthesis

Meta-ethnography is a systematic and a rigorous way to synthesise results from qualitative research studies (Noblit et al. 1988). A meta-ethnography was performed to understand the perspectives of informal caregivers caring for individuals with stroke on community healthcare services and primary care (Pindus et al. 2018). The meta-ethnography revealed the caregiver's need for communication and quality of information to enhance post-discharge care, education, and training to care for individuals with stroke. In addition, caregivers expressed their frustrations with the delay in the patient's rehabilitation therapy and lack of continuity of care following stroke hospitalisation. The meta-ethnography also revealed that involving patients and caregivers within the first year after stroke promotes self-management of the patient's condition. Meta-ethnography is powerful, as it provides potential patient- and family-centred solutions to manage the individual's health and well-being.

Quality Appraisal of Qualitative Research

Well-established guidelines proposed by Walsh and Downe (2006) or the Critical Appraisal Skills Programme (Kuper et al. 2008) can be utilised to appraise the quality of qualitative research. Systematic reviews and meta-ethnographic reviews using qualitative research have adopted these guidelines to determine the credibility of results obtained from qualitative studies (Krishnan et al. 2017a, Pindus et al. 2018). These tools assist in appraising the quality of the studies by assessing the research question, sampling, data collection approaches, analysis, interpretation, and presentation of the results.

Mixed Methods Design

Integrating and drawing inferences from more than one method to answer a single research question is known as mixed methods design. Both qualitative and quantitative methods can be used in the same research project (Creswell and Clark 2017). Methods can be combined from the same research paradigm, e.g., focus groups and observation (Morse 2009). The combination of different methods provides better understanding of the research question. Mixed methods has many advantages that include triangulation of the research results, where the weakness of one method is often counterbalanced by the strengths of the other. For instance, a study mixed both qualitative and quantitative research methods to test the feasibility of a caregiver coping program that included psycho-educative interventions (Pihet and Kipfer 2018). This mixed methods study utilised the convergent parallel design, where the quantitative and qualitative data were collected concurrently, analysed separately, and interpreted together (Creswell and Creswell 2017). Qualitative semi-structured interviews with informal caregivers were conducted to understand the impact and acceptability of the psycho-educative interventions from the perspectives of informal caregivers (Pihet and Kipfer 2018). Using qualitative methods in this study's context enhanced the knowledge of the benefits of the intervention. For example, caregivers mentioned that the group format of the intervention was significantly helpful to reduce depression amongst themselves. Evidence from the qualitative research also provides patient-centred evidence to modify or retain some parts of the intervention or the whole intervention itself. For instance, the quantitative results of Pihet's study revealed that some strategies such as 'reframing' were difficult to implement. However, the results from the qualitative interview highlighted that the 'reframing' strategy in fact enhanced the caregiver's skill to control their negative emotions. The quality of mixed methods can be evaluated by utilising established quality assessment tools such as the Health Care Practice R&D Unit Evaluation tool for mixed methods studies (Long et al. 2002) or Mixed Methods Appraisal Tool (Pace et al. 2012). A scoping review exploring the needs of stroke survivors from the caregivers' perspectives used the Mixed Methods Appraisal Tool to evaluate the quality of mixed methods (Krishnan et al. 2017a).

Future Directions

Understanding the role of caregivers and involving them in the patient's continuity of care will decrease care fragmentation and increase quality. A scoping review revealed that only a limited number of photovoice-based articles are published in rehabilitation and disability related journals (Lal et al. 2012). This could be attributed to limited knowledge of the methodology amongst rehabilitation professionals. Future work must focus on identifying the burden and needs specific to the caregiver population. Very few studies have explored the impact of caregiving on 'sandwich generations' (Barker et al. 2017). Future work using qualitative methodology must explore the needs of this cohort across various disease process and must include caregivers in designing interventions. Perceptions of the sandwich generation must also be incorporated whilst evaluating the implementation of a program or intervention in healthcare settings and communities. Caregivers of lesbian, gay, bisexual, and transgender adults have unique experiences that may be overlooked by the healthcare community (Price 2010), a goal for future research. Another understudied area involves the needs and expectations of male caregivers.

References

Barker, K. L., Minns Lowe, C. J. & Toye, F. 2017. 'It is a big thing': Exploring the impact of osteoarthritis from the perspective of adults caring for parents – The sandwich generation. *Musculoskeletal Care*, 15, 49–58.

Bernard, H. R., Killworth, P., Kronenfeld, D. & Sailer, L. 1984. The problem of informant accuracy: The validity of retrospective data. *Annual Review of Anthropology*, 13, 495–517.

Bernard, H. R., Wutich, A. & Ryan, G. W. 2016. *Analyzing Qualitative Data: Systematic Approaches*, Sage publications, Thousand Oaks, CA.

Boucher, N. A., Bull, J. H., Cross, S. H., Kirby, C., Davis, J. K. & Taylor, D. H., Jr. 2018. Patient, caregiver and taxpayer knowledge of palliative care and views on a model of community-based palliative care. *J Pain Symptom Manage*, 56(6), 951–956.

Cameron, J. I. & Gignac, M. A. 2008. 'Timing it right': A conceptual framework for addressing the support needs of family caregivers to stroke survivors from the hospital to the home. *Patient Educ Couns*, 70, 305–314.

Cameron, J. I., Naglie, G., Silver, F. L. & Gignac, M. A. 2013. Stroke family caregivers' support needs change across the care continuum: A qualitative study using the timing it right framework. *Disabil Rehabil*, 35, 315–324.

Cannell, C. F. & Kahn, R. L. 1968. Interviewing. In Peter H. Rossi, James D. Wright, and Andy B. Anderson (Eds.) *The Handbook of Social Psychology*, 2, 526–595.

Castleberry, A. 2014. NVivo 10 [software program]. Version 10. QSR International; 2012. American *Journal of Pharmaceutical Education*, 78(1), 25.

Chan, Z. C., Fung, Y.-L. & Chien, W.-T. 2013. Bracketing in phenomenology: Only undertaken in the data collection and analysis process. *The Qualitative Report*, 18, 1–9.

Charmaz, K. 2000. Grounded theory: Objectivist and constructivist methods, In Norman K. Denzin and Yvonne S. Lincoln (Eds.) *Handbook of Qualitative Research*.

Cherry, C. O., Chumbler, N. R., Richards, K., Huff, A., Wu, D., Tilghman, L. M. & Butler, A. 2017. Expanding stroke telerehabilitation services to rural veterans: A qualitative study on patient experiences using the robotic stroke therapy delivery and monitoring system program. *Disabil Rehabil Assist Technol*, 12, 21–27.

Clark, I. N., Tamplin, J. D. & Baker, F. A. 2018. Community-dwelling people living with dementia and their family caregivers experience enhanced relationships and feelings of well-being following therapeutic group singing: A qualitative thematic analysis. *Front Psychol*, 9, 1332.

Creswell, J. W. & Clark, V. L. P. 2017. *Designing and Conducting Mixed Methods Research*, Sage publications, Los Angeles, CA.

Creswell, J. W. & Creswell, J. D. 2017. *Research Design: Qualitative, Quantitative, and Mixed Methods Approaches*, Sage publications, Los Angeles, CA.

Danzl, M. M., Hunter, E. G., Campbell, S., Sylvia, V., Kuperstein, J., Maddy, K. & Harrison, A. 2013. 'Living with a ball and chain': The experience of stroke for individuals and their caregivers in rural Appalachian Kentucky. *J Rural Health*, 29, 368–382.

Dionne-Odom, J. N., Taylor, R., Rocque, G., Chambless, C., Ramsey, T., Azuero, A., Ivankova, N., Martin, M. Y. & Bakitas, M. A. 2018. Adapting an early palliative care intervention to family caregivers of persons with advanced cancer in the rural deep south: A qualitative formative evaluation. *J Pain Symptom Manage*, 55, 1519–1530.

Doekhie, K. D., Strating, M. M. H., Buljac-Samardzic, M., Van De Bovenkamp, H. M. & Paauwe, J. 2018. The different perspectives of patients, informal caregivers and professionals on patient involvement in primary care teams. A qualitative study. *Health Expect*, 21(6), 1171–1182.

Egerod, I., Andersson, A. E., Fagerdahl, A. M. & Knudsen, V. E. 2017. Images of suffering depicted in diaries of family caregivers in the acute stage of necrotising soft tissue infection: A content analysis. *Intensive Crit Care Nurs*, 41, 57–62.

El-Jawahri, A., Traeger, L., Shin, J. A., Knight, H., Mirabeau-Beale, K., Fishbein, J., Vandusen, H. H., Jackson, V. A., Volandes, A. E. & Temel, J. S. 2017. Qualitative study of patients' and caregivers' perceptions and information preferences about hospice. *J Palliat Med*, 20, 759–766.

Family Caregiver Alliance 2016. Caregiver Statistics: Work and Caregiving.

Faucher, M. A. & Garner, S. L. 2015. A method comparison of photovoice and content analysis: Research examining challenges and supports of family caregivers. *Appl Nurs Res*, 28, 262–267.

Ferrell, B. R. & Kravitz, K. 2017. Cancer care: Supporting underserved and financially burdened family caregivers. *J Adv Pract Oncol*, 8, 494–500.

Friese, S. 2014. *Qualitative data analysis with ATLAS. ti*, Sage, Los Angeles, CA.

Gage-Bouchard, E. A., Lavalley, S., Mollica, M. & Beaupin, L. K. 2017. Cancer communication on social media: Examining how cancer caregivers use facebook for cancer-related communication. *Cancer Nurs*, 40, 332–338.

Gillick, M. R. 2013. The critical role of caregivers in achieving patient-centered care. *Jama*, 310, 575–576.

Glaser, B. G. & Strauss, A. L. 2017. *Discovery of Grounded Theory: Strategies for Qualitative Research*, Routledge, New York.

Grossman, M. R., Zak, D. K. & Zelinski, E. M. 2018. Mobile apps for caregivers of older adults: Quantitative content analysis. *JMIR Mhealth Uhealth*, 6, e162.

Haines, K. J., Denehy, L., Skinner, E. H., Warrillow, S. & Berney, S. 2015. Psychosocial outcomes in informal caregivers of the critically ill: A systematic review. *Crit Care Med*, 43, 1112–1120.

Hallberg, L. R. 2006. The 'core category' of grounded theory: Making constant comparisons. *Int J Qual Stud Health Well-Being*, 1, 141–148.

Hsieh, H.-F. & Shannon, S. E. 2005. Three approaches to qualitative content analysis. *Qualitative Health Research*, 15, 1277–1288.

Kalocsai, C., Amaral, A., Piquette, D., Walter, G., Dev, S. P., Taylor, P., Downar, J. & Gotlib Conn, L. 2018. 'It's better to have three brains working instead of one': A qualitative study of building therapeutic alliance with family members of critically ill patients. *BMC Health Serv Res*, 18, 533.

Kitwood, T. & Bredin, K. 1992. Towards a theory of dementia care: Personhood and well-being. *Ageing Soc*, 12, 269–287.

Kleinpell, R., Vasilevskis, E. E., Fogg, L. & Ely, E. W. 2016. Exploring the association of hospice care on patient experience and outcomes of care. *BMJ Support Palliat Care*, 1–6.

Krishnan, S., Pappadis, M. R., Weller, S. C., Fisher, S. R., Hay, C. C. & Reistetter, T. A. 2018. Patient-centered mobility outcome preferences according to individuals with stroke and caregivers: A qualitative analysis. *Disabil Rehabil*, 40, 1401–1409.

Krishnan, S., Pappadis, M. R., Weller, S. C., Stearnes, M., Kumar, A., Ottenbacher, K. J. & Reistetter, T. A. 2017a. Needs of stroke survivors as perceived by their caregivers: A scoping review. *Am J Phys Med Rehabil*, 96, 487–505.

Krishnan, S., York, M. K., Backus, D. & Heyn, P. C. 2017b. Coping with caregiver burnout when caring for a person with neurodegenerative disease: A guide for caregivers. *Arch Phys Med Rehabil*, 98, 805–807.

Krueger, R. A. & Casey, M. A. 2014. *Focus Groups: A Practical Guide for Applied Research*, Sage Publications, Thousand Oaks, CA.

Kuper, A., Lingard, L. & Levinson, W. 2008. Critically appraising qualitative research. *BMJ*, 337, a1035–a1035.

Lal, S., Jarus, T. & Suto, M. J. 2012. A scoping review of the Photovoice method: Implications for occupational therapy research. *Can J Occup Ther*, 79, 181–190.

Long, A., Godfrey, M., Randall, T., Brettle, A. & Grant, M. 2002. HCPRDU Evaluation tool for mixed methods studies.

McSwiggan, L. C., Marston, J., Campbell, M., Kelly, T. B. & Kroll, T. 2017. Information-sharing with respite care services for older adults: A qualitative exploration of carers' experiences. *Health Soc Care Community*, 25, 1404–1415.

Moberg, J. Y., Larsen, D. & Brodsgaard, A. 2017. Striving for balance between caring and restraint: Young adults' experiences with parental multiple sclerosis. *J Clin Nurs*, 26, 1363–1374.

Mori, H., Fukuda, R., Hayashi, A., Yamamoto, K., Misago, C. & Nakayama, T. 2012. Characteristics of caregiver perceptions of end-of-life caregiving experiences in cancer survivorship: In-depth interview study. *Psycho-oncology*, 21, 666–674.

Morse, J. M. 2009. Mixing qualitative methods. Sage Publications, Los Angeles, CA.

National Alliance for Caregiving and AARP Public Policy Institute 2015. Caregiving in the United States 2015.

Noblit, G. W., Hare, R. D. & Hare, R. 1988. *Meta-Ethnography: Synthesizing Qualitative Studies*. Sage Publications.

Pace, R., Pluye, P., Bartlett, G., Macaulay, A. C., Salsberg, J., Jagosh, J. & Seller, R. 2012. Testing the reliability and efficiency of the pilot Mixed Methods Appraisal Tool (MMAT) for systematic mixed studies review. *Int J Nurs Stud*, 49, 47–53.

Parker, K. & Patten, E. 2013. The sandwich generation. *Pew Research Center Social Demographic Trends Project RSS*, 30.

Pharr, J. R., Dodge Francis, C., Terry, C. & Clark, M. C. 2014. Culture, caregiving, and health: Exploring the influence of culture on family caregiver experiences. *ISRN Public Health*, 2014.

Pihet, S. & Kipfer, S. 2018. Coping with dementia caregiving: A mixed-methods study on feasibility and benefits of a psycho-educative group program. *BMC Geriatr*, 18, 209.

Pindus, D. M., Mullis, R., Lim, L., Wellwood, I., Rundell, A. V., Abd Aziz, N. A. & Mant, J. 2018. Stroke survivors' and informal caregivers' experiences of primary care and community healthcare services – A systematic review and meta-ethnography. *PLoS One*, 13, e0192533.

Price, E. 2010. Coming out to care: Gay and lesbian carers' experiences of dementia services. *Health Soc Care Community*, 18, 160–168.

Richardson, V. E., Fields, N., Won, S., Bradley, E., Gibson, A., Rivera, G. & Holmes, S. D. 2017. At the intersection of culture: Ethnically diverse dementia caregivers' service use. *Dementia (London)*, 1471301217721304.

Riekkola Carabante, J., Rutberg, S., Lilja, M. & Isaksson, G. 2017. Spousal caregivers' experiences of participation in everyday life when living in shifting contexts. *Scand J Occup Ther*, 1–9.
Ritchie, J. & Spencer, L. 1994. Qualitative data analysis for applied policy research by Jane Ritchie and Liz Spencer. In A. Bryman and R. G. Burgess (Eds.) *Analysing qualitative data'*, 173–194.
Saillard, E. K. 2011. Systematic versus interpretive analysis with two CAQDAS packages: NVivo and MAXQDA. Forum Qualitative Sozialforschung/Forum: Qualitative Social Research, 2011.
Schaepe, C. & Ewers, M. 2018. 'I see myself as part of the team' – Family caregivers' contribution to safety in advanced home care. *BMC Nurs*, 17, 40.
Schoenmakers, B., Buntinx, F. & Delepeleire, J. 2010. Factors determining the impact of care-giving on caregivers of elderly patients with dementia. A systematic literature review. *Maturitas*, 66, 191–200.
Schulz, R., Beach, S. R., Friedman, E. M., Martsolf, G. R., Rodakowski, J. & James, A. E., 3rd 2018. Changing structures and processes to support family caregivers of seriously ill patients. *J Palliat Med*, 21, S36–S42.
Sokolowski, R. 2000. *Introduction to Phenomenology*, Cambridge University Press.
Spendelow, J. S., Adam, L. A. & Fairhurst, B. R. 2017. Coping and adjustment in informal male carers: A systematic review of qualitative studies. *Psychol Men Masc*, 18, 134.
Starks, H. & Trinidad, S. B. 2007. Choose your method: A comparison of phenomenology, discourse analysis, and grounded theory. *Qual Health Res*, 17, 1372–1380.
Strauss, A. L. 1987. *Qualitative Analysis for Social Scientists*, Cambridge University Press.
Teno, J. M., Clarridge, B. R., Casey, V., Welch, L. C., Wetle, T., Shield, R. & Mor, V. 2004. Family perspectives on end-of-life care at the last place of care. *JAMA*, 291, 88–93.
Tong, A., Sainsbury, P. & Craig, J. 2007. Consolidated criteria for reporting qualitative research (COREQ): A 32-item checklist for interviews and focus groups. *Int J Qual Health Care*, 19, 349–357.
Walker, D.-M. 2014. *An Introduction to Health Services Research: A Practical Guide*, Sage.
Walsh, D. & Downe, S. 2006. Appraising the quality of qualitative research. *Midwifery*, 22, 108–119.
Wang, C., Burris, M. A. & Ping, X. Y. 1996. Chinese village women as visual anthropologists: A participatory approach to reaching policymakers. *Soc Sci Med*, 42, 1391–1400.
Washington, K. T., Mcelroy, J., Albright, D., Oliver, D. P., Lewis, A., Meadows, S. & Elliott, S. 2015. Experiences of sexual and gender minorities caring for adults with non-AIDS-related chronic illnesses. *Social Work Res*, 39, 71–81.
Womack, J. L., Lilja, M., Dickie, V. & Isaksson, G. 2018. Occupational Therapists' Interactions With Older Adult Caregivers: Negotiating Priorities and Expertise. *OTJR Occupation Participation Health*, 39(1), 48–55.

18

Multiple Sclerosis

Yvonne C. Learmouth

CONTENTS

Introduction

Multiple sclerosis (MS) is a non-traumatic, chronic disease, which affects the brain, brain stem, spinal cord, and optic nerves. Worldwide, the disease affects an estimated 2.5 million people, and there is epidemiological evidence of a growing prevalence of the disease (Benito-León 2011), especially among women (Sellner et al. 2011). MS is typically diagnosed between the second and fourth decade of life. The pathogenesis of MS is unknown, but is believed to be linked with multifactorial interactions between factors including: genetics and epigenetics, infection including Epstein-Barr virus, nutrition and smoking, climate and sunlight exposure, or other environmental influences (Hedström et al. 2016a, 2016b: Rhead et al. 2016; Olsson et al. 2017). The factors leading to MS result in a loss of immune homeostasis and the development of unregulated pathologic inflammatory responses directly affecting the central nervous system (CNS). Accumulated damage leads to myelin loss, axonal loss and gliosis, and progressive, often severe neurological dysfunction. The disease is complicated by a dependent relationship between neuroinflammation and neurodegeneration, and the autoimmune model of pathogenesis results in an immunotherapy approach as the primary clinical management strategy (Baranowski et al. 1997). The progressive damage to the CNS, which eventually becomes unresponsive to immunotherapy, is associated with increasing disability in MS and this underscores the need to emphasise other management strategies to counteract the decline in CNS function.

There is growing evidence to suggest that exercise is a countermeasure to the declining CNS function (Motl and Sandroff 2018) and more than two decades of evidence acknowledging the benefits, safety, and feasibility of exercise in persons with MS (Kinnett-Hopkins et al. 2017a). The most recent evidence of exercise being a countermeasure to CNS decline is based on associations between physical fitness and physical activity and exercise training affect in relation to cognitive decline (Motl and Sandroff 2018). There is growing rationale that physical fitness and exercise training represent a behavioural approach for slowing, preventing, or possibly reversing the CNS decline (Motl and Sandroff 2018). The benefits of physical activity and exercise, which include improvements in fatigue, cognition, depression, mobility disability, cardiorespiratory fitness, muscular strength and endurance, balance and gait, and improved quality of life has led to physical activity being considered one of the best therapeutic strategies for comprehensive MS care (Vollmer et al. 2012), and guidelines have been developed for physical activity in persons with MS (Latimer-Cheung et al. 2013a). The safety of physical activity is evident from a systematic review of exercise training studies in MS, where it is established that exercise is associated with a slight decrease in the risk of relapse, and that the risk of adverse events associated with exercise training is comparable with that which is reported in healthy populations (Pilutti et al. 2014b). Thus, exercise seems feasible as a powerful clinical management strategy in MS as it is: (1) a countermeasure to the declining CNS function associated with the disease, (2) a countermeasure to the physical and cognitive symptoms, and (3) a safe strategy when used appropriately.

An important 4th dimension to determining the feasibility of exercise as a clinical management strategy in MS is the acknowledgement of its use by the patient and public (Brett et al. 2014). Such evidence will emerge from qualitative interaction with persons with MS and other members of the MS community (e.g., healthcare providers). Quantitative studies report that persons with MS engage in less physical activity than the general population (Kinnett-Hopkins et al. 2017a), and this questions the feasibility of exercise as an effective management strategy. Persons with MS cannot benefit from the potential CNS protection or symptom management offered by exercise if they are not engaging. There are a number of reasons why this might be, for example:

1. Persons with MS are not aware of exercise as a management strategy for their disease.
2. Persons with MS require assistance to access exercise.
3. Persons with MS require exercise that is appropriate for them.
4. Persons with MS may require information on exercise.

The MS community (e.g., healthcare professionals) may play a role in exercise promotion. Qualitative inquiry might unlock the missing information for researchers to improve access to and improve the content of exercise interventions to allow more persons with MS to benefit from exercise. This further might help to establish if the aforementioned reasons explain exercise behaviour in persons with MS. To date, the qualitative research on exercise in MS has not been gathered and systematically reviewed. Such an endeavour is timely considering the growing acceptance and methodological underpinnings of qualitative review (Chenail 2011). This chapter offers a philosophical attempt to collectively communicate the known qualitative literature related to the topic of exercise in association with MS. The contents will allow those less versed in qualitative methodology the opportunity to incorporate the collective views and opinions of the MS community into research and clinical recommendations. This is an important undertaking considering that rehabilitation through management strategies such as exercise is considered a highly effective approach for improving outcomes in persons with MS (Kraft 1999; Vollmer et al. 2012; Coote 2014).

Within this chapter, we will first discuss review studies and the important research groups which have focussed the opinions of the MS community on the topic of physical activity and exercise. This will be followed by an in depth discussion of key areas of qualitative inquiry from original research studies which have been undertaken in persons with MS or those involved in the MS community. The chapter includes a discussion of study quality limitations with the existing research and highlights approaches which can be taken to incorporate past research results into future inquiry and clinical strategies. We highlight that physical activity and exercise are often discussed in unison within the literature, and we acknowledge that these are separate constructs (Box 18.1). Within this review we will discuss both physical activity and exercise.

BOX 18.1 DEFINITIONS OF PHYSICAL ACTIVITY, EXERCISE, AND FITNESS

Physical activity

Any bodily movement produced by contraction of skeletal muscles that results in a substantial increase in energy expenditure over resting levels

Exercise

A subset of physical activity that is planned, structured, and repetitive with the objective of improving or maintaining physical fitness

American College of Sports Medicine (2013)

Method

The systematic review was undertaken following key steps from the literature (Walsh and Downe 2005; Erwin et al. 2011; Learmonth and Motl 2016), and this allowed us to collate and understand the various themes and topics gathered through qualitative research on topics related to exercise in persons with MS. Three main steps were followed to ensure a systematic approach was taken to gathering, reviewing, and presenting the current research. Step 1 included selection and appraisal of studies and adopting the quality assessment criteria. Step 2 included gathering data and themes from the studies to allow comparison and synthesis. Finally, in step 3, the studies were appraised, and the relationships between and key finding within the studies were established.

Search Strategy

Four major research databases were searched without limit: PsycINFO, PubMed, CINAHL, and Web of Science. The key terms searched involved 'Multiple Sclerosis' AND 'Qualitative' AND 'physical activity OR exercise'. A manual search was conducted on the reference list of the included studies and by citation tracking using Google Scholar.

Inclusion and Exclusion Criteria

Original research studies and relevant review studies were included if they were written in English, examined qualitative inquiry with people with a diagnosis of MS or persons involved with persons with MS (e.g., carers or healthcare professionals of persons with MS), and examined physical activity or exercise. The original research studies had to be primarily qualitative in nature or report qualitative results as part of a mixed-methods design. If more than one study reported findings from the same research project then we included the study that reported most prevalently on physical activity and/or exercise. Review articles were included to provide a framework for which to base this chapter upon and were included if they were written in English and examined qualitative inquiry on persons with MS in relation to physical activity or exercise On identification of studies, the inclusion/exclusion criteria were applied to the abstracts of the identified studies.

Quality Assessment

To standardise our qualitative review, and further allow for critical appraisal of the relevant literature, we determined the quality of each study using the McMaster Critical review form (Letts et al. 2007a), and associated guidelines (Letts et al. 2007b), for qualitative research. The McMaster review form contains 25 items. Twenty-four items incorporate a nominal scale (Yes or No/Not assessed). The items address study background (one item), study design (three items), sampling (three items), data collection (six items), data analysis (five items), trustworthiness (five items), and conclusions (one item). The scores from the 24 items are summed, and the overall score provides a quantifiable assessment of study quality. The study design item provides descriptive information on the methodology and was not included in the scoring criteria.

Original research studies were scored based on whether each category of the McMaster Qualitative review form was met (Table 18.1). Scores of 0–24 were obtained from summation of all items, with higher scores indicating higher methodological

TABLE 18.1

Quality Assessment Scoring Criteria, adapted from McMaster Critical Review Form for Qualitative Research

Criteria	Scoring
Background	
1 Was the study purpose stated clearly?	Y/N
2 Was the relevant background literature reviewed?	Y/N
Study Design	
3a What was the design?	Not scored
3b Was a theoretical perspective identified?	Y/N
3c What method(s) were used?	Not scored
Sampling	
4a Was the process of purposeful sampling described?	Y/N
4b Was sampling done until redundancy was reached?	Y/N/NA
4c Was informed consent obtained?	Y/N/NA
Data Collection	
5a Was there clear and complete description of site?	Y/N
5b Was there clear and complete description of the participants?	Y/N
5c Was there clear and complete description of the researcher's credentials?	Y/N
5d Was there clear and complete description of the role of researcher and relationship with participants?	Y/N
5e Was there identification (bracketing) of assumptions of researcher?	Y/N
5f Was procedural rigour used in data collection strategies?	Y/N/NA
Data Analysis	
6a Was data analysis inductive?	Y/N/NA
6b Were findings consistent with and reflective of data?	Y/N
6c Was the decision trail developed and the rules reported?	Y/N/NA
6d The process of transforming data into themes/codes was described adequately?	Y/N/NA
6e Did a meaningful picture of the phenomenon under study emerge?	Y/N
Trustworthiness	
7a Was triangulation reported for sources?	Y/N
7b Was triangulation reported for methods?	Y/N
7c Was triangulation reported for researchers?	Y/N
7d Was triangulation reported for theories?	Y/N
7e Was member checking used to verify findings?	Y/N/NA
Conclusions	
8a Were the conclusions appropriate given the study methods and results?	Y/N
8b Do the findings contribute to theory development and future of practice/research?	Y/N
TOTAL (1 point for each Y response)	

Source: Letts, L. et al. *Critical Review Form - Qualitative Studies* (*Version 2.0*), McMaster University, Hamilton, Canada, 2007; *Guidelines for Critical Review Form: Qualitative Studies* (*Version 2.0*), McMaster University, Hamilton, Canada, 2007.

Note: Y; yes, N; no, NA; not assessed.

quality (Thorpe et al. 2012). There is no current literature indicating what cut-off scores are indicative of overall study quality (i.e., moderate quality or high quality), as such, we rated studies with scores of 12 or less points to be of lower quality. A similar method where higher scores indicate higher quality has been used in relevant past work (Learmonth and Motl 2016). Original studies were assessed for quality by two researchers (see Acknowledgements).

Data Gathering and Analysis

A standardised form was used to extract data from the original research studies as follows: authors, publication, year published and country of origin, study design, data collection method (i.e., individual interview or focus group) participant characteristics (i.e., sex, age (mean, SD, range) and race), clinical characteristics of participants (i.e., time since MS diagnosis (mean years, SD and range), MS type, disability level (outcome assessment used and result), mobility aid usage (where more than one aid was reportedly used, the mobility aid of higher dependency, i.e., wheelchair rather than cane, is reported) (these data were applicable for persons with MS only), information on any associated intervention, theme area (e.g., *the wider MS community, opinions on exercise associated with an exercise intervention,* and *moving when you have MS*), and description of associated intervention.

Results

The search strategy was highly specific and yielded a total of 161 studies (Figure 18.1). After removing seven duplicate studies, articles were read in full and, at this stage, 88 publications were removed, reasons for removal of studies included the following:

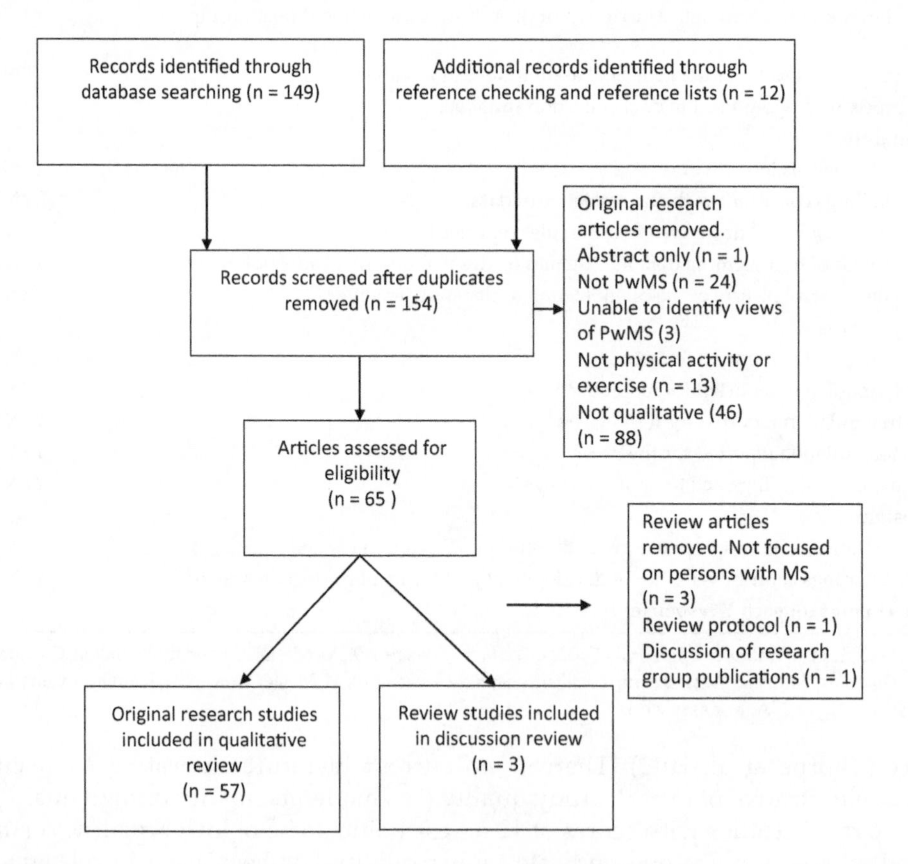

FIGURE 18.1
Literature selection process (PRISMA flow diagram). PRISMA = Preferred Reporting Items for Systematic Reviews and Meta-analyses. (From Moher, D. et al. *PLoS Med*, 151, 2009.)

studies published as abstracts only, studies not including persons with MS, views of persons with MS not being clear (e.g., when studies included views of participants with a variety of difference healthcare conditions), studies not focused on physical activity or exercise, studies not written in English, and studies not including qualitative methodology (i.e., data were not collected using interviews or focus groups). There were 65 articles of interest, and this comprised eight review articles that were of direct interest and 57 original research studies which were eligible for qualitative review.

Research Groups

It is notable that there have been key research groups around the world who have brought us much information related to the thoughts and opinions of the MS community. Research from Europe led by Professor Susan Coote has explored the views of Irish people who have MS about community exercise programmes and the design of web-based exercise interventions (Toomey and Coote 2013; Clarke and Coote 2015; Casey et al. 2016). The North America research led by Professor Robert Motl has determined a variety of topics ranging from factors important in exercise engagement, the relationship between relapse and exercise, the meaning of exercise, and the role of healthcare providers in the promotion of exercise to Americans who have MS (Dlugonski et al. 2012; Learmonth et al. 2015, 2017a, 2017b, 2018a, 2018b; Chiu et al. 2016; Kinnett-Hopkins et al. 2017a; Adamson et al. 2018). Elsewhere in North America, research led by Professors Marcia Finlayson and Matthew Plow have researched topics related to the relationships between carers and persons with MS regarding exercise, the opinions of exercise computer games (e.g., exergaming), and leaflet-based exercise interventions in Americans and Canadians with MS (Plow and Finlayson 2014; Plow et al. 2014; Fakolade et al. 2018). However one of the first, and in many researchers opinions most patient- and community-focused research groups, have produced research in New Zealand, the group originally led by Professor Leigh Hale and Dr. Cath Smith have inspired many other qualitative researchers. The research undertaken in New Zealand has gathered important data on the influence of fatigue in exercise participation, the delivery of long term community physical activity intervention, and the importance of motivation towards exercise (Smith et al. 2009, 2011, 2013a, 2013b, 2015; Mulligan et al. 2013; Hall-McMaster et al. 2016a, 2016b).

Review Articles

Eight review articles have been published on the broader topic of physical activity and/or exercise in persons with MS and which have included articles of qualitative inquiry (Hale et al. 2012; Christensen et al. 2016; Dennett et al. 2016; Learmonth and Motl 2016; Newitt et al. 2016; Ploughman 2017; Williams et al. 2017). However, only three review articles focus specifically on persons with MS (Christensen et al. 2016; Learmonth and Motl 2016; Ploughman 2017). A summary of the aim, the original studies included in the review, and outcome of these review articles are provided in Table 18.2. The review studies have been undertaken since 2016, and this reflects the overall increase in qualitative research on the topic of physical activity in MS. All three reviews aim to identify the general topics surrounding participation in physical activity and exercise in persons with MS. In two studies (Christensen et al. 2015; Learmonth and Motl 2016), the authors took a critical review of the literature, and this critical review allowed the authors to appraise the quality of the literature overall and between original studies. In the third review

TABLE 18.2

Aim, Included Articles, Summary of Finding, and Conclusions from Relevant Review Articles

Author (Date)	Aim	Included Articles	Themes	Implications for Rehabilitation/ Conclusions
Christensen et al. (2016)	To identify factors influencing the intention to exercise and the execution of exercise among persons with multiple sclerosis	9 (Borkoles et al. 2008; Kasser 2009; Plow et al. 2009; Kayes et al. 2011; Smith et al. 2011, 2013b; Dlugonski et al. 2012; Learmonth et al. 2013; Mulligan et al. 2013)	Social Support Professional support • Exercise-supporting strategies • Exercise program • Exercise setting • Professional relationships Outcome Expectations • Changes in symptoms • General well-being • Previous experiences	Social support, professional support, and outcome expectations are potential facilitators and barriers for the intention to exercise and the execution of exercise among PwMS. Health professionals specialising in MS rehabilitation can influence the intention and the execution of physical exercise among PwMS when there exists a personal and supportive patient-professional relationship. Outcome expectations may impact the motivational and volitional phases of physical exercise
Learmonth and Motl (2016)	To evidence of the perceived determinants and consequences of physical activity and exercise based on qualitative research in multiple sclerosis	19 (Dodd et al. 2006; Borkoles et al. 2008; Elsworth et al. 2009; Kasser 2009; Plow et al. 2009; Smith et al. 2009, 2011, 2013b; Schneider and Young 2010; Kayes et al. 2011; Aubrey and Demain 2012; Brown et al. 2012; Dlugonski et al. 2012; Giacobbi et al. 2012; Learmonth et al. 2013; Normann et al. 2013; VanRuymbeke and Schneider 2013; Plow and Finlayson 2014; van der Linden et al. 2014)	Consequences of physical activity and exercise participation • Beneficial consequence • Adverse consequence Perceived determinants of physical activity and exercise participation • Barriers • Facilitators	Physical activity and exercise behaviour in people with MS is subject to a number of modifiable determinants. Healthcare professionals working to promote physical activity and exercise in those with MS should choose to endorse the positive benefits of participation. Future physical activity interventions for those with MS may be improved by incorporating behavioural management strategies.

(*Continued*)

TABLE 18.2 (*Continued*)

Aim, Included Articles, Summary of Finding, and Conclusions from Relevant Review Articles

Author (Date)	Aim	Included Articles	Themes	Implications for Rehabilitation/ Conclusions
Ploughman (2017)	To consolidate the evidence examining the barriers to physical activity among people with MS, describe innovative methods to overcome barriers, whilst discussing the physical therapist's role as the physical activity promotion specialist	9 (Borkoles et al. 2008; Kayes et al. 2011; Brown et al. 2012; Dlugonski et al. 2012; Plow et al. 2014; Learmonth et al. 2015; Hall-McMaster et al. 2016b; Hundza et al. 2016; Ploughman 2017) Note the 9 included articles were discussed by the authors alongside 12 quantitative studies	Barriers • MS-related impairment and disability • Attitudes and outlook • Fatigue • Knowledge/perceived benefits of exercise • Logistical factors: finances, support, and accessibility	In order to increase levels of physical activity among people with MS in the long-term, physical therapists' reach must extend beyond the patient-provider relationship as they take on the roles of coach and community liaison. Physical therapists, other health team members, and volunteers are more likely to be successful in breaking the barriers to physical activity in MS by working together. Physical therapists employing tailored and combined approaches using tools (education, motivational interviewing, exercise practice, and problem-solving) will address a wider range of barriers concurrently.

(Ploughman 2017), the authors included both quantitative and qualitative research and no critical appraisal was undertaken.

Learmonth and Motl (2016) aimed to identify the *perceived determinants and consequences of physical activity and exercise*, and through inclusion of 19 original studies they identified *beneficial consequences, adverse consequences, barriers*, and *facilitators*. Ploughman (2017) aimed to *examine the barriers to physical activity and methods to overcome barriers*, whilst Christensen et al. (2016) aimed to *identify factors influencing the intention to exercise*.

In terms of barriers to physical activity and exercise, Learmonth and Motl (2016) categorised barriers based upon the environmental factors: the environment and social influences, and personal factors: health condition and cognitive and behavioural areas (Table 18.3). They identified that access to facilities, advice from healthcare professionals, fatigue, and fear and apprehension were some of the most important barriers. Ploughman (2017) categorised barriers from the evidence as related to: impairment/disability, attitude/outlook, fatigue, and knowledge/perceived benefits and established that MS-related impairment and disability and attitude and outlook seemed to be the more common barriers perceived by persons with MS. In terms of facilitators to physical activity and exercise, Learmonth and Motl (2016) categorised facilitators upon the same factors as for barriers (Table 18.3). They identified that the type of exercise modality, access to physical activity services, social influences, exercise appropriateness for physical capabilities, and feeling accomplished were some of the most important factors. Christensen et al. (2016) identified factors related to the intention to and execution of exercise as: professional support, social support, and outcome expectations.

Key messages from these reviews tell us of the important role healthcare professionals have in physical activity and exercise among persons with MS. For example *health professionals specialising in* MS rehabilitation can influence the intention and the execution of physical exercise among persons with MS (Christensen et al. 2016). Recommendations on how healthcare professionals can meet this end include: *endorsing the positive benefits of exercise participation* (Learmonth and Motl 2016), *take on the role of coach and community liaison, and work together with other healthcare professionals* (Ploughman 2017). The three reviews further noted the importance of increasing motivation towards exercise and provided some recommendations on strategies to achieve motivation. For example, the promotion of *outcome expectations* (Christensen et al. 2016), *incorporation of behavioural management strategies* (Learmonth and Motl 2016), and *education and motivational interviewing* (Ploughman 2017) might all result in increased participation. Finally, the reviews established that participation in physical activity and exercise is *subject to a number of modifiable determinants* (Learmonth and Motl 2016), and that a *tailored and combined approach* (Ploughman 2017) may be needed to increase participation.

Original Papers

The views of 57 different groups were included in the review of original research groups. Studies were conducted globally, and all were published in peer-reviewed rehabilitation journals between 2006 and 2018. We categorised the different studies based on three themes to allow for discussion and comparison. These areas were: (1) the wider MS community, and this included views and opinions from individuals involved in the MS community, but who did not have MS (i.e., healthcare providers and carers); (2) opinions on exercise (from persons with MS) associated with an exercise intervention; and (3) keeping moving when you have MS, and this involved opinions on persons with MS on the realities of exercise when you have MS. Gathering opinions from the entire MS community represents an

TABLE 18.3

Determinants of Physical Activity and Exercise Behaviour in MS

Facilitators			
Environmental		**Personal**	
Environment	**Social Influences**	**Health Condition**	**Cognitive and Behavioural**
Minimal or no disabled facilities (Borkoles et al. 2008; Elsworth et al. 2009; Plow et al. 2009; Brown et al. 2012; VanRuymbeke and Schneider 2013; van der Linden et al. 2014)	Social exclusion (Borkoles et al. 2008; Kasser 2009; Smith et al. 2009; Aubrey and Demain 2012; Learmonth et al. 2013; Plow and Finlayson 2014; van der Linden et al. 2014)	Fatigue (Dodd et al. 2006; Borkoles et al. 2008; Smith et al. 2009, 2011; Kayes et al. 2011; Brown et al. 2012; Dlugonski et al. 2012; van der Linden et al. 2014)	Fear and apprehension (Borkoles et al. 2008; Kayes et al. 2011; Smith et al. 2011, 2013a; Brown et al. 2012; Learmonth et al. 2013; Plow and Finlayson 2014)
Inappropriate exercise for level of physical ability (Aubrey and Demain 2012; Normann et al. 2013; Plow and Finlayson 2014)	Minimal or conflicting advice on physical activity and exercise from healthcare professionals (Smith et al. 2009, 2011, 2013b; Schneider and Young 2010; Kayes et al. 2011; Aubrey and Demain 2012; Brown et al. 2012; Learmonth et al. 2013)	Symptom fluctuations (Kasser 2009; Kayes et al. 2011; Brown et al. 2012; VanRuymbeke and Schneider 2013; van der Linden et al. 2014)	Poor self-management (Kasser 2009; Smith et al. 2009, 2011; Schneider and Young 2010; Plow and Finlayson 2014)
Lack of disabled parking (Kayes et al. 2011; Brown et al. 2012; Learmonth et al. 2013)	Limited finances (Borkoles et al. 2008; Brown et al. 2012; van der Linden et al. 2014)	Lack of personal knowledge about physical activity and exercise for those with MS (Plow et al. 2009; Aubrey and Demain 2012; Smith et al. 2013a)	Loss of self-control (Borkoles et al. 2008; Smith et al. 2009, 2011; Brown et al. 2012)
Public transport inflexibility (Brown et al. 2012; van der Linden et al. 2014)	Dependence on others (Brown et al. 2012; Giacobbi et al. 2012)	Pain (Dodd et al. 2006; Elsworth et al. 2009; Dlugonski et al. 2012)	Frustrations with limitations (Borkoles et al. 2008; Kayes et al. 2011; Smith et al. 2011)
Inappropriate information at diagnosis (Brown et al. 2012; Plow and Finlayson 2014)	Family distractions (Plow et al. 2009; Plow and Finlayson 2014)	Symptom progression (Kasser 2009)	Time-management (Plow et al. 2009; Dlugonski et al. 2012; Plow and Finlayson 2014)
Lack of physical activity and exercise opportunities (Learmonth et al. 2013; van der Linden et al. 2014)	Social stress (Smith et al. 2013b)	Medication (Giacobbi et al. 2012)	Low confidence (Plow et al. 2009; Smith et al. 2011; Learmonth et al. 2013)
Inappropriate temperature and climate	Vague exercise explanation from exercise leaders (Dodd et al. 2006)	MS-related surgery (Giacobbi et al. 2012)	Apathy towards home or independent exercise (Aubrey and Demain 2012; Giacobbi et al. 2012; van der Linden et al. 2014)
Need for a personal programme (Smith et al. 2011)	Negative attitudes from others with MS (Aubrey and Demain 2012)	Non-MS-related musculoskeletal problems (Dodd et al. 2006)	Low illness acceptance (Plow et al. 2009; Brown et al. 2012)
one on one support		Forgetting to exercise (Dodd et al. 2006)	Programme interruptions (Giacobbi et al. 2012; Plow and Finlayson 2014)

(*Continued*)

TABLE 18.3 (*Continued*)

Determinants of Physical Activity and Exercise Behaviour in MS

Facilitators			
Environmental		Personal	
Environment	**Social Influences**	**Health Condition**	**Cognitive and Behavioural**
			Depression (Borkoles et al. 2008; Kayes et al. 2011) Reliance on mobility aid and home adaptations (Kayes et al. 2011; van der Linden et al. 2014) Derision towards exercise (Kasser 2009) Uncommitted (Kasser 2009)

Facilitators			
Environmental		Personal	
Environment	**Social Influences**	**Health Condition**	**Cognitive and Behavioural**
Type of exercise modality (Smith et al. 2009, 2011, 2013a; Brown et al. 2012; Learmonth et al. 2013; Plow and Finlayson 2014; van der Linden et al. 2014) Community programme or venue (Elsworth et al. 2009; Kasser 2009; Learmonth et al. 2013; Smith et al. 2013a; Plow and Finlayson 2014) Increased frequency of classes (Dodd et al. 2006; Borkoles et al. 2008; Kasser 2009; Aubrey and Demain 2012; Van Ruymbeke and Schneider 2013; van der Linden et al. 2014) Accessible disabled friendly environments (Dodd et al. 2006; Brown et al. 2012; Learmonth et al. 2013; Smith et al. 2013a; VanRuymbeke and Schneider 2013)	MS role models and peer support social acceptance (Dodd et al. 2006; Borkoles et al. 2008; Elsworth et al. 2009; Kasser 2009; Smith et al. 2011, 2013a; Aubrey and Demain 2012; Brown et al. 2012; Dlugonski et al. 2012; Learmonth et al. 2013; VanRuymbeke and Schneider 2013; van der Linden et al. 2014) Coaches/leaders who are knowledgeable in MS (Dodd et al. 2006; Smith et al. 2009; Kayes et al. 2011; Aubrey and Demain 2012; Learmonth et al. 2013; Normann et al. 2013; Smith et al. 2013a; VanRuymbeke and Schneider 2013; van der Linden et al. 2014) Coaches/leaders who are friendly and motivating (Dodd et al. 2006;	Appropriate exercise for physical capabilities (Smith et al. 2009, 2011, 2013a; Brown et al. 2012; Dlugonski et al. 2012; Learmonth et al. 2013; Plow and Finlayson 2014; van der Linden et al. 2014) Rest periods allowing for Fatigue (Smith et al. 2009, 2011; Schneider and Young 2010; Kayes et al. 2011; Dlugonski et al. 2012; Normann et al. 2013; Plow and Finlayson 2014) Fatigue management awareness (Smith et al. 2009; Kayes et al. 2011)	Accomplishment (Dodd et al. 2006; Elsworth et al. 2009; Kasser 2009; Plow et al. 2009; Schneider and Young, 2010; Kayes et al. 2011; Smith et al. 2011, 2013a; Brown et al. 2012; Dlugonski et al. 2012; Learmonth et al. 2013; Plow and Finlayson 2014; van der Linden et al. 2014) Self-management (Kasser 2009; Plow et al. 2009; Smith et al. 2009, 2011; Schneider and Young 2010; Aubrey and Demain 2012; Dlugonski et al. 2012; Learmonth et al. 2013) Self-choice in physical activity and exercise (Dodd et al. 2006; Kasser 2009; Plow et al. 2009; Smith et al. 2011, 2013b; Aubrey and Demain 2012; Dlugonski et al. 2012; Learmonth et al. 2013; Plow and Finlayson 2014; van der Linden et al. 2014)

(*Continued*)

TABLE 18.3 (*Continued*)

Determinants of Physical Activity and Exercise Behaviour in MS

Facilitators			
Environmental		Personal	
Environment	Social Influences	Health Condition	Cognitive and Behavioural
Appropriate temperature (Smith et al. 2011; Brown et al. 2012; Plow and Finlayson 2014) Verbal, written and visual instruction (Smith et al. 2009, 2013a; Normann et al. 2013) Good public transportation availability (Kayes et al. 2011; Brown et al. 2012) Time-flexibility (Dodd et al. 2006; Dlugonski et al. 2012) Personal exercise programme (Aubrey and Demain, 2012; Normann et al. 2013) Quiet exercise areas (Smith et al. 2011) Public awareness of MS (Brown et al. 2012)	Plow et al. 2009; Smith et al. 2009, 2013a; Brown et al. 2012; VanRuymbeke and Schneider 2013; van der Linden et al. 2014) Coaches/leaders who are challenging, progressive and provide feedback (Learmonth et al. 2013; Smith et al. 2013a; Plow and Finlayson 2014) Ongoing healthcare professional input (Dodd et al. 2006; Elsworth et al. 2009; Plow et al. 2009; Aubrey and Demain 2012; Giacobbi et al. 2012; Normann et al. 2013; Smith et al. 2013a) Time with family (Borkoles et al. 2008; Schneider and Young 2010; Smith et al. 2013a; Plow and Finlayson 2014) Social accountability (Kasser 2009; Smith et al. 2011; Plow and Finlayson 2014) Assistance from others (Elsworth et al. 2009; Normann et al. 2013) Email/phone communication (Schneider and Young 2010; Smith et al. 2011) Early advise (at time of diagnosis) from healthcare professionals (Normann et al. 2013) Affordability (Dodd et al. 2006)		Awareness of improvement (Plow et al. 2009; Schneider and Young 2010; Kayes et al. 2011; Smith et al. 2011; Dlugonski et al. 2012; VanRuymbeke and Schneider 2013; van der Linden et al. 2014) Learning coping strategies (Borkoles et al. 2008; Plow et al. 2009; Smith et al. 2009, 2011, 2013b; Brown et al. 2012) Previous exercise experiences (Borkoles et al. 2008; Kayes et al. 2011; Smith et al. 2011) Feeling safe (Smith et al. 2011; Brown et al. 2012; VanRuymbeke and Schneider 2013) Time-management (Kasser, 2009; Schneider and Young 2010; Kayes et al. 2011) Activity diary (Plow et al. 2009; Smith et al. 2013b) Self-determination (Dlugonski et al. 2012; van der Linden et al. 2014) Commitment (Plow et al. 2009; van der Linden et al. 2014) Low anxiety (Aubrey and Demain 2012)

Source: Recreated from Learmonth, Y.C., and Motl, R.W., *Disabil. Rehabil.*, 38, 1227–1242, 2016.

example of consumer-based participatory research, as it enables the research community to learn from the consumer of exercise interventions and the role of exercise within life of persons with MS.

Theme 1: The Wider MS Community

> 'It is not enough to say, "you need to exercise", you have to help the client create a plan that takes into account the specific, contextual issues operating in the context of a person's life', study participant, occupational therapist (Learmonth et al. 2018a).

We must engage with the wider MS community of patients, carers, and healthcare professionals to identify mechanisms to improve exercise participation in persons with MS, and researchers have begun to engage healthcare professionals and carers in conversation surrounding exercise for persons with MS. Studies have been conducted between 2013 and 2017. In six of these studies (Toomey and Coote 2013; Forsberg et al. 2015; Horton et al. 2015; Fakolade et al. 2018; Giunti et al. 2018; Held Bradford et al. 2018), views of persons with MS were also gathered, and, where applicable, these will be discussed in subsequent sections of this chapter.

From the wider MS community, the views of at least four fitness facility managers (Anderson et al. 2017), 34 physiotherapists (Smith et al. 2013a; Toomey and Coote 2013; Forsberg et al. 2015; Giunti et al. 2018; Held Bradford et al. 2018; Learmonth et al. 2018a), one sports trainer (Giunti et al. 2018), 15 occupational therapists (Smith et al. 2013a; Giunti et al. 2018; Learmonth et al. 2018a), 2 'exercise buddies' who were paid carers trained by physiotherapists (Toomey and Coote 2013), and 16 neurologists have been gathered. Views of 27 family carers (Horton et al. 2015; Fakolade et al. 2018) have also been gathered.

All of the studies were primarily qualitative in method and gathered data via interviews or focus groups. Table 18.4 provides study information, participant information, quality score, main thematic findings, and a summary of the authors main conclusions or relevant points.

To recruit participants, the researchers used either purposive (Anderson et al. 2017; Giunti et al. 2018), purposeful (Fakolade et al. 2018; Held Bradford et al. 2018; Learmonth et al. 2018a), or convenience (Smith et al. 2013a; Toomey and Coote 2013; Forsberg et al. 2015; Horton et al. 2015) sampling. Data were collected via one to one in-person interviews (Toomey and Coote 2013; Horton et al. 2015; Anderson et al. 2017), telephone interviews (Held Bradford et al. 2018), focus groups (Fakolade et al. 2018; Giunti et al. 2018), or a combination of interviews and focus groups (Smith et al. 2013a; Forsberg et al. 2015; Learmonth et al. 2018a). Four of the studies gathered further data via surveys in addition to the interviews or focus groups (Anderson et al. 2017; Fakolade et al. 2018; Giunti et al. 2018; Held Bradford et al. 2018). To analyse the data, analysis was described as *thematic analysis* in most of the studies (Smith et al. 2013a; Toomey and Coote 2013; Anderson et al. 2017; Giunti et al. 2018; Learmonth et al. 2018a), three research groups described the use of *content-constant comparison* (Forsberg et al. 2015; Fakolade et al. 2018; Held Bradford et al. 2018), and one used *hierarchical content analysis* (Horton et al. 2015).

TABLE 18.4

Summary of Each Study, Participant Characteristics, Associated Intervention, Quality Score and Inclusion of the Consequences or Determinants of Physical Activity and Exercise Participation. Note all Participants Persons with MS Unless Otherwise Noted

Study/ Country of Study	Study Aim (Abbreviated)	Design/Data Collection Method/ Analytical Approach/ Theoretical Perspective/ Sampling Method	N/Sex/Age (Mean, SD and Range)/Race	Mean Years Diagnosed (SD)/ Years Diagnose Rang e)/Disease Type/Disability Severity/Mobility Device Use	Associated Intervention Description	Quality Score	Area/ Theme	Main Themes Emerging in Study	Main Clinical Points/ Conclusion
Adamson et al. (2018) USA	To understand how persons with MS describe the roles of PA and exercise as part of daily life with MS, relapses, and disability identity.	Design; Qualitative data col: interviews Analysis: interpretative pheno-menological analysis Sampling: purposeful	N: 15 Sex: 14 F, 1 M Age: 48.4 (±13.7) 30–70 Race; 10 white, 1 Latina, 2 American Indian, 2 black	Diag: unreported Type: unreported Disability: EDSS 4.7 (±1.4)	None	18	Moving with MS	PA has a paradoxical role in MS relapse PA has a role in guilt and empowerment Defiance of disability (disability preventer, disability eraser)	PA should be promoted carefully as it occupies many important and sometimes conflicting roles in the life of an individual with MS.
Anderson et al. (2017) UK	To identify potential barriers to exercise provision by the fitness industry for people with neurological disease (pwND).	Design: Mixed methods Data col: Surveys and interviews Analysis: thematic content analysis Theory: none Sampling method: purposeful	Fitness facility managers N: 4 interviews Age: unreported Sex: unreported Race: unreported	NA	None	14	Wider MS community	Exercise for people with neurological conditions Disabled vs able-bodied/ similarities Disabled vs able-bodied/ differences Equality Benefits of exercise for people with neurological conditions Gym accessibility for people with neurological conditions Barriers to exercise for people with neurological conditions Encouraging people with neurological conditions to exercise in a gym	Ensuring the provision of specially trained staff to support pwND to exercise in gyms may be the main barrier to provision for this population. Investigation into the standard training of fitness professionals combining the expertise of neurological physiotherapists with that of fitness professionals to meet the needs of for people with neurological conditions would be advantageous

(Continued)

TABLE 18.4 (*Continued*)

Summary of Each Study, Participant Characteristics, Associated Intervention, Quality Score and Inclusion of the Consequences or Determinants of Physical Activity and Exercise Participation. Note all Participants Persons with MS Unless Otherwise Noted

Study/ Country of Study	Study Aim (Abbreviated)	Design/Data Collection Method/ Analytical Approach/ Theoretical Perspective/ Sampling Method	N/Sex/Age (Mean, SD and Range)/Race	Mean Years Diagnosed (SD)/ Years Diagnose Rang e)/Disease Type/Disability Severity/Mobility Device Use	Associated Intervention Description	Quality Score	Area/ Theme	Main Themes Emerging in Study	Main Clinical Points/ Conclusion
								Role of health sector Deterrents to providing for pwND Conscious vs unconscious discrimination Not being actively inclusive vs being inclusive	
Aubrey and Demain (2012) UK	Establish how a community-based exercise group is perceived to influence MS self-management.	Design: Qualitative Data col: Focus group Analysis: Thematic analysis Theory: None Sampling: Convenience	N: 25, Sex: 14 F Age: 62.2 (±14.8), 32–85 Race: unreported	Diag.: 17.4 (±12.5), Type: unreported Disability: unreported Mob. device; 16 WC, 1 Wa, 6 Ca, 2 None.	Ongoing fortnightly MS group exercise class	16	Intervention opinion: Moving with MS	Camaraderie: taking action; understanding MS and the role of exercise; exercising outside the environment.	Exercise providers need to have an understanding of MS to ensure appropriate exercise prescription. Exercise is an opportunity for PwMS to increase self- efficacy and reducing feelings of helplessness associated with the nature of MS. The group dynamics and the support of peers foster a positive attitude towards MS and enable people to learn management strategies from each other. However, the group format makes it difficult to meet the variety of participant exercise needs.

(*Continued*)

TABLE 18.4 (*Continued*)

Summary of Each Study, Participant Characteristics, Associated Intervention, Quality Score and Inclusion of the Consequences or Determinants of Physical Activity and Exercise Participation. Note all Participants Persons with MS Unless Otherwise Noted

Study/ Country of Study	Study Aim (Abbreviated)	Design/Data Collection Method/ Analytical Approach/ Theoretical Perspective/ Sampling Method	N/Sex/Age (Mean, SD and Range)/Race	Mean Years Diagnosed (SD)/ Years Diagnose Rang e)/Disease Type/Disability Severity/Mobility Device Use	Associated Intervention Description	Quality Score	Area/ Theme	Main Themes Emerging in Study	Main Clinical Points/ Conclusion
Borkoles et al. (2008) UK	Examine the lived experiences of people diagnosed with MS in relation to exercise.	Design: Qualitative Data col: Face interview Analysis: Interpretative phenomenology Theory: None Sampling: Purposive	N: 7 Sex: 4 F Age: 47.1 (±19.1), 34–65 Race: unreported	Diag.: 16.3 (±9.1), Type: unknown, Disability (EDSS): all 4–6, Mob. Dev: unreported	None	14	Moving with MS	Functional limitations to exercise; the effect of previous exercise experience; views of others; environmental and social barriers to exercise	The wider exercise experience narratives were related to concerns about safety, dependability on others to overcome the challenges, and potential environmental hazards. The loss of spontaneous opportunities to exercise because of these actual and perceived barriers was key to this population. This research highlighted the need to rethink the health and social service arrangements in relation to exercise provision for individuals with MS.

(*Continued*)

TABLE 18.4 (*Continued*)

Summary of Each Study, Participant Characteristics, Associated Intervention, Quality Score and Inclusion of the Consequences or Determinants of Physical Activity and Exercise Participation. Note all Participants Persons with MS Unless Otherwise Noted

Study/ Country of Study	Study Aim (Abbreviated)	Design/Data Collection Method/ Analytical Approach/ Theoretical Perspective/ Sampling Method	N/Sex/Age (Mean, SD and Range)/Race	Mean Years Diagnosed (SD)/ Years Diagnose Rang e)/Disease Type/Disability Severity/Mobility Device Use	Associated Intervention Description	Quality Score	Area/ Theme	Main Themes Emerging in Study	Main Clinical Points/ Conclusion
Brown et al. (2012) Canada	Identify factors that facilitate or impede participation in aquatic fitness (AF) programs by individuals with MS	Design: Qualitative Data col: Focus group Analysis: Thematic content analysis Theory: Person Environment educational Model (Strong et al. 1999) Sampling: convenience & snowball	N: 8 Sex: 5 F Age: 42–66 Race; unreported	Diag.: 16.9 (±10.6), Type: 2 RR, 6 PP Disability: unreported Mob. Device: unreported	None	12	Moving with MS	The benefits of AF encourage continued participation; The environment must be accessible and tailored to the needs of those with MS; The ability to get to and from the pool influences participation; Pool staff attitudes and knowledge are important for facilitating AF participation; Lack of one-on-one support may restrict participation in AF programs.	People with MS encounter various barriers to participation in AF programs, including lack of transportation, need for one-on-one support, inaccessible pool environments, and fitness professionals' lack of knowledge about MS. As fear can prevent MS patients from initiating participation in AF programs, support from clinicians is needed to help patients begin and continue these programs.
Casey et al. (2016) Ireland	To investigate what PwMS want from a web-based resource that encourages physical activity	Design: Qualitative Data col: Focus groups & interviews Analysis: Thematic analysis Theory: None Sampling: Convenience	N: 33 Age: 30–79 Sex: 20 F, 13 M Race: unreported	Diag: unreported Type: unreported Disability: PDDS 3.09 (2.04) 0–7 Mob. device: Wheelchair 4, cane 9, unknown 7, none 13	None	15	Intervention opinion	Content – important information to include; Presentation – varying format, different abilities; Interactivity – build a sense of community; Reach the audience – let people know.	The data suggest that PwMS want a variety of information from a variety of sources and that this information is to be both stratified and interactive. These results will be used to inform the development of the 'Activity Matters' website which will aim to enable PwMS to become more physically active.

(*Continued*)

TABLE 18.4 (*Continued*)

Summary of Each Study, Participant Characteristics, Associated Intervention, Quality Score and Inclusion of the Consequences or Determinants of Physical Activity and Exercise Participation. Note all Participants Persons with MS Unless Otherwise Noted

Study/ Country of Study	Study Aim (Abbreviated)	Design/Data Collection Method/ Analytical Approach/ Theoretical Perspective/ Sampling Method	N/Sex/Age (Mean, SD and Range)/Race	Mean Years Diagnosed (SD)/ Years Diagnose Rang e)/Disease Type/Disability Severity/Mobility Device Use	Associated Intervention Description	Quality Score	Area/ Theme	Main Themes Emerging in Study	Main Clinical Points/ Conclusion
Chard (2017) US	To identify the individual and social experiences underlying the initiation and satisfaction with aquatic exercise among persons with MS.	Design: Qualitative Data col: Telephone interview Analysis: Thematic analysis Theory: None Sampling: Convenience	N: 45 Sex: 35 F, 10 M Age: 55.0 (9.4) Race: 40 non-Hispanic white	Diag: 16.3 (9.0) Type: 30 RR, 15 unreported Disability: unreported Mob. device: unreported	Attendance at aquatic exercise	13	Moving with MS: Intervention opinion	Initiating a program; Information sources; Role of exercise history; Class fit and a sense of belonging.	Providers could play a stronger role in emphasising the feasibility and benefits of aquatic programs. In addition, persons with MS should be encouraged to try local MS and more generalised aquatic programs in order to identify a program matching their social and physical goals
Chiu et al. (2016) US	To identify what are psychosocial factors which initiate and maintain physical activity over time among African Americans with MS.	Design: qualitative Data col: Focus groups & interviews Analysis: semantic coding analysis Theory: HAPA Sampling: purposeful	N: 18 Sex: 14 F 4 M Age: 27–61 Race; African Americans	Diag: 7.8 (5.6) Type: 17 PP, 1 SP Disability: unreported Mob. Device: unreported	None	19	Moving with MS	Acceptance and control of MS; benefits of physical activity; self-defined enjoyable physical activity; autonomous motivation; social support to engage in physical activity; physical activity self-efficacy; self-monitoring of physical activity level and changes; resilience coping	Example key findings: Participants who showed acceptance of MS and recognised immediate and long-term effects of engaging in self-defined enjoyable PA may have more motivation to engage in PA. Interventions that continue to develop these psychosocial adjustment of PA participation, along with self-monitoring of PA and its effects of daily functioning, could enhance adherence to physical activity,

(*Continued*)

TABLE 18.4 (*Continued*)

Summary of Each Study, Participant Characteristics, Associated Intervention, Quality Score and Inclusion of the Consequences or Determinants of Physical Activity and Exercise Participation. Note all Participants Persons with MS Unless Otherwise Noted

Study/ Country of Study	Study Aim (Abbreviated)	Design/Data Collection Method/ Analytical Approach/ Theoretical Perspective/ Sampling Method	N/Sex/Age (Mean, SD and Range)/Race	Mean Years Diagnosed (SD)/ Years Diagnose Rang e)/Disease Type/Disability Severity/Mobility Device Use	Associated Intervention Description	Quality Score	Area/ Theme	Main Themes Emerging in Study	Main Clinical Points/ Conclusion
									social support can positively affect African Americans with MS to engage in PA; interventions must incorporate friends, family, and healthcare professionals who are physically active or have related PA knowledge for MS disease strategies. Strategies to increase positive coping and resilience will help individuals resume PA after relapses and improve perseverance to engage in PA.
Clarke and Coote (2015) Ireland	To explore the perceptions of people with multiple sclerosis of a community-based, group exercise programme.	Design: qualitative Data col: focus groups Analysis: thematic analysis Theory: none Sampling: convenience	N:14 pwMS Sex: unreported Age: 53.9 (13.0) Race: unreported	Diag: 10.3 (10.9) Type: 11 RR, 3 SP Disability: < = 5.5 Mob. Device: 14 cane	Community-based group exercise group	16	Intervention opinion: Moving with MS	Psychological benefits, physical benefits, and knowledge gained	The qualitative analysis supports the findings of the main trial confirming positive effects of community exercise interventions by reducing the impact of MS and fatigue and improving participation.

(*Continued*)

TABLE 18.4 (*Continued*)

Summary of Each Study, Participant Characteristics, Associated Intervention, Quality Score and Inclusion of the Consequences or Determinants of Physical Activity and Exercise Participation. Note all Participants Persons with MS Unless Otherwise Noted

Study/ Country of Study	Study Aim (Abbreviated)	Design/Data Collection Method/ Analytical Approach/ Theoretical Perspective/ Sampling Method	N/Sex/Age (Mean, SD and Range)/Race	Mean Years Diagnosed (SD)/ Years Diagnose Rang e)/Disease Type/Disability Severity/Mobility Device Use	Associated Intervention Description	Quality Score	Area/ Theme	Main Themes Emerging in Study	Main Clinical Points/ Conclusion
Crank et al. (2017) UK	To undertake a qualitative investigation of exercise perceptions and experiences in PwMS before, during, and after participation in a personally tailored program designed to promote long-term maintenance of self-directed exercise	Design: qualitative Data col: focus groups and interviews Analysis: framework analysis Theory: none Sampling: purposive convenience	N: 33 Sex: 26 F, 7 M Age: 47.6 (7.9) Race: unreported	Diag: FG participants: 8.8 (7.0), Interview participants: 9.7 (3.5) Type: unreported Disability: FG participants: 3.8 (1.0–6.0), Interview participants: 3.0 (1.5–6.5) Mob. Device: unreported	Personally tailored supervised and self-directed exercise program	14	Intervention opinion: Moving with MS	The transition to inactivity; lack of knowledge and confidence; positive exercise experiences; perspectives on exercise adherence	Perceptions of improved posture, ability to overcome everyday difficulties, acute mood enhancements during and after exercise, and increased opportunities for social interaction were among the reported benefits of exercise participation. Despite the provision of a personally tailored exercise plan and use of cognitive behavioural strategies, self-directed exercise continued to present challenges to PwMS, and the importance of seeking cost-effective ways to maintain motivational support was implicit in participant responses.

(*Continued*)

TABLE 18.4 (*Continued*)

Summary of Each Study, Participant Characteristics, Associated Intervention, Quality Score and Inclusion of the Consequences or Determinants of Physical Activity and Exercise Participation. Note all Participants Persons with MS Unless Otherwise Noted

Study/ Country of Study	Study Aim (Abbreviated)	Design/Data Collection Method/ Analytical Approach/ Theoretical Perspective/ Sampling Method	N/Sex/Age (Mean, SD and Range)/Race	Mean Years Diagnosed (SD)/ Years Diagnose Rang e)/Disease Type/Disability Severity/Mobility Device Use	Associated Intervention Description	Quality Score	Area/ Theme	Main Themes Emerging in Study	Main Clinical Points/ Conclusion
Dixon-Ibarra et al. (2017) US	To describe the development, implementation, and evaluation of a physical activity programme.	Design: mixed methods Data col: focus groups Analysis: content analysis Theory: SCT Sampling: convenience	N: 8 in FG Sex: 6 F 2 M Age: 56 (10.8) Race: unreported	Diag: 8.4 (7.4) Type: 7 RR, 1 SP Disability: unreported Mob. Device: 2 walker, 3 cane, 1 wheelchair, 1 scooter, 3 no device	Health Education programme (participant own choice of physical activity separate from this intervention)	17	Intervention opinion: Moving with MS	Outcome Evaluation: Experiences with physical activity and SCT during the program; Process and resource feasibility dose received- satisfaction: General program experience; Context: Barriers to program participation; Dose received-exposure: Educational tools	Focus group data provided valuable feedback for future iterations of the program including critiques on the delivery, content, and group support provided. Outcome evaluation showed increases in self-efficacy (survey), improvements in theoretical constructs (focus groups), and increased physical activity (focus groups). Results show that health promotion programs for persons with MS can improve physical activity and related constructs.

(Continued)

TABLE 18.4 (*Continued*)

Summary of Each Study, Participant Characteristics, Associated Intervention, Quality Score and Inclusion of the Consequences or Determinants of Physical Activity and Exercise Participation. Note all Participants Persons with MS Unless Otherwise Noted

Study/ Country of Study	Study Aim (Abbreviated)	Design/Data Collection Method/ Analytical Approach/ Theoretical Perspective/ Sampling Method	N/Sex/Age (Mean, SD and Range)/Race	Mean Years Diagnosed (SD)/ Years Diagnose Rang e)/Disease Type/Disability Severity/Mobility Device Use	Associated Intervention Description	Quality Score	Area/ Theme	Main Themes Emerging in Study	Main Clinical Points/ Conclusion
Dlugonski et al. (2012) USA	To better understand the adoption and maintenance of physical activity from the perspective of women with MS.	Design: Qualitative Data col: Face interview Analysis: inductive coding Theory: SCT Sampling area: purposeful	N: 11 Sex: 11 F Age: 42.9 (±10.2), 29–58 Race: unreported	Diag.: unreported, Type: unreported Disability (PDDS): 4 Normal, 4 Mild, 3 Moderate, Mob. Device: 11 none	None	18	Moving with MS	Meaning of physical activity (subthemes: Being 'normal'; Savouring current health/level of Functioning); Motives for physical activity (subthemes: 'Feel Good'; Enjoyment of the activity; Sense of accomplishment; Weight control; Maintenance of physical function); Strategies for engaging in physical activity (subthemes: Make physical activity a priority; Create a flexible routine; Management of disease-specific barriers; Build a social support network)	Researchers and clinicians working to promote physical activity among women with MS might consider teaching skills related to prioritising physical activity, assisting in the development of social support networks, and encouraging participants to explore their personal meanings for physical activity.

(*Continued*)

TABLE 18.4 (*Continued*)

Summary of Each Study, Participant Characteristics, Associated Intervention, Quality Score and Inclusion of the Consequences or Determinants of Physical Activity and Exercise Participation. Note all Participants Persons with MS Unless Otherwise Noted

Study/ Country of Study	Study Aim (Abbreviated)	Design/Data Collection Method/ Analytical Approach/ Theoretical Perspective/ Sampling Method	N/Sex/Age (Mean, SD and Range)/Race	Mean Years Diagnosed (SD)/ Years Diagnose Rang e)/Disease Type/Disability Severity/Mobility Device Use	Associated Intervention Description	Quality Score	Area/ Theme	Main Themes Emerging in Study	Main Clinical Points/ Conclusion
Dodd et al. (2006) Australia	Explore the perceptions of adults with multiple sclerosis about the positive and negative effects of a progressive resistance strengthening programme.	Design: Qualitative Data col: Face interview Analysis: Thematic analysis Theory: None Sampling: Convenience	N: 9, Sex: 7 F, Age: 45.6 (±13.4), 35–61 Race: 7 Caucasian	Diag.: 6 (±4.12), Type: unreported, Disability (MSIS-29): psychological mean = 34.9 (±17.3), physical mean = 25.3 (±9.9) Mob. Device: 9 none	10 week group-based progressive resistance training	15	Intervention opinion: Moving with MS	Positive outcomes physical; Positive outcomes psychological; Positive outcomes social; Extrinsic factors important for programme completion; Intrinsic factors important for programme completion	The results of this study suggest that progressive resistance strength training is a feasible fitness option for some people with multiple sclerosis. Factors perceived to be important for programme completion suggest that choosing encouraging leaders with knowledge of exercise, and exercising in a group may contribute to programme success.
Elsworth et al. (2009) UK	Determine the opinions of pwND on factors facilitating their physical activity participation.	Design: Qualitative Data col: Focus group Analysis: Categorical content analysis Theory: Implementation Sampling: Purposeful	N: 7 Sex: unreported Age: unreported Race: unreported	Diag.: unreported, Type: unreported, Disability: unreported, Mob. device unreported	None	11	Moving with MS	Opinions of physical activity; barriers to physical activity; actors that would encourage increased physical activity involvement	Individuals with neurological conditions wish to participate in a range of activities that they enjoy in a community setting, and prefer to exercise with the support of health and fitness professionals with expertise relevant to their condition.

(*Continued*)

TABLE 18.4 (*Continued*)

Summary of Each Study, Participant Characteristics, Associated Intervention, Quality Score and Inclusion of the Consequences or Determinants of Physical Activity and Exercise Participation. Note all Participants Persons with MS Unless Otherwise Noted

Study/ Country of Study	Study Aim (Abbreviated)	Design/Data Collection Method/ Analytical Approach/ Theoretical Perspective/ Sampling Method	N/Sex/Age (Mean, SD and Range)/Race	Mean Years Diagnosed (SD)/ Years Diagnose Rang e)/Disease Type/Disability Severity/Mobility Device Use	Associated Intervention Description	Quality Score	Area/ Theme	Main Themes Emerging in Study	Main Clinical Points/ Conclusion
									A general preference to exercising in groups of individuals with similar disabilities, rather than with able-bodied individuals, was evident. Emotional issues such as embarrassment and informational issues relating to knowledge of professionals were highlighted as particular concerns that may act as barriers to participation.
Fakolade et al. (2018) Canada	To explore shared perceptions of caregiver/ care-recipient dyads affected by moderate-to-severe MS-related disability about PA.	Design: qualitative Data col: focus group Analysis: constant comparison Theory: none Sampling: purposeful	N: 23 pwms, 12 carers Sex: pwms 16 F, 7 M – carers 6 M, 5 F Age: pwms 54.6 (9.8) 37–71, carers 57 (13.8) 38–79 Race: unreported	Diag: 14.7 (9.0) Type: 12 RR. 5PP, 2 SP Disability: MSWS-12 68.4 (16.7) Mob. device: unreported	None	16	Wider MS community: Moving with MS	PA is a continuum; cycle of disengagement; cycle of adjustment.	The caregiver/care-recipient dyad is an important juncture for focusing PA interventions in persons with moderate-to-severe MS.

(*Continued*)

TABLE 18.4 (*Continued*)

Summary of Each Study, Participant Characteristics, Associated Intervention, Quality Score and Inclusion of the Consequences or Determinants of Physical Activity and Exercise Participation. Note all Participants Persons with MS Unless Otherwise Noted

Study/ Country of Study	Study Aim (Abbreviated)	Design/Data Collection Method/ Analytical Approach/ Theoretical Perspective/ Sampling Method	N/Sex/Age (Mean, SD and Range)/Race	Mean Years Diagnosed (SD)/ Years Diagnose Rang e)/Disease Type/Disability Severity/Mobility Device Use	Associated Intervention Description	Quality Score	Area/ Theme	Main Themes Emerging in Study	Main Clinical Points/ Conclusion
Fasczewski et al. (2018) USA	To explore physical activity motivation and benefits with a sample of highly active pwMS.	Design: mixed methods Data col: survey & telephone interview Analysis: thematic analysis Theory: SDT Sampling: convenience	N: 15 (8 did interviews) Sex: 7 F, 1 M Age: 43.5 (10.05) 29–61 Race: unreported	Diag: 7 (4.34) 1–13 Type: total 15 RR Disability: unreported Mob. device: unreported	None	16	Moving with MS	Motivational strategies used to maintain physical activity; benefits and impact of PA.	Interventions aimed at increasing long-term physical activity adherence should focus on increasing autonomy and competence for physical activity in the individual and promoting potential increased quality of life outcomes from physical activity participation.
Forsberg et al. (2015) Sweden	To describe experiences of using Nintendo Wii Fit for balance exercise, from the perspectives of patients with MS and their physiotherapists (PT).	Design: qualitative Data col: interviews and focus groups Analysis: content-constant comparative Theory: none Sampling: convenience	N: 24 (15 PwMS, 9 PT) Sex: 9 F, 6 M (PwMS). F8. M1 (PT). Age: PwMS 52.60 (12.13) 32–73, Race: unreported	Diag: Type: Disability: Mob. device:	Home-based computer exercise programme	16	Wider MS community: Intervention opinion	Experiences from exercising using Wii; Effects related to the intervention; Perceptions of usability	Patients with MS and their PT considered Wii Fit exercises to be fun, challenging, and self-motivating. Exercising with Wii games can address balance impairments in MS, and can be performed at home as well as in rehabilitation settings.

(*Continued*)

TABLE 18.4 (*Continued*)

Summary of Each Study, Participant Characteristics, Associated Intervention, Quality Score and Inclusion of the Consequences or Determinants of Physical Activity and Exercise Participation. Note all Participants Persons with MS Unless Otherwise Noted

Study/ Country of Study	Study Aim (Abbreviated)	Design/Data Collection Method/ Analytical Approach/ Theoretical Perspective/ Sampling Method	N/Sex/Age (Mean, SD and Range)/Race	Mean Years Diagnosed (SD)/ Years Diagnose Rang e)/Disease Type/Disability Severity/Mobility Device Use	Associated Intervention Description	Quality Score	Area/ Theme	Main Themes Emerging in Study	Main Clinical Points/ Conclusion
Giacobbi et al. (2012) USA	To evaluate perceptions of quality of life after a 4-month progressive resistance training program for pwMS. A second purpose was to examine participants' views about factors that facilitated or impeded exercise behaviour.	Design: Mixed methods Data col: Face then telephone interview Analysis: Constant comparative Theory: PAD Sampling: Convenience	N: 8 Sex: 8 F Age: 49.9 (±6.9), 40–61 Race: unreported.	Diag.: 8.8 (±6.1), Type: unreported, Disability: unreported Mob. device: unreported	16 week, instructor one on one, progressive resistance training.	19	Moving with MS	Perceived physical responses to the intervention; Psychosocial responses to the intervention; Facilitators and barriers to exercise behaviour	Supervised resistance training may promote perceived improvement in physical ability (i.e., standing, walking, balance, endurance, strength and daily tasks) and psychosocial changes (i.e., social impact, energy / vigour, emotional responses and confidence) in women with RR MS.
Giunti et al. (2018)[a] Switzerland	To (1) explore MS-specific needs for MS mobile health (mHealth) solutions for PA, (2) detect perceived obstacles and facilitators for mHealth solutions from pwMS and healthcare professionals, and (3) understand the motivational aspects behind adoption of mHealth solutions for MS.	Design: mixed methods Data col: focus groups & surveys Analysis: thematic analysis Theory: none Sampling: purposeful	N: 24 (12 PwMS, 12 HCPs) Sex: 6 F 6 M (PwMS), 6 F 6 M (HCP) Age: PwMS 34–62, HCPs 26–64 Race: unreported	Diag: Type: 7 RR, 2 PP, 3 SP Disability: (EDSS) <4.5 Mob. device: unreported	Physiotherapy at a specialist neurological rehabilitation centre	15	Wider MS community; Intervention opinion: Moving with MS	MS-related barriers and facilitators; mHealth design considerations; general motivational aspects	mHealth solutions for increasing PA in persons with MS hold promise. Allowing for realistic goal setting and positive feedback, whilst minimising usability burdens, seems to be critical for the adoption of such apps. Fatigue management is especially important in this population; more attention should be brought to this area.

(*Continued*)

TABLE 18.4 (*Continued*)

Summary of Each Study, Participant Characteristics, Associated Intervention, Quality Score and Inclusion of the Consequences or Determinants of Physical Activity and Exercise Participation. Note all Participants Persons with MS Unless Otherwise Noted

Study/ Country of Study	Study Aim (Abbreviated)	Design/Data Collection Method/ Analytical Approach/ Theoretical Perspective/ Sampling Method	N/Sex/Age (Mean, SD and Range)/Race	Mean Years Diagnosed (SD)/ Years Diagnose Rang e)/Disease Type/Disability Severity/Mobility Device Use	Associated Intervention Description	Quality Score	Area/ Theme	Main Themes Emerging in Study	Main Clinical Points/ Conclusion
Hall-McMaster et al. (2016a) NZ	To investigate thoughts about PA motivation.	Design: qualitative Data col: think aloud interview Analysis: inductive thematic analysis Theory: none Sampling: convenience	N: 1 Sex: 1 M Age: 70 Race: unreported	Diag: 5 Type: unreported Disability: unreported Mob. device: 1 Wheelchair	None	10	Moving with MS	Positive thinking as Norman's way to fight against MS; coping with MS by choosing to think positively; using positivity to maintain control; and using PA to think positively; goals give a positive purpose to Norman's engagement in PA; viewing PA as a necessity for goal achievement; and goals providing determination.	Positive thinking and purposeful goals were central to high PA motivation in our case study of one individual with MS.
Hall-McMaster et al. (2015b) NZ	To investigate in-depth the role of positive thinking in physical activity motivation.	Design: qualitative Data col: think aloud interview Analysis: inductive thematic analysis Theory: none Sampling: convenience	N: 4 Sex: 2 F 2 M Age: 46–70 Race: unreported	Diag: 2–11 Type: unreported Disability: unreported Mob. device: 3 none, 1 wheelchair	None	13	Moving with MS	Thoughts about purpose, self-efficacy, the past, and reinforcement through positive thinking.	The present findings support the potential of thought-based strategies to increase PA motivation. Thus, we conclude that positive thinking and related thought-based strategies may serve as useful tools to enhance motivation for PA in the MS community.

(*Continued*)

TABLE 18.4 (*Continued*)

Summary of Each Study, Participant Characteristics, Associated Intervention, Quality Score and Inclusion of the Consequences or Determinants of Physical Activity and Exercise Participation. Note all Participants Persons with MS Unless Otherwise Noted

Study/ Country of Study	Study Aim (Abbreviated)	Design/Data Collection Method/ Analytical Approach/ Theoretical Perspective/ Sampling Method	N/Sex/Age (Mean, SD and Range)/Race	Mean Years Diagnosed (SD)/ Years Diagnose Rang e)/Disease Type/Disability Severity/Mobility Device Use	Associated Intervention Description	Quality Score	Area/ Theme	Main Themes Emerging in Study	Main Clinical Points/ Conclusion
Held Bradford et al. (2018) USA	To describe the behavioural decisions used by persons with MS and physical therapists to maximise gait and balance following outpatient physical therapy.	Design: mixed Data col: telephone surveys + interviews Analysis: content-constant comparative Theory: SCT Sampling: purposeful quota	N: 12 (7 pwMS, 5 Phys) Sex: 6 F, 1 M (pwMS), 4 F (Phys), 1 M (Phys) Age: pwMS 54.43 (±10.74) 41–67 Race: unreported	Diag: unreported Type: 6 RR, 1 SP Disability: (PDDS) 4.29, (±0.95), 3–6 Mob. device: 2 walker, 4 cane, 2 none	None	18	Wider MS community: Moving with MS	Person with MS core theme: Challenging self by pushing, but respecting limits; Person with MS theme: Resolving uncertainty; Person with MS supporting: Action: Setting goals and building routines and resilience; Physical therapist core theme: Finding the right fit; Physical therapist supporting theme 1 : Seeing similarities and getting to know differences; Physical therapist supporting theme 2: Developing a partnership and plan for empowerment and self-management; Keeping their lived world large; Overarching theme: Keeping their lived world large, or participation in valued life roles.	Participants have a shared goal of maximising gait and balance so persons with MS can participate in valued life roles. Understanding the differences in the behavioural decisions and optimising skill sets in shared .decision-making and self-management may enhance the therapeutic partnership and engagement in gait- and balance-enhancing behaviours.

(*Continued*)

TABLE 18.4 (*Continued*)

Summary of Each Study, Participant Characteristics, Associated Intervention, Quality Score and Inclusion of the Consequences or Determinants of Physical Activity and Exercise Participation. Note all Participants Persons with MS Unless Otherwise Noted

Study/ Country of Study	Study Aim (Abbreviated)	Design/Data Collection Method/ Analytical Approach/ Theoretical Perspective/ Sampling Method	N/Sex/Age (Mean, SD and Range)/Race	Mean Years Diagnosed (SD)/ Years Diagnose Rang e)/Disease Type/Disability Severity/Mobility Device Use	Associated Intervention Description	Quality Score	Area/ Theme	Main Themes Emerging in Study	Main Clinical Points/ Conclusion
Horton et al. (2015) Canada	To investigate the exercise experiences of individuals with MS and the extent to which these experiences affect, or are affected by, their spousal relationship.	Design: qualitative Data col: interviews Analysis: hierarchical content analysis Theory: none Sampling: convenience	N: 10 (5 pwMS, 5 spouses) Sex: 5 F, 5 M Age: pwms 57.5 (11.6) 45–70, spouses 56.8 (11.7) 44–69 Race: unreported	Diag: 44 (12.0) Type: unreported Disability: EDSS 4–6 Mob. device: unreported	None	16	Wider MS community: Moving with MS	Maintaining independence, overcoming isolation, and negotiating if exercise is worth it.	Rather than an inexorable downward decline in physical ability that is common with MS, participants spoke of a positive reversal in physical function, which has had far-reaching implications for multiple aspects of their lives, including their psychological outlook, their sense of independence, overcoming isolation, and their relationship with their spouse, all of which are identified in the literature as notable aspects of life affected by the disease.

(*Continued*)

TABLE 18.4 (*Continued*)

Summary of Each Study, Participant Characteristics, Associated Intervention, Quality Score and Inclusion of the Consequences or Determinants of Physical Activity and Exercise Participation. Note all Participants Persons with MS Unless Otherwise Noted

Study/ Country of Study	Study Aim (Abbreviated)	Design/Data Collection Method/ Analytical Approach/ Theoretical Perspective/ Sampling Method	N/Sex/Age (Mean, SD and Range)/Race	Mean Years Diagnosed (SD)/ Years Diagnose Rang e)/Disease Type/Disability Severity/Mobility Device Use	Associated Intervention Description	Quality Score	Area/ Theme	Main Themes Emerging in Study	Main Clinical Points/ Conclusion
Hundza et al. (2016) Canada	To examine the facilitators for, and barriers to, participation in physical activity pwND.	Design: cross sectional mixed methods Data col: interviews Analysis: inductive data-driven approach Theory: none Sampling: purposeful	N: 30 (15 stroke, 11 MS, 4 incomplete spinal cord injury) Sex: stroke 8 F 7 M, MS 7 F 4 M, incomplete spinal cord injury M4 Age: 58.6 (11.7) 23–78 Race: unreported	Diag: 11.40 (9.90) Type: 3 RR, 1 PP, 7 SP Disability: unreported Mob. device: pwms 5 none, 2 walker, 4 cane	None	14	Moving with MS	'Dealt a new set of cards'. (2) 'Influence of interactions between conditions and context'	The presence of similar barriers and facilitators across the clinical groups suggests that rehabilitation assessment and treatment as well as support and services to promote valued forms of physical activity could be organised and delivered based on limitations in mobility and functioning rather than clinical diagnosis.
Kasser (2009) USA	To explore the meaning of exercise in the lives of individuals with MS and describe the motivational basis that contributed to their exercise involvement.	Design: Qualitative Data col: Face interview Analysis: Thematic analysis Theory: SCT Sampling: Purposive Convenience	N: 12, Sex: 10 F Age: 46.3 (±7.3), 32–55, Race: unreported.	Diag.: 9.9 (±7.2), Type: 7 RR, 2 PP, 3 SP, Disability: unreported Mob. device: 1 WC, 2 Ca, 9 none.	Ongoing, instructor group exercise program	16	Intervention opinion: Moving with MS	Exercising to maintain function and health: Enhanced exercise self-efficacy: Feelings of hope and optimism	Participants appreciated the constant of exercise and the support of others in light of the highly variable and changing nature of their MS. The exercise program provided a personal, physical, and social venue from which participants could learn about their own strengths, needs, and confidence capabilities.

(*Continued*)

TABLE 18.4 (*Continued*)

Summary of Each Study, Participant Characteristics, Associated Intervention, Quality Score and Inclusion of the Consequences or Determinants of Physical Activity and Exercise Participation. Note all Participants Persons with MS Unless Otherwise Noted

Study/ Country of Study	Study Aim (Abbreviated)	Design/Data Collection Method/ Analytical Approach/ Theoretical Perspective/ Sampling Method	N/Sex/Age (Mean, SD and Range)/Race	Mean Years Diagnosed (SD)/ Years Diagnose Rang e)/Disease Type/Disability Severity/Mobility Device Use	Associated Intervention Description	Quality Score	Area/ Theme	Main Themes Emerging in Study	Main Clinical Points/ Conclusion
Kayes et al. (2011) NZ	To explore the barriers and facilitators to engagement in physical activity from the perspective of pwMS.	Design: Qualitative Data col: Face interview Analysis: Grounded theory Theory: None Sampling: Purposeful	N: 10 Sex: 7 F Age: 44.3 (±6.6), 34–53 Race: 9 Caucasian, 1 Māori.	Diag.: 8.8 (±4.9), Type: 4 RR, 3 PP, 3 SP, Disability (GNDS): mean = 17.1 (±10) Mobility dev. 3 WC, 1 walker, 2 cane, 4 none.	None	14	Moving with MS	Beliefs about physical activity; related emotional responses; and the role of fatigue in the decision to take part in physical activity.	For people with MS, the decision to engage in physical activity (or not) is complex, fluid, and individual; made more complex by the unpredictable nature of MS. Rehabilitation professionals attempting to engage people with MS in a physical activity programme should consider adopting an individualised approach to barrier management which takes into account personal beliefs and perceptions regarding physical activity engagement.

(Continued)

TABLE 18.4 (*Continued*)

Summary of Each Study, Participant Characteristics, Associated Intervention, Quality Score and Inclusion of the Consequences or Determinants of Physical Activity and Exercise Participation. Note all Participants Persons with MS Unless Otherwise Noted

Study/ Country of Study	Study Aim (Abbreviated)	Design/Data Collection Method/ Analytical Approach/ Theoretical Perspective/ Sampling Method	N/Sex/Age (Mean, SD and Range)/Race	Mean Years Diagnosed (SD)/ Years Diagnose Rang e)/Disease Type/Disability Severity/Mobility Device Use	Associated Intervention Description	Quality Score	Area/ Theme	Main Themes Emerging in Study	Main Clinical Points/ Conclusion
Kersten et al. (2014) Germany	To conduct an exercise-based patient education program in order to ensure participants training management beyond the project.	Design: quasi experimental Data col: intervention and interview Analysis: content analysis Theory: none Sampling: convenience	N: 15 Sex: 12 F 3 M Age: 48.1 (9.2) Race: unreported	Diag: 10.9 (7.7) Type: 8 RR, 3 PP, 4 SP Disability: EDSS 4 (1.5) Mob. device: unreported	Exercise education and then home exercise programme	15	Intervention opinion: Moving with MS	Motivation: Training & therapeutic management: Training barriers: Knowledge interrogation regarding training theory: Knock-out criteria: Quality of Life: Subjective attitude towards physical exercise: Criticism and tips for further patient education programs	Qualitative analyses showed improved self-confidence and identified training strategies and barriers. This pilot study provides evidence that PwMS are able to acquire good knowledge about physical exercise and apply this knowledge successfully in training management. Exercise-based patient
Kersten et al. (2015) NZ	To test the feasibility and acceptability of an implementation intention strategy (if-then plans) increasingly used in health psychology to bridge the goal intention-action gap in rehabilitation with people with neurological conditions who are experiencing difficulties with mobility.	Design: qualitative Data col: Focus group, interview and intervention Analysis: thematic analysis Theory: none Sampling: convenience	N: 20 (10 pwms, 10 stroke) Sex: 14 F 6 M Age: 48–87 Race: 1 Chinese, 18 NZ European, 1 European	Diag: unreported Type: unreported Disability: unreported Mob. device: unreported	Exercise goal setting using 'if-then' plans.	13	Intervention opinion	Rehabilitation in context: Encapsulating the usefulness of the if-then strategy in thinking about the patient in the context of complexity; usefulness of home-based rehabilitation: perceived need for a few more sessions	education seems to be a feasible option to maintain or improve patients' integral constitution concerning physical and mental health.

(*Continued*)

TABLE 18.4 (*Continued*)

Summary of Each Study, Participant Characteristics, Associated Intervention, Quality Score and Inclusion of the Consequences or Determinants of Physical Activity and Exercise Participation. Note all Participants Persons with MS Unless Otherwise Noted

Study/ Country of Study	Study Aim (Abbreviated)	Design/Data Collection Method/ Analytical Approach/ Theoretical Perspective/ Sampling Method	N/Sex/Age (Mean, SD and Range)/Race	Mean Years Diagnosed (SD)/ Years Diagnose Rang e)/Disease Type/Disability Severity/Mobility Device Use	Associated Intervention Description	Quality Score	Area/ Theme	Main Themes Emerging in Study	Main Clinical Points/ Conclusion
Kinnett-Hopkins (2017b) USA	To examine the interpretations of physical activity, exercise, and sedentary behaviour by persons with multiple sclerosis.	Design: qualitative Data col: interview Analysis: thematic analysis Theory: none Sampling: purposeful	N: 53 Sex: 42 F 1 1M Age: 55.3 (9.4) 31–70 Race: 53 Caucasian	Diag: unreported Type: unreported Disability: EDSS 4.09 (1.51) 1–6, Mob. device: unreported	None	13	Moving with MS	Physical activity -consistent definition, -ambiguous definition: Exercise -consistent definition, -ambiguous definition: Sedentary behaviour -consistent definition, -in-consistent definition, ambiguous definition	Results highlight the need to provide and utilise consistent definitions for accurate understanding, proper evaluation and communication of physical activity, exercise, and sedentary behaviours among persons with multiple sclerosis. The application of consistent definitions may minimise ambiguity, alleviate the equivocality of findings in the literature, and translate into improved communication about these behaviours in multiple sclerosis.
Learmonth et al. (2013) UK	To explore the experiences and views of people moderately affected with MS following participation in a 12-week exercise programme.	Design: Qualitative Data col: Focus group Analysis: General inductive Theory: None	N: 14 Sex: 10 F Age: 52.1 (±8), 40–68 Race: 14 Caucasian.	Diag.: 14.8 (±6.3), Type: unreported, Disability (EDSS): 6.1 (±0.4) Mob. device: unreported	Group community-based exercise class	16	Intervention opinion	The benefits of the class, helping them to overcome barriers to exercise.	People moderately affected with MS feel group exercise offers symptom improvement and social benefits. MS-related symptoms and a lack of service options may prevent those with MS exercising.

(*Continued*)

TABLE 18.4 (*Continued*)

Summary of Each Study, Participant Characteristics, Associated Intervention, Quality Score and Inclusion of the Consequences or Determinants of Physical Activity and Exercise Participation. Note all Participants Persons with MS Unless Otherwise Noted

Study/ Country of Study	Study Aim (Abbreviated)	Design/Data Collection Method/ Analytical Approach/ Theoretical Perspective/ Sampling Method	N/Sex/Age (Mean, SD and Range)/Race	Mean Years Diagnosed (SD)/ Years Diagnose Rang e)/Disease Type/Disability Severity/Mobility Device Use	Associated Intervention Description	Quality Score	Area/ Theme	Main Themes Emerging in Study	Main Clinical Points/ Conclusion
									Physiotherapists should work alongside exercise professionals to establish exercise services for those with MS.
Learmonth et al. (2015) USA	To explore the meanings, motivations, and outcomes of physical activity in wheelchair users with MS.	Design: qualitative Data col: interviews Analysis: thematic analysis Theory: none Sampling: purposeful	N: 15 Sex: 12 F 3 M Age: 52 (8.8) Race: unreported	Diag: 10–15 Type: 7 RR, 2 PP, 6 SP Disability: Mob. device: 15 wheelchair	None	19	Moving with MS	Everyday experiences: Physical activity and exercise experiences	Physical activity and exercise are important components of comprehensive MS care and patient self-management. Physical activity and exercise for those with advanced MS who are wheelchair users should be part of everyday life and should incorporate adaptive strategies and accessible facilities. The integration of behavioural change constructs into physical activity and exercise interventions might overcome negative personal beliefs and promote successful initiation and maintenance of physical activity and exercise.

(*Continued*)

TABLE 18.4 (*Continued*)

Summary of Each Study, Participant Characteristics, Associated Intervention, Quality Score and Inclusion of the Consequences or Determinants of Physical Activity and Exercise Participation. Note all Participants Persons with MS Unless Otherwise Noted

Study/ Country of Study	Study Aim (Abbreviated)	Design/Data Collection Method/ Analytical Approach/ Theoretical Perspective/ Sampling Method	N/Sex/Age (Mean, SD and Range)/Race	Mean Years Diagnosed (SD)/ Years Diagnose Rang e)/Disease Type/Disability Severity/Mobility Device Use	Associated Intervention Description	Quality Score	Area/ Theme	Main Themes Emerging in Study	Main Clinical Points/ Conclusion
Learmonth et al. (2016) USA	To explore the needs and wants of pwMS regarding exercise promotion through healthcare providers.	Design: qualitative Data col: interviews Analysis: thematic analysis Theory: SCT Sampling: convenience	N: 50 Sex: 33 F 17 M Age: 49.2 (10.3) Race: unreported	Diag: 13.0 (8.4) Type: 41 RR, 1 PP, 5 SP, 3 Ben Disability: EDSS ≤5.5 Mob. device: unreported	None	16	Moving with MS	Information and knowledge on the benefits of exercise and exercise prescription: Materials to allow home and community exercise; Tools for initiating and maintaining exercise behaviour	Patients with MS frequently interact with healthcare providers and are generally unsatisfied with exercise promotion during interactions. Healthcare providers can address the low uptake of exercise among persons with MS by acting upon the identified unmet needs involving materials, knowledge and behaviour change strategies for exercise.
Learmonth et al. (2017a) USA	To identify the desired and preferred format and source of exercise information for pw MS that can be delivered through healthcare providers.	Design: Qualitative Data col: Interview Analysis: Thematic Analysis Theory: None Sampling: Purposeful	N: 50 Sex: 33 F 17 M Age: 49.2 (10.3) Race: unreported	Diag: 13.0 (8.40) Type: 41 RR, 1 PP, 5 SP, 3 Ben Disability: 3.50 (2.00) Mob. device: unreported	None	17	Moving with MS	Approach for receiving exercise promotion: Ideal person for promoting exercise	Based on the views and opinions of participants in our study, it is clear that we must ensure that healthcare providers are prepared to provide exercise information to patients, research and develop exercise promotion material in print media, and establish credible electronic sources of exercise promotion for persons with MS.

(*Continued*)

TABLE 18.4 (*Continued*)

Summary of Each Study, Participant Characteristics, Associated Intervention, Quality Score and Inclusion of the Consequences or Determinants of Physical Activity and Exercise Participation. Note all Participants Persons with MS Unless Otherwise Noted

Study/ Country of Study	Study Aim (Abbreviated)	Design/Data Collection Method/ Analytical Approach/ Theoretical Perspective/ Sampling Method	N/Sex/Age (Mean, SD and Range)/Race	Mean Years Diagnosed (SD)/ Years Diagnose Rang e)/Disease Type/Disability Severity/Mobility Device Use	Associated Intervention Description	Quality Score	Area/ Theme	Main Themes Emerging in Study	Main Clinical Points/ Conclusion
Learmonth et al. (2017b) USA	To explore the needs of healthcare providers for promoting exercise behaviour among pwMS.	Design: Qualitative Data col: Interview Analysis: Thematic analysis Theory: SCT Sampling: Purposeful	N: 44 HPs (13 Neuro, 10 OT, 11 Phys, 10 nurses Sex: F = 30, M = 14 Age: 49.7 (±12.8) Race:	NA	None	17	Wider MS community	Opportunities for exercise promotion: Healthcare provider education on exercise for persons with MS; Patient tools/strategies	Providers in MS healthcare consider the patient-provider interaction within the healthcare system, healthcare team, and clinical appointment as a novel opportunity for exercise promotion. Such an opportunity requires education of healthcare providers and provision of tools and strategies for exercise promotion among persons with MS
Learmonth et al. (2018)[b] USA	To understand experiences of persons with MS who participated in a feasibility research study of a home-based exercise intervention grounded in current physical activity guidelines and supplemented with behavioural change modules.	Design: Qualitative Data col: Interview Analysis: Thematic analysis Theory: SCT Sampling: Convenience	N = 18 Sex: 18 F Age: 50 (10) Race: 14 White, 4 Black	Diag: unreported Type: 18 RR Disability: 1* (IQR 0–2.5) Mobility device: none	Home-based exercise following current exercise guidelines for persons with MS	20	Intervention opinion	Enrolment and assessment: Improvement in the design and delivery of the exercise programme components	The current physical activity guidelines for persons with MS are acceptable to persons with MS and rehabilitation professionals should prescribe these guidelines as appropriate. Consideration should be made to the use of individualised recruitment methods to optimise participation of persons with MS in exercise interventions.

(*Continued*)

TABLE 18.4 (*Continued*)

Summary of Each Study, Participant Characteristics, Associated Intervention, Quality Score and Inclusion of the Consequences or Determinants of Physical Activity and Exercise Participation. Note all Participants Persons with MS Unless Otherwise Noted

Study/ Country of Study	Study Aim (Abbreviated)	Design/Data Collection Method/ Analytical Approach/ Theoretical Perspective/ Sampling Method	N/Sex/Age (Mean, SD and Range)/Race	Mean Years Diagnosed (SD)/ Years Diagnose Rang e)/Disease Type/Disability Severity/Mobility Device Use	Associated Intervention Description	Quality Score	Area/ Theme	Main Themes Emerging in Study	Main Clinical Points/ Conclusion
									Rehabilitation professionals should combine behaviour change approaches with exercise interventions to optimise exercise participation in persons with MS.
Mulligan et al. (2013) NZ	To report on an innovative program, entitled the 'Blue Prescription approach', in which physical therapists work collaboratively with persons with a disability to promote community-based physical activity participation.	Design: qualitative Data col: interview Analysis: general inductive analysis Theory: none Sampling: convenience	N: 27 Sex: 23 F 4 M Age: 51 (11.1) 34–71 Race: 2 European, 24 White, 1 Maori	Diag: 15.48 (9.66) Type: 9 RR, 3 PP, 8 SP, 7 unknown Disability: unreported Mob. device: 6 wheelchair, 3 walker	Community-based PA. collaboration between physio-therapists and pwMS (Blue Prescription)	11	Intervention opinion: Moving with MS	Content and pragmatics of Blue Prescription: Interactions required for delivery of Blue Prescription: Improvements and refinements to the Blue Prescription approach	Evidence indicated that the Blue Prescription approach can provide a collaborative and flexible way for physical therapists to work with individuals with MS, to increase participation in community-based physical activity. To further develop the approach, there is a need to address issues related to the use of standardised measures and develop strategies to train physical therapists in collaborative approaches for promotion of physical activity.

(*Continued*)

TABLE 18.4 (*Continued*)

Summary of Each Study, Participant Characteristics, Associated Intervention, Quality Score and Inclusion of the Consequences or Determinants of Physical Activity and Exercise Participation. Note all Participants Persons with MS Unless Otherwise Noted

Study/ Country of Study	Study Aim (Abbreviated)	Design/Data Collection Method/ Analytical Approach/ Theoretical Perspective/ Sampling Method	N/Sex/Age (Mean, SD and Range)/Race	Mean Years Diagnosed (SD)/ Years Diagnose Rang e)/Disease Type/Disability Severity/Mobility Device Use	Associated Intervention Description	Quality Score	Area/ Theme	Main Themes Emerging in Study	Main Clinical Points/ Conclusion
									The integration of self-help and professional help provided by the Blue Prescription approach appeared to result in successful promotion of physical activity in persons with MS. Additional testing is required to examine its efficacy in other healthcare systems, in conditions beyond MS, and in terms of its economic impact.
Normann et al. (2013) Norway	To investigate how PwMS perceive movement during single sessions of physiotherapy.	Design: Qualitative Data col: Face interview Analysis: Content analysis Theory: None Sampling: Purposeful	N: 12 Sex: 9 F Age: 48 (±13.5), 31–81, Race: unreported.	Diag.: 8.8 (±6.4), Type: 7 RR, 2 PP, 3 SP, Disability (EDSS): 3.6 disability, Mob. Device: 7 none, 2 Ca, 1 Wa, 3 WC	1 day session (≤1.5 hours) of PT assessment, consultation, and exercise advice	20	Intervention opinion: Moving with MS	Knowledge of body part interactions and consequences for AD: Insight into limitations and possibilities of ADL	Contextualised perceptions of improvements in movement may strengthen the person's sense of ownership and sense of agency and thus promote autonomy and self-encouragement. The findings underpin the

(Continued)

TABLE 18.4 (*Continued*)

Summary of Each Study, Participant Characteristics, Associated Intervention, Quality Score and Inclusion of the Consequences or Determinants of Physical Activity and Exercise Participation. Note all Participants Persons with MS Unless Otherwise Noted

Study/ Country of Study	Study Aim (Abbreviated)	Design/Data Collection Method/ Analytical Approach/ Theoretical Perspective/ Sampling Method	N/Sex/Age (Mean, SD and Range)/Race	Mean Years Diagnosed (SD)/ Years Diagnose Rang e)/Disease Type/Disability Severity/Mobility Device Use	Associated Intervention Description	Quality Score	Area/ Theme	Main Themes Emerging in Study	Main Clinical Points/ Conclusion
									importance of contextualised perceptions of movement based on exploration of potential for change, as an integrated part of information and communication in the healthcare for PwMS.
Palacios-Ceña et al. (2016) Spain	To explore the experiences of multiple sclerosis patients who performed a virtual home-exercise programme using Kinect.	Design: qualitative Data col: interviews Analysis: convenience Theory: none Sampling: convenience	N: 24 Sex: 13 F 11 M Age: 36.69 (8.13) 20–60 Race: unreported	Diag: 9.68 (6.76) Type: 16 RR, 5 PP, 3 SP Disability: EDSS 3.9 (0.6) 3–5 Mob. device: unreported	Home-based computer exercise programme	14	Intervention opinion	Regaining previous capacity and abilities; sharing the disease; adapting to the new treatment; comparing oneself	The patients' experiences gathered in this study highlight perceptions of unexpected improvement, an eagerness to improve, and the positive opportunity of sharing treatment with their social entourage thanks to the games. These results can be applied to future research using video consoles, by individualising and adapting the games to the patient's abilities, and by developing a new field in rehabilitation.

(Continued)

TABLE 18.4 (*Continued*)

Summary of Each Study, Participant Characteristics, Associated Intervention, Quality Score and Inclusion of the Consequences or Determinants of Physical Activity and Exercise Participation. Note all Participants Persons with MS Unless Otherwise Noted

Study/ Country of Study	Study Aim (Abbreviated)	Design/Data Collection Method/ Analytical Approach/ Theoretical Perspective/ Sampling Method	N/Sex/Age (Mean, SD and Range)/Race	Mean Years Diagnosed (SD)/ Years Diagnose Rang e)/Disease Type/Disability Severity/Mobility Device Use	Associated Intervention Description	Quality Score	Area/ Theme	Main Themes Emerging in Study	Main Clinical Points/ Conclusion
Paul et al. (2014) UK	To explore the effectiveness and participant experience of web-based physiotherapy for pwMS.	Design: qualitative Data col: intervention Analysis: thematic analysis Theory: none Sampling: convenience	N: 30 Sex: 24 F 6 M Age: 51.7 (11.2) Race: unreported	Diag: 12.70 (9.05) Type: 17 RR, 4 PP, 5 SP, 2 Ben, 2 Unknown Disability: EDSS 5.9 (0.5) 5–6.5 Mob. device: unreported	Home-based computer physiotherapy and exercise programme	14	Intervention opinion	Use of the website: Physical and psychological change: Web-based physiotherapy as a mode of delivery: Future plans	Web-based physiotherapy is a feasible method of delivering physiotherapy and is acceptable to people moderately affected with MS. All participants rated the web-based physiotherapy programme as good or excellent and would be happy to use it again in the future.
Ploughman (2012) Canada	To describe the factors influencing healthy aging from the perspective of the older person with MS in order to build curricula for MS self-management programs.	Design: qualitative Data col: interview Analysis: thematic framework analysis Theory: none Sampling: purposeful	N: 18 Sex: 14 F 4 M Age: 66.5 (6.7) 56–80 Race: unreported	Diag: unreported Type: 3 RR 2 PP 10 SP 1 Ben 2 Unknown Disability: unreported Mob. device: 8 wheelchair, 5 walker, 5 none	None	14	Moving with MS	Finances: Social support: Strategies to stay healthy: The MS experience: Healthcare interactions	Healthcare, social engagement, lifestyle, and independence make critical contributions to health-related quality of life among older people with MS. This contribution depends on less-commonly addressed factors: financial flexibility, mental and cognitive health, resilience and social support. Strategies that target factors are important components of a comprehensive approach to rehabilitation and self-management of MS.

(Continued)

TABLE 18.4 (*Continued*)

Summary of Each Study, Participant Characteristics, Associated Intervention, Quality Score and Inclusion of the Consequences or Determinants of Physical Activity and Exercise Participation. Note all Participants Persons with MS Unless Otherwise Noted

Study/ Country of Study	Study Aim (Abbreviated)	Design/Data Collection Method/ Analytical Approach/ Theoretical Perspective/ Sampling Method	N/Sex/Age (Mean, SD and Range)/Race	Mean Years Diagnosed (SD)/ Years Diagnose Rang e)/Disease Type/Disability Severity/Mobility Device Use	Associated Intervention Description	Quality Score	Area/ Theme	Main Themes Emerging in Study	Main Clinical Points/ Conclusion
Plow et al. (2009) USA	Identify facilitators and barriers to physical activity (PA), and explore the utility of SCT and Transactional Model of Stress and Coping (TMSC) in understanding PA behaviour among pwMS.	Design: Qualitative Data col: Face interview Analysis: General Inductive Theory: SCT Sampling: Purposeful	N: 13 Sex: 11 F Age: 46.7 (±13.4), 18–61 Race: unreported.	Diag.: 12.2 (±14.1) Type: 9 RR, 2 SP, 2 Unk Disability (MSFC): Range -1.2–0.78. Mob. device: 8 none, 7 unreported	16 week group wellness (behavioural intervention) and home DIY exercise	16	Moving with MS	Self-efficacy: Outcome expectations: Self-regulation: Physical environment: Social environment: Primary appraisal: Secondary appraisal: Coping style	Results from this pilot study suggest that PA interventions will need to implement multiple strategies that target self-efficacy, social environment and coping styles. We found SCT and TMSC useful in understanding PA behaviour amongst persons with MS: however, a limitation to these theories is that they are not explicit in the relationship between health and cognitions. Future research will need to explore how to incorporate models of health and function into existing behaviour change theories.

(*Continued*)

TABLE 18.4 (*Continued*)

Summary of Each Study, Participant Characteristics, Associated Intervention, Quality Score and Inclusion of the Consequences or Determinants of Physical Activity and Exercise Participation. Note all Participants Persons with MS Unless Otherwise Noted

Study/ Country of Study	Study Aim (Abbreviated)	Design/Data Collection Method/ Analytical Approach/ Theoretical Perspective/ Sampling Method	N/Sex/Age (Mean, SD and Range)/Race	Mean Years Diagnosed (SD)/ Years Diagnose Rang e)/Disease Type/Disability Severity/Mobility Device Use	Associated Intervention Description	Quality Score	Area/ Theme	Main Themes Emerging in Study	Main Clinical Points/ Conclusion
Plow et al. (2014) USA	To (i) examine the potential of the intervention to improve psychosocial constructs and stages of change placement, (ii) describe participants' perceived motivators, barriers, and strategies for engaging in an exercise program, and (iii) identify strategies to better target and tailor the print-based intervention in future research.	Design: Data col: questionnaire and interview Analysis: Issue-focused analysis Theory: None Sampling: Convenience	N: 30 (14) Sex: 30 F Age: 47.5 (9.5) Race: 10 'racial minority'	Diag: 9 (7) Type: 30 RR Disability: PDDS 2.5 (1.57) 1–5 Mob. device: 10 cane	Pamphlet-based PA home programme	12	Intervention opinion: Moving with MS	Barriers: Action plan goals	Fatigue, pain, and lack of time were the commonly cited barriers to engage in the PA program: whereas the pamphlets, phone calls and action planning were cited as motivators. Participants used fatigue management strategies, enlisted social support, and modified their environment to routinely engage in the PA program. Strategies were identified to improve the PA intervention in future research.

(Continued)

TABLE 18.4 (*Continued*)

Summary of Each Study, Participant Characteristics, Associated Intervention, Quality Score and Inclusion of the Consequences or Determinants of Physical Activity and Exercise Participation. Note all Participants Persons with MS Unless Otherwise Noted

Study/ Country of Study	Study Aim (Abbreviated)	Design/Data Collection Method/ Analytical Approach/ Theoretical Perspective/ Sampling Method	N/Sex/Age (Mean, SD and Range)/Race	Mean Years Diagnosed (SD)/ Years Diagnose Rang e)/Disease Type/Disability Severity/Mobility Device Use	Associated Intervention Description	Quality Score	Area/ Theme	Main Themes Emerging in Study	Main Clinical Points/ Conclusion
Plow and Finlayson (2014) US	To examine the usability of Nintendo Wii Fit to promote physical activity in pwMS.	Design: Qualitative Data col: Telephone interviews Analysis: Inductive thematic Theory: Occupational well-being (Doble and Santha 2008) Sampling: Purposeful	N: 30 Sex: 23 F Age: 43.2 (±9.3), range unreported, Race: unreported.	Diag.: 9 (±6.8), Type: unreported, Disability (PDDS): 8 none, 7 mild, 14 moderate, 1 unknown. Mob. device: 1 Ca, 28 none, 1 unknown.	Home-based computer exercise programme	15	Intervention opinion	Reflecting on my abilities (i.e., Wii Fit provided feedback that encouraged participants to reflect on their health and function): Fitting into one's narrative (i.e., participants who used Wii Fit regularly described themselves as exercisers and that Wii Fit met their needs to engage in exercise): Convenient and fun to play (i.e., many participants described having fun whilst playing Wii and the advantages of using Wii Fit in their home vs going to gym): Novel technology, but same old exercise barriers (i.e., barriers described for using Wii Fit were	Improving the usability and customisability of commercially available exergaming technology could be of benefit to people with disabling conditions. Rehabilitation professionals need to consider patients' functional level, surrounding environment and preferences when prescribing a Wii Fit-based exercise programme.

(*Continued*)

TABLE 18.4 (*Continued*)

Summary of Each Study, Participant Characteristics, Associated Intervention, Quality Score and Inclusion of the Consequences or Determinants of Physical Activity and Exercise Participation. Note all Participants Persons with MS Unless Otherwise Noted

Study/ Country of Study	Study Aim (Abbreviated)	Design/Data Collection Method/ Analytical Approach/ Theoretical Perspective/ Sampling Method	N/Sex/Age (Mean, SD and Range)/Race	Mean Years Diagnosed (SD)/ Years Diagnose Rang e)/Disease Type/Disability Severity/Mobility Device Use	Associated Intervention Description	Quality Score	Area/ Theme	Main Themes Emerging in Study	Main Clinical Points/ Conclusion
								similar to barriers for engaging in a typical exercise programme): Usability issue (i.e., difficulties in learning to use Wii Fit and inability to customise exercises to meet the functional level of the participant).	
Salminen et al. (2014) Finland	To investigate the helpful components of rehabilitation from the point of view of pwMS.	Design: qualitative Data col: focus group & interview Analysis: inductive content analysis Theory: none Sampling: convenience	N: 68 Sex: 46 F 22 M Age: 47.0 (9.10) 28–61 Race: unreported	Diag: median = 12, 0–33 Type: 27 RR, 16 PP, 22 SP, 3 unknown Disability: EDSS 5.50 (1.30) 4–8 Mob. device: unreported	Community-based exercise group	15	Intervention opinion: Moving with MS	Rehabilitee him/herself; structures of everyday life; information; activity physical environment; social relationships; support	The findings show that helpful rehabilitation for people with MS is not a set of mechanistic interventions, but requires good social relationships and support.

(*Continued*)

TABLE 18.4 (*Continued*)

Summary of Each Study, Participant Characteristics, Associated Intervention, Quality Score and Inclusion of the Consequences or Determinants of Physical Activity and Exercise Participation. Note all Participants Persons with MS Unless Otherwise Noted

Study/ Country of Study	Study Aim (Abbreviated)	Design/Data Collection Method/ Analytical Approach/ Theoretical Perspective/ Sampling Method	N/Sex/Age (Mean, SD and Range)/Race	Mean Years Diagnosed (SD)/ Years Diagnose Rang e)/Disease Type/Disability Severity/Mobility Device Use	Associated Intervention Description	Quality Score	Area/ Theme	Main Themes Emerging in Study	Main Clinical Points/ Conclusion
Schneider and Young (2010) Canada	To explore the lived experiences of women living with multiple sclerosis and their perceived barriers to accessing physical activity.	Design: Qualitative Data col: Face interview Analysis: Thematic content analysis Theory: None Sampling: Purpose snowball	N: 7 Sex: 7 F Age: 50.4 (±5.2), 41–55 Race: 7 Caucasian.	Diag.: 6.1 (±2.9) 2–9, Type: 4 RR, 3 PP Disability: unreported Mob. device: 1 WC, 6 none	None	14	Moving with MS	Self-management, treatments, and personal attitude	The findings highlight the stated importance of informative dialogue with a physician at the time of diagnosis, as physicians have the potential to do much more for these women than just prescribe medications. Acknowledging the key importance of doctors' role in assisting MS patients with the day-to-day management of their condition is essential, if physicians hope to have a beneficial impact on these women's overall quality of life.
	fatigue perceptions in people with multiple sclerosis.	Interpretative description Theory: None Sampling: Purposeful		Mob. device: 10 none				tiredness: Exercise outcomes	control over fatigue' and promote 'listening to your body', in order to maximise the benefits of exercise intervention for individuals with MS-related fatigue.

(Continued)

TABLE 18.4 (*Continued*)

Summary of Each Study, Participant Characteristics, Associated Intervention, Quality Score and Inclusion of the Consequences or Determinants of Physical Activity and Exercise Participation. Note all Participants Persons with MS Unless Otherwise Noted

Study/ Country of Study	Study Aim (Abbreviated)	Design/Data Collection Method/ Analytical Approach/ Theoretical Perspective/ Sampling Method	N/Sex/Age (Mean, SD and Range)/Race	Mean Years Diagnosed (SD)/ Years Diagnose Rang e)/Disease Type/Disability Severity/Mobility Device Use	Associated Intervention Description	Quality Score	Area/ Theme	Main Themes Emerging in Study	Main Clinical Points/ Conclusion
Smith et al. (2009) NZ	To explore the influence of an 8-week exercise programme on	Design: Qualitative Data col: Face interview Analysis:	N: 10 Sex: 8 F, 2 M Age: 46.4 (±10.9), 32–61 Race: unreported.	Diag.: 13.1 (±14.6) Type: 10 RR Disability: unreported,	8 week DIY (physio-therapist suggested) aerobic exercise	17	Intervention opinion: Moving with MS	Perceived control: Listening to your body: Reaching the edge: Nature of	Healthcare professionals need to be cognisant of strategies which may enhance 'perceived
Smith et al. (2011) NZ	To describe the experiences of pwMS-related fatigue, who engaged in community-based exercise activities in order to discover how fatigue influenced their exercise participation.	Design: Qualitative Data col: Face interview Analysis: Thematic analysis Theory: None Sampling: Purposeful	N: 9 Sex: 9 F Age: range 28–70 Race: unreported.	Diag.: unreported Type: RR 5, SP 3, 1 unknown Mob. device: unreported	Weekly self-guided exercise	16	Intervention opinion: Moving with MS	Wellness philosophy: Related goal: Belief that control is possible; Feeling safe; Feeling supported; Defining self; Managing limits; Satisfied with trade-offs; Self-integrity	Identification of factors influencing perceived control over fatigue will assist healthcare providers when facilitating community exercise choices for people with MS.

(*Continued*)

TABLE 18.4 (*Continued*)

Summary of Each Study, Participant Characteristics, Associated Intervention, Quality Score and Inclusion of the Consequences or Determinants of Physical Activity and Exercise Participation. Note all Participants Persons with MS Unless Otherwise Noted

Study/ Country of Study	Study Aim (Abbreviated)	Design/Data Collection Method/ Analytical Approach/ Theoretical Perspective/ Sampling Method	N/Sex/Age (Mean, SD and Range)/Race	Mean Years Diagnosed (SD)/ Years Diagnose Rang e)/Disease Type/Disability Severity/Mobility Device Use	Associated Intervention Description	Quality Score	Area/ Theme	Main Themes Emerging in Study	Main Clinical Points/ Conclusion
Smith et al. (2013a) NZ	To investigate experiences of participating in a feasibility trial of a novel physiotherapy intervention (Blue Prescription).	Design: Qualitative Data col: Face interview Analysis: General inductive Theory: Transtheoretical (Prochaska and Velicer 1997) Sampling: Convenience	N: 27, Sex: 23 F, 4 M Age: 51 (±11.1), 34–71 Race: 26 Caucasian, 1 Māori.	Diag.: 15.8 (±10.3), Type: 8RR, 3PP, 7SP, 9 unknown Disability: unreported, Mob dev.: 7WC, 2 Wa, 8 Ca, 10 none.	Community based PA. collaboration between physio-therapists and pwMS (Blue prescription)	14	Intervention opinion: Moving with MS	'Support' (subthemes: 'The therapeutic relationship': 'The Blue Prescription approach': 'Supporting themselves): Motivation to participate: Improving the Blue Prescription approach	The Blue Prescription Intervention was perceived by participants to be supportive, motivating and enabling when attempting to increase levels of PA. Participants with multiple sclerosis who were ready to adopt higher levels of PA appeared to be more receptive to the Blue Prescription intervention than those who were not. Frequently used outcome measures might require further development or refinement in order to make better sense to people with multiple sclerosis living in New Zealand.

(*Continued*)

TABLE 18.4 (*Continued*)

Summary of Each Study, Participant Characteristics, Associated Intervention, Quality Score and Inclusion of the Consequences or Determinants of Physical Activity and Exercise Participation. Note all Participants Persons with MS Unless Otherwise Noted

Study/ Country of Study	Study Aim (Abbreviated)	Design/Data Collection Method/ Analytical Approach/ Theoretical Perspective/ Sampling Method	N/Sex/Age (Mean, SD and Range)/Race	Mean Years Diagnosed (SD)/ Years Diagnose Rang e)/Disease Type/Disability Severity/Mobility Device Use	Associated Intervention Description	Quality Score	Area/ Theme	Main Themes Emerging in Study	Main Clinical Points/ Conclusion
Smith et al. (2013b) NZ	To describe the experiences of four groups of healthcare providers who facilitate exercise interventions for people with MS-related fatigue.	Design: Qualitative Data Col: Focus Groups & Interviews Analysis: Thematic analysis Theory: None Sampling: Purposeful	N: 15 (6 PT, 3 OT, 3 Support worker, 3 Neuro) Sex: unreported Age: unreported Race: unreported	Diag: Type: Disability: Mob. device:	None	13	Wider MS community	Nature of fatigue: Professional challenges (Subthemes: • Barriers to implementation • Stirring conflict • Modifying roles): Demanding creativity (Subthemes: • Challenging science • Mind-body)	The nature of fatigue and professional challenges influenced clinician practice by 'demanding creativity' with regard to exercise prescription and advice. Healthcare providers are encouraged to consider strategies of active listening and careful observation when providing individualised exercise programs for people with MS-related fatigue. In addition, recognition and understanding of the complex nature of fatigue by the interdisciplinary team might facilitate more positive exercise experiences for this population.
Smith et al. (2015) NZ	To better understand how MS-related fatigue	Design: qualitative	N: 18 Sex 18 M Age: 36–68	Diagnosed: 3 yrs–21 yrs Type: 10 RR, 5 PP, 3 SP	None	13	Moving with MS	Emotional responses to fatigue and exercise Self-regulation	exercise engagement and achieve greater self-efficacy. Healthcare

(*Continued*)

TABLE 18.4 (*Continued*)

Summary of Each Study, Participant Characteristics, Associated Intervention, Quality Score and Inclusion of the Consequences or Determinants of Physical Activity and Exercise Participation. Note all Participants Persons with MS Unless Otherwise Noted

Study/ Country of Study	Study Aim (Abbreviated)	Design/Data Collection Method/ Analytical Approach/ Theoretical Perspective/ Sampling Method	N/Sex/Age (Mean, SD and Range)/Race	Mean Years Diagnosed (SD)/ Years Diagnose Rang e)/Disease Type/Disability Severity/Mobility Device Use	Associated Intervention Description	Quality Score	Area/ Theme	Main Themes Emerging in Study	Main Clinical Points/ Conclusion
	influences exercise participation.	Data col: interviews (2 telephone, 16 face to face) Analysis: thematic analysis Theory: none Sampling: purposeful	Race: 17 Caucasian, 1 Maori	Disability: unreported Mob. device: unreported				processes in response to fatigue and exercise. Subthemes: Complex expressions of fatigue; Engaging in exercise and goal adjustment; exercise engagement and achieve greater self-efficacy.	professionals might consider introducing goal readjustment strategies to help men with MS-related fatigue retain perceived control over exercise engagement and achieve greater self-efficacy.
Sweet et al. (2013) Canada	To examine the preferred sources and methods for acquiring physical activity information of individuals with MS using the Comprehensive Model of Information Seeking. A secondary objective was to explore the barriers and facilitators to physical activity information seeking	Design: qualitative Data col: focus group and telephone interview Analysis: thematic analysis Theory: Comprehensive Model of Information Seeking Sampling: convenience	N: 21 Sex: 13 F, 8M Age: 48.9 (14.2) 18–80 Race: unreported	Diag: 12.4 (9.92) Type: 9 RR, 5 PP, 4 SP, 3 Unknown Disability: EDSS 4.63 (2.19) Mob. device: 9 none, 12 unknown	None	15	Moving with MS	Antecedents: Information carrier factors: Content and tools to deliver physical activity messages: Information seeking actions	Healthcare professionals, National MS Societies, and peers should work together to deliver specific and relevant physical activity messages the MS population.

(*Continued*)

TABLE 18.4 (*Continued*)

Summary of Each Study, Participant Characteristics, Associated Intervention, Quality Score and Inclusion of the Consequences or Determinants of Physical Activity and Exercise Participation. Note all Participants Persons with MS Unless Otherwise Noted

Study/ Country of Study	Study Aim (Abbreviated)	Design/Data Collection Method/ Analytical Approach/ Theoretical Perspective/ Sampling Method	N/Sex/Age (Mean, SD and Range)/Race	Mean Years Diagnosed (SD)/ Years Diagnose Rang e)/Disease Type/Disability Severity/Mobility Device Use	Associated Intervention Description	Quality Score	Area/ Theme	Main Themes Emerging in Study	Main Clinical Points/ Conclusion
Thomas et al. (2017) UK Note: Full qualitative results in preparation.	To test the feasibility of conducting a definitive trial of the effectiveness and cost-effectiveness of Mii-vitaliSe: a home-based, physiotherapist-supported Nintendo Wii intervention.	Design: mixed method Data col: semi structured interview Analysis: thematic analysis Theory: SCT Sampling: convenience	N: 30 Sex: 27 F 3 M Age: 49.3 (8.7) 33–65 Race: all Caucasian	Diag: 0–16 Type: 21 RR 1 PP 5 SP 1 Ben 2 Unknown Disability: unreported Mob. device: unreported	Home-based computer exercise programme	14	Intervention opinion: Moving with MS	Acceptability of study design: Acceptability of the Mii-vitaliSe intervention – participants	Most study participants were positive about Mii-vitaliSe, which was seen to be an activity levels. Materials and physiotherapy contact time were acceptable.
Toomey and Coote (2013) Ireland	To explore the development, implementation, and outcome of a new model of care has used Exercise Buddies (paid professional carers) to exercise with PwMS under the direction of community physiotherapists.	Design: qualitative Data col: semi structured interview Analysis: thematic analysis Theory: none Sampling: convenience	N: 9 (2 PwMS 1 spouse, 2 phys, 2 exercise buddys with their supervisor) Sex: unreported Age: unreported Race: unreported	Diag: 15+ Type: unreported Disability: unreported Mob. device: unreported	Home-based buddy exercise programme	15	Wider MS community	Physical and psychological benefits for PwMS and physical and psychological benefits for carers emerged. Within communication difficulties, themes of defining roles & expectations and feedback & communication during implementation emerged. A subtheme of Insufficient training of buddies emerged within the theme of Defining roles and expectations.	The Exercise Buddy system is a home-based intervention delivered at a community level, and has potential as a model of care with both physical and psychological benefits reported for PwMS and their carers. Issues discussed mostly related to communication and training. These need to be addressed for future successful development.

(*Continued*)

TABLE 18.4 (*Continued*)

Summary of Each Study, Participant Characteristics, Associated Intervention, Quality Score and Inclusion of the Consequences or Determinants of Physical Activity and Exercise Participation. Note all Participants Persons with MS Unless Otherwise Noted

Study/ Country of Study	Study Aim (Abbreviated)	Design/Data Collection Method/ Analytical Approach/ Theoretical Perspective/ Sampling Method	N/Sex/Age (Mean, SD and Range)/Race	Mean Years Diagnosed (SD)/ Years Diagnose Rang e)/Disease Type/Disability Severity/Mobility Device Use	Associated Intervention Description	Quality Score	Area/ Theme	Main Themes Emerging in Study	Main Clinical Points/ Conclusion
Van der Linden et al. (2014) UK	To explore the feasibility, efficacy, and the participants' experiences of a Pilates programme for pwMS who use a wheelchair.	Design: Mixed methods Data col: Face interview Analysis: Thematic analysis Theory: None Sampling: Purposeful	N: 10. Sex: unclear Age: unclear Race: unreported.	Diag.: unreported Type: unreported Disability: unreported, Mob. device: 10 WC	12 week group-based wheelchair Pilates	16	Intervention opinion	Participation in targeted Pilates classes; Perceived benefits of Pilates program; No perceived benefits: Negative effects; Difficulty identifying change; Small changes that are valued; Class content and structure; Views relating to home exercise; Negative views regarding exercise classes not targeted at people with MS: Barriers to participation; Attitudes towards continuing Pilates	Group-based core stability exercise or Pilates for people with MS who use wheelchair is a feasible and safe way of exercising for this patient group. Pilates exercises for people moderately to severely affected by MS resulted in a decrease in back and shoulder pain and improvement in sitting balance. Future appropriately powered randomised controlled studies into Pilates for people with MS reliant on wheelchair are warranted.

(*Continued*)

TABLE 18.4 (*Continued*)

Summary of Each Study, Participant Characteristics, Associated Intervention, Quality Score and Inclusion of the Consequences or Determinants of Physical Activity and Exercise Participation. Note all Participants Persons with MS Unless Otherwise Noted

Study/ Country of Study	Study Aim (Abbreviated)	Design/Data Collection Method/ Analytical Approach/ Theoretical Perspective/ Sampling Method	N/Sex/Age (Mean, SD and Range)/Race	Mean Years Diagnosed (SD)/ Years Diagnose Rang e)/Disease Type/Disability Severity/Mobility Device Use	Associated Intervention Description	Quality Score	Area/ Theme	Main Themes Emerging in Study	Main Clinical Points/ Conclusion
Van Ruymbeke and Schneider (2013) Canada	To identify the effects of physical activity on the lives of those living with MS and to determine their perception of their overall well-being with a focus on physical, emotional, and social determinants of health.	Design: Qualitative Data col: Face interview Analysis: thematic analysis Theory: None Sampling: Purposeful	N: 6 Sex: 6 F Age 64.5 (±unreported) Range unreported	Diag.: unreported, Disability: unreported. Type: 2 RR, 2 PP, 1 Benign, 1 unknown Disability: unreported Mob. device: 2 WC, 4 unknown	None (inclusion criteria required they exercised twice per week)	10	Moving with MS	Group atmosphere: Everyday activities as exercise	Participants identified that being in a group atmosphere and having a competent and motivating program facilitator are key aspects of any exercise program. Likewise, the idea that everyday activities and tasks can be used as a means of physical activity also was mentioned by many participants.

Note: Data are described as mean and standard deviation unless otherwise noted *.

Demographic details of whole sample reported, unable to differentiate interviewed MS sample from larger sample.

Data col: data collection method, Analysis: analytical approach, Theory: theoretical perspective, F: female, Diag: years diagnosed, Type: disease type, Disability: disability severity, Mob. Dev. mobility device used (highest dependency recorded), WC: wheelchair, Wa: walker, Ca: cane/single point assistance, RR: relapsing remitting MS, PP: primary progressive MS, SP: secondary progressive MS, Ben: benign MS, EDSS: Expanded Disability Status Scale, PDDS: patient determined disease steps, MSIS-29: MS Impact Scale-29, GNDS: Guys Neurological Disability Scale, MSFC: Multiple Sclerosis Functional Composite, PwMS: people with Multiple Sclerosis, Phys: physical therapist/physiotherapist, OT: occupational therapist, Neuro: neurologist, NA: not applicable, HCPs: healthcare practitioners, AF: aqua fitness.

[a] *Giunti*: PwMS age median = 43.5, (IQR = 40.25–50), HCPs age median = 40 (IQR = 28–53.25), EDSS median = 4 (IQR = 3.75–5.12), and years since diagnosis median = 17 (IQR = 10.50–21.50).

[b] *Learmonth*: EDSS median = 1 (IQR = 0–2.5).

Participants

The opinions of a total of 106 people involved in the MS community were gathered in the interviews or focus groups. Demographic and clinical data were not always reported for participants and reported data can be seen in Table 18.4. Four studies reported the age, sex, and time in clinical practice for their healthcare professional participants (Forsberg et al. 2015; Giunti et al. 2018; Held Bradford et al. 2018; Learmonth et al. 2018a), overall average age was around 42 years, overall there were 48 female and 22 male healthcare professionals, and overall the average time in clinical practice was around 15 years. In the one study which included fitness centre managers (Anderson et al. 2017), detail on age and sex was not reported. The two studies who included carers (Horton et al. 2015; Fakolade et al. 2018) reported the age of carers to be around 56 years, and there were opinions from 20 female and 7 male carers.

Quality Assessment

For studies including the wider MS community, quality assessment scores ranged from 13 to 18 (Table 18.4), suggesting reasonable study quality. All of the studies reported the study purpose and provided a relevant review of the literature. Two studies identified a theoretical perspective (Held Bradford et al. 2018; Learmonth et al. 2018a), and in both cases this was social cognitive theory, based on the work of Bandura (2004). The process of sampling was discussed in all studies, and sampling was continued until redundancy in five studies (Anderson et al. 2017; Fakolade et al. 2018; Giunti et al. 2018; Held Bradford et al. 2018; Learmonth et al. 2018a), and all studies reported receiving participants consent for participation. In terms of data collection, no studies provided a clear description of where the research took place, although one study described telephone interviews (Held Bradford et al. 2018). Six studies gave clear and complete descriptions of the participants (Smith et al. 2013a; Forsberg et al. 2015; Horton et al. 2015; Fakolade et al. 2018; Held Bradford et al. 2018; Learmonth et al. 2018a), and, in one study, authors provided a clear description of the researchers credentials (Learmonth et al. 2018a). Only one study provided a clear and complete description of the relationship between researchers and participants (Fakolade et al. 2018), no study clearly provided researchers assumptions, and procedural rigour was described in all except one study (Giunti et al. 2018).

For data analysis, all studies used inductive analysis, and all studies' findings reflected the data. Most studies (Smith et al. 2013a; Toomey and Coote 2013; Forsberg et al. 2015; Fakolade et al. 2018; Giunti et al. 2018; Held Bradford et al. 2018; Learmonth et al. 2018a) reported following a decision trail to analyse data, all studies described their process for transforming data into themes, and all studies resulted in a meaningful picture of the topic of interest. To ensure trustworthiness in the data, all studies reported triangulation of sources and methods, and five studies reported triangulation of researchers (Smith et al. 2013a; Toomey and Coote 2013; Fakolade et al. 2018; Giunti et al. 2018; Learmonth et al. 2018a), no study used triangulation of theories, and member checking was used to verify findings in five studies (Forsberg et al. 2015; Horton et al. 2015; Fakolade et al. 2018; Held Bradford et al. 2018; Learmonth et al. 2018a). In relation to conclusions, all studies reported appropriate conclusions which are relevant to clinical and research practice for MS care, however, one study (Thomas et al. 2017) provided limited qualitative results (as part of results for a feasibility trial) and therefore full conclusions could not be made at this time.

Appraisal of Studies

In relation to the conclusions from the papers, it is noteworthy to comment upon the general aims of studies, their main findings and conclusions are listed in Table 18.4. There were two main subthemes within the theme of *the wider MS community*, and these comprised opinions from (1) healthcare and fitness professionals and (2) carers.

Healthcare and Fitness Professionals

The one study which explicitly gathered opinions from (fitness facility) managers (Anderson et al. 2017) aimed to identify barriers to persons with neurological conditions (including MS) towards accessing exercise, and the researchers concluded that specially trained exercise staff and training of fitness professionals in this area is a priority. Studies of healthcare professionals (Smith et al. 2013a; Toomey and Coote 2013; Giunti et al. 2018; Held Bradford et al. 2018; Learmonth et al. 2018a) have mainly aimed to understand the experiences of healthcare providers delivering a specific physiotherapy or exercise intervention to persons with MS (Smith et al. 2013a; Toomey and Coote 2013; Giunti et al. 2018; Held Bradford et al. 2018), and these studies conclude the patient provider relationship is critical for success in exercise interventions, and that creativity is required by clinicians to deliver interventions which address patients' needs. One study (Learmonth et al. 2018a) had a wider aim to explore the needs of healthcare providers for promoting exercise, the authors concluded that the patient provider role is critical, but that healthcare providers require specific training to provide tools and strategies for increased exercise promotion in patients with MS.

> The healthcare system, the healthcare team, and the clinical appointment represent opportunities for the promotion of exercise behaviour among persons with MS. We further identified that such opportunities require education of healthcare providers and the development and provision of tools and strategies for behaviour change. (Learmonth et al. 2018a)

Opinions from Carers

Two studies gathered views of carers, one study highlighted the importance of integrating an exercise approach which is relevant to both the person with MS and carer (Fakolade et al. 2018), whilst in the other study, the carers spoke of the many far reaching benefits they noted from participation in exercise by the person with MS whom they cared for (Horton et al. 2015). These studies indicate that carers are aware of changing behaviours (i.e., participation in physical activity and exercise), and both studies identify that both the carer and person with MS might work together learn about the importance of physical activity and exercise. These studies highlight the importance of healthcare providers to educate both the person with MS and the carer of physical activity and exercise.

> Participants shared their experiences with finding other options or modifying existing types of activities so they could continue being active [together, both person with MS and carer]. Throughout this process, people with Multiple Sclerosis (PwMS) also reported working collaboratively with their family caregivers to problem-solve and identify ways to ensure continuous participation in physical activity (PA). (Fakolade et al. 2018).

Summary

Taken together, the opinions of the wider MS community suggest that there is an important relationship between healthcare professionals and persons with MS, and this relationship offers an opportunity to better understand the exercise behaviours of persons with MS and to promote exercise overall. The research also suggests that training may be required for healthcare and fitness professionals involved in the MS community, it is important that there are professionals available to persons with MS who are knowledgeable in both exercise and MS. Finally, it is important that the role of the carer in the MS community is addressed and provided with a greater voice in research, as carers play a pivotal role in the health behaviours of persons with MS.

Theme 2: Opinions on Exercise Associated with Exercise Interventions

> 'I think the reasons (for exercising) are the same [as for everyone else], but I think now because of this condition it's much more valuable – the benefit is going to be much greater. I know if I don't exercise I'm just going to get worse and worse... got to do it because I know I need to. I've got to do it today, tomorrow, and every day.' Study participant with MS (Kasser 2009)

For over 25 years, researchers have been establishing the effect of exercise and physical activity during research-focused exercise interventions (Kinnett-Hopkins et al. 2017a). This offers a good opportunity to gather opinions from these research participants. Many studies have gathered opinions of persons with MS who are involved in an exercise or physical activity intervention associated with the research team.

Opinions from some 570 persons with MS reported in 26 studies (Dodd et al. 2006; Kasser 2009; Smith et al. 2009, 2011, 2013b; Aubrey and Demain 2012; Learmonth et al. 2013; Mulligan et al. 2013; Normann et al. 2013; Kersten et al. 2014, 2015; Paul et al. 2014; Plow and Finlayson 2014; Plow et al. 2014; Salminen et al. 2014; van der Linden et al. 2014; Clarke and Coote 2015; Forsberg et al. 2015; Casey et al. 2016; Palacios-Ceña et al. 2016; Chard 2017; Crank et al. 2017; Dixon-Ibarra et al. 2017; Thomas et al. 2017; Giunti et al. 2018; Learmonth et al. 2018b) are included. It is notable that data gathered during these studies would also be applicable to other topics discussed in this chapter. Equally, there are studies which will be discussed elsewhere that recruited persons with MS for an exercise or physical activity intervention, but subsequent qualitative publications had an aim which was not to generate opinions on the intervention, and these studies will be highlighted appropriately.

The research was conducted globally by several groups of researchers in North America (Kasser 2009; Plow and Finlayson 2014; Plow et al. 2014; Chard 2017; Dixon-Ibarra et al. 2017; Learmonth et al. 2018b), Europe (Aubrey and Demain 2012; Normann et al. 2013; Kersten et al. 2014; Paul et al. 2014; Salminen et al. 2014; van der Linden et al. 2014; Clarke and Coote 2015; Forsberg et al. 2015; Casey et al. 2016; Palacios-Ceña et al. 2016; Crank et al. 2017; Thomas et al. 2017; Giunti et al.2018), and Oceania (Dodd et al. 2006; Smith et al. 2009, 2011, 2013b; Mulligan et al. 2013; Kersten et al. 2015). Studies were conducted between 2006 and 2018. All of the studies were primarily qualitative in method and gathered data via interviews or focus groups. Table 18.4 provides study information, participant information, associated information, quality score, main thematic findings, and a summary of the authors main conclusions or relevant points.

To recruit participants for studies, the most common recruitment process was convenience sampling used by 15 research teams (Dodd et al. 2006; Smith et al.2009, 2013b; Aubrey and Demain 2012; Learmonth et al. 2013; Mulligan et al. 2013; Kersten et al. 2014, 2015; Paul et al. 2014; Plow et al. 2014; Salminen et al. 2014; Clarke and Coote 2015; Forsberg et al. 2015; Casey et al. 2016; Palacios-Ceña et al. 2016; Chard 2017; Dixon-Ibarra et al. 2017; Learmonth et al. 2018b), other sampling approaches included purposive sampling (Smith et al. 2011; Normann et al. 2013; Thomas et al. 2017), purposive-convenience (Kasser 2009; Crank et al. 2017), and purposeful (Plow and Finlayson 2014; van der Linden et al. 2014; Giunti et al. 2018). Data were collected via one-to-one interviews in 12 studies (Dodd et al. 2006; Kasser 2009; Smith et al. 2009; Aubrey and Demain 2012; Mulligan et al. 2013; Normann et al. 2013; Kersten et al. 2014; Paul et al. 2014; Plow and Finlayson 2014; Plow et al. 2014; van der Linden et al. 2014; Palacios-Ceña et al. 2016), with some groups adopting telephone interviews for some of their participants (van der Linden et al. 2014; Chard 2017; Thomas et al. 2017; Learmonth et al. 2018b). Research groups also conducted focus groups (Learmonth et al. 2013; Clarke and Coote 2015; Dixon-Ibarra et al. 2017) or a combination of focus groups and interviews (Smith et al. 2011, 2013b; Salminen et al. 2014; Forsberg et al. 2015; Kersten et al. 2015; Casey et al. 2016; Crank et al. 2017) to gather data from participants. Most studies described using a *content* or *thematic analysis* except for one study which used a *framework analysis* (Crank et al. 2017) and another study which described using an *issue-focused analysis* approach.

Participants

570 persons with MS took part in the interviews or focus groups. Demographic and clinical data were not always reported for participants and reported data can be seen in Table 18.4. For the 466 persons for whom age was reported, mean age of participants was 50 years, and of the 536 people for whom sex was reported, 408 (~75%) participants were female. Some studies reported time since diagnoses, type of MS, disability level (most commonly expressed via the Expanded Disability Status Scale [EDSS] [Kurtzke 1983] or the self-reported EDSS (Ratzker et al. 1997]), and race. Of the 159 persons for whom mean time since diagnosis was recorded, this was 11.6 years, and of the of 379 persons for whom type of MS was reported, 220 had relapsing remitting MS, 41 had primary progressive MS, and 68 had secondary progressive MS. Of the 196 participants for whom EDSS was reported, the mean EDSS was 4.5, and disability was more generally described for 95 participants in studies, with 18 having no disability, 27 mild disability, 52 medium disability, and 55 high levels of disability. Two studies reported race where 40 participants were white and 15 were black.

Quality Assessment

For studies undertaken related to an exercise or physical activity intervention, quality assessment scores ranged from 11 to 20 (Table 18.4), suggesting a fairly wide range of quality. All of the studies reported the study purpose and provided a relevant review of the literature.

Four studies identified a theoretical perspective (Kasser 2009; Plow and Finlayson 2014; Thomas et al. 2017; Learmonth et al. 2018b), and these theoretical perspectives were social cognitive theory (Kasser 2009; Thomas et al. 2017; Learmonth et al. 2018b) and the theory of occupational well-being (Plow et al. 2009). The process of sampling was discussed in all studies, and sampling was continued until redundancy in 13 studies (Smith et al. 2011, 2013b; Aubrey and Demain 2012; Learmonth et al. 2013; Normann et al. 2013; Kersten et al. 2014, 2015; Paul et al. 2014; Salminen et al. 2014; van der Linden et al. 2014; Palacios-Ceña et al. 2016; Chard 2017; Thomas et al. 2017; Giunti et al. 2018). Four studies did not clearly indicate that informed consent was taken from participants (Kasser 2009; Plow et al. 2009; Mulligan et al. 2013; Plow and Finlayson 2014). In terms of data collection, six studies provided a clear description of where the research took place (Dodd et al. 2006; Normann et al. 2013; Paul et al. 2014; Palacios-Ceña et al. 2016; Thomas et al. 2017; Learmonth et al. 2018b). Almost all studies gave a reasonably clear description of participants except for two studies (van der Linden et al. 2014; Giunti et al. 2018), and in 11 studies authors provided a clear description of the researchers credentials (Plow et al. 2009; Smith et al. 2009; Aubrey and Demain 2012; Learmonth et al. 2013; Normann et al. 2013; Salminen et al. 2014; van der Linden et al. 2014; Kersten et al. 2015; Crank et al. 2017; Dixon-Ibarra et al. 2017; Learmonth et al. 2018b). Nine studies provided a clear and complete description of the relationship between researchers and participants (Dodd et al. 2006; Kasser 2009; Smith et al. 2011; Learmonth et al. 2013; Normann et al. 2013; Paul et al. 2014; van der Linden et al. 2014; Clarke and Coote 2015; Learmonth et al. 2018b), no study clearly provided researchers assumptions. Procedural rigour was described in 16 studies (Dodd et al. 2006; Kasser 2009; Plow et al. 2009; Aubrey and Demain 2012; Learmonth et al. 2013; Mulligan et al. 2013; Normann et al. 2013; Smith et al. 2013b; Kersten et al. 2014, 2015; Plow and Finlayson 2014; Salminen et al. 2014; Clarke and Coote 2015; Forsberg et al. 2015; Casey et al. 2016; Learmonth et al. 2018b).

For data analysis, almost all studies stated used inductive analysis except for three (Kasser 2009; Normann et al. 2013; Paul et al. 2014), all studies' findings reflected the data. Some of the studies (Smith et al. 2009; Normann et al. 2013; Plow and Finlayson 2014; Salminen et al. 2014; van der Linden et al. 2014; Clarke and Coote 2015; Forsberg et al. 2015; Casey et al. 2016; Crank et al. 2017; Dixon-Ibarra et al. 2017; Giunti et al. 2018; Learmonth et al. 2018b) reported following a decision trail to analyse data, most studies clearly indicated the process used for transforming data into themes except for five studies (Dodd et al. 2006; Kersten et al. 2014, 2015; Paul et al. 2014; Plow and Finlayson 2014), and all studies resulted in a meaningful picture of the topic of interest. To ensure trustworthiness in the data, nine studies reported triangulation of sources and methods (Smith et al. 2009, 2011, 2013b; Aubrey and Demain 2012; van der Linden et al. 2014; Forsberg et al. 2015; Dixon-Ibarra et al. 2017; Giunti et al. 2018; Learmonth et al. 2018b), and 14 studies reported triangulation of researchers (Dodd et al. 2006; Kasser 2009; Smith et al. 2009; Normann et al. 2013; Kersten et al. 2014, 2015; Paul et al. 2014; Plow and Finlayson 2014; Forsberg et al. 2015; Casey et al. 2016; Crank et al. 2017; Dixon-Ibarra et al. 2017; Giunti et al. 2018; Learmonth et al. 2018b), no study reported triangulation of theories, member checking was used to verify findings in nine studies (Dodd et al. 2006; Kasser 2009; Smith et al. 2011; Aubrey and Demain 2012; Normann et al. 2013; Kersten et al. 2014; Casey et al. 2016; Crank et al. 2017; Dixon-Ibarra et al. 2017). In relation to conclusions, all studies reported appropriate conclusions which are relevant to clinical and research practice for MS care, one study, which provided results of both quantitative and qualitative outcomes, indicated further reporting of in-depth qualitative data will occur in the future (Thomas et al. 2017).

Appraisal of Studies

The main findings and conclusion from the studies related to *opinions on exercise associated with exercise interventions* are listed in Table 18.4. There were three main subthemes within this these, and these comprised opinions on: (1) group-based exercise interventions, (2) home- and individual-based exercise interventions, and (3) interventions and new technology.

Group-Based Exercise Interventions

Interventions which participants with MS have included community group classes (Aubrey and Demain 2012; Learmonth et al. 2013; Smith et al. 2013a; Salminen et al. 2014; van der Linden et al. 2014; Clarke and Coote 2015; Chard 2017; Dixon-Ibarra et al. 2017), and perhaps the strongest conclusions from these studies suggested that participants experienced many physical and psychological benefits, with most participants enjoying the social aspect of community group classes. Similar reports were heard from participants who took part in group-based exercise where the setting was in university or clinic settings (Dodd et al. 2006; Kasser 2009; Giunti et al. 2018). For example, participants perceived that the group settings were good for peer support and were an important factor in participants completing their exercise programme. However, participants occasionally commented that group exercise didn't allow for 1:1 instruction or a personalised exercise plan, and therefore some participants may have also liked to have individualised exercises based on their personal needs alongside group activities.

> Many participants described the exercise groups as generating a sense of camaraderie. They viewed this as instrumental in fostering a positive attitude towards managing their MS. On the negative side, several of the more able members explicitly stated the MS group exercise was not intense enough for them. It was also suggested that the routines should be varied to keep people's attention (Aubrey and Demain 2012).

Studies also reported that there were numerous knowledge gains, and physical and psychological benefits perceived by participants from taking part in a group exercise intervention, and these were summarised in many studies, for example, (Dodd et al. 2006; Kasser 2009; Learmonth et al. 2013; van der Linden et al. 2014; Clarke and Coote 2015) and are depicted in Figure 18.2.

The importance of group exercise is perhaps clarified best from qualitative research. The voices of participants speak of the peer support, knowledge gained, and other psychological and physical benefits of group exercise. These opinions further suggest that the true value of a whole intervention is greater than the sum of its parts (i.e., the prescribed exercises, the social interaction, and the knowledge gains).

Home- and Individual-Based Exercise Interventions

Home-based, or exercises chosen by participants to be completed unsupervised and individually in a home or community setting, are also popular in the literature (Plow et al. 2009; Smith et al. 2009, 2011; Mulligan et al. 2013; Kersten et al. 2014, 2015; Paul et al. 2014;

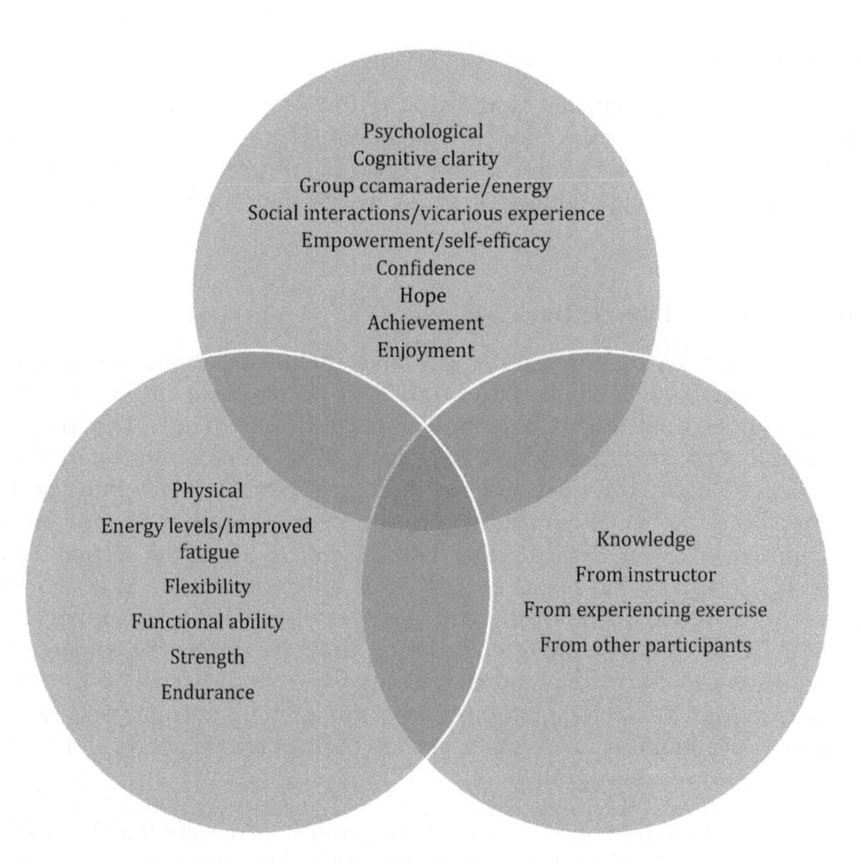

FIGURE 18.2
Perceived benefits from participation in exercise interventions.

Plow and Finlayson 2014; Forsberg et al. 2015; Palacios-Ceña et al. 2016; Crank et al. 2017; Thomas et al. 2017; Learmonth et al. 2018b). These exercise programmes were researcher- or physiotherapist-led in-person delivered (Smith et al. 2009, 2011; Mulligan et al. 2013; Kersten et al. 2014, 2015; Crank et al. 2017), delivered via phone or video calls, or delivered via mail-outs from researchers (Plow et al. 2009; Learmonth et al. 2018b). From these studies, the importance of the relationship between the exercise provider and the client is wanted. For example, the exercise provider provides an appropriate interactive information source, motivation, and social support. In Chard et al.'s study (Chard 2017), participant satisfaction with the exercise programme was heavily influenced by their relationship with the instructor:

> They described their satisfaction as stemming from having a 'good' instructor, i.e., someone who was appropriately enthusiastic, inclusive, and able to offer exercise modifications to accommodate ability level (Chard 2017).

Thus, the importance of the relationship between the healthcare provider and person with MS is underscored once again. The importance of this provider-patient relationship is also evident from negative narratives by participants. For example, poor instruction from exercise providers may results in attrition from exercise. In one study, participants narrative indicates the importance of instructor knowledge on MS symptoms (Aubrey and Demain 2012), and this theme was echoed in a number of studies:

> It was important to participants that the physiotherapist was specialised in neurology and had an appreciation of the range of symptoms PwMS may present with and how to prescribe exercises for this group. In other examples of exercise prescription, participants had negative experiences that they attributed to the lack of the instructors' knowledge about MS, inadequate levels of supervision, and exercise programmes which were too difficult (Aubrey and Demain 2012).

One study has determined participants opinion of a home-based intervention which was based on the current physical activity guidelines for persons with MS (Learmonth et al. 2018b). These guidelines involve two 30 minute sessions of aerobic exercise and two sessions of resistance exercises per week. The study participants found the guidelines to be appropriate for themselves and perceived that they were appropriate for others with MS. The participants noted that they would like to see a variety of exercise options to meet these physical activity guidelines.

Interventions and New Technology

Website and online interventions designed for research purposes are growing in popularity, and to date one study has reported qualitative findings from a website hosted intervention (Paul et al. 2014), and a more recent study has gathered participants opinions on what their preferred content would be for a specific website and online intervention (Casey et al. 2016). Comments from participants indicate that online web-based and mobile health technology to encourage exercise should be convenient, customisable to the participants needs, and motivating. A sociability aspect was also deemed important, and it would seem that participants would like access to knowledge from healthcare providers and access to peer support from other persons with MS who were also using the programme.

> Participants explained how the web resource might build a sense of community and peer support amongst users. Also, for those not actively involved in their local or regional MS Society's, that the website could act as a bridge to contact other PwMS (Casey et al. 2016).

Studies have also gathered qualitative data from participants who completed computer console-based exercise programmes, known as exergaming (Plow and Finlayson 2014; Forsberg et al. 2015; Palacios-Ceña et al. 2016; Thomas et al. 2017). The novelty of exercising using a computer game was clear in all studies, further, some participants found that the exercise regime was in line with their own goals (Plow and Finlayson 2014). However, it was not clear if this form of intervention was suitable to all participants, as in most cases, participants indicated that they would have preferred a more individualised exercise programme.

> In contrast to some participants thinking it was too difficult to use or that the board was too small, others felt it was not enough of a challenge, as they were not getting a workout (Plow and Finlayson 2014).

Many of the benefits described by participants in the group-based interventions (Figure 18.2) were similar for those in the individual interventions, in particular the physical benefits. However, the psychological benefits related to group camaraderie and social interaction were not discussed by participants who had less outside interaction with others who had MS.

To some extent, participants told researchers that they preferred a bespoke exercise programme, and this translated to needing an exercise programme appropriate for their personal interests, fitness or exercise experiences, and disabilities.

Summary

The views of participants who have told researchers about their experiences with exercise interventions have all generally been positive. There was much benefit from both group and individual exercise interventions, and these included discussions and comments on the physical and psychological benefits and increased knowledge. The importance of social interaction was also evident, with participants telling researchers of the pleasure of interacting with other people, whether this be with other persons with MS taking part in a group exercise programme or interacting with exercise leaders or coaches who were most commonly healthcare professionals. Future research should aim to harness some of these psychosocial benefits by perhaps including a social component in the design of exercise interventions. It is important to highlight that individual and home-based exercise is accepted by persons with MS, and that they particularly liked the perceived individual approach, and this too should be harnessed in future research where programmes designed for personal interest and ability might offer good acceptance and clinical applicability. Furthermore, there is evidence indicating that persons with MS accept the current physical activity guidelines for persons with MS (Latimer-Cheung et al. 2013a).

Theme 3: Moving When You Have MS

> Individuals specifically described fear of future impairment/disability as motivation for engaging in exercise with the negative impact on body image during the acute relapse feeding that fear. 'Move it or lose it' was a commonly used expression to describe motivations for exercising in the context of disability (Adamson et al. 2018).

The relationship between the person with MS and exercise is discussed in this theme entitled *balancing MS and exercise*. Despite the many known benefits of exercise and physical activity in persons with MS, persons with MS are still physically inactive in comparison with the general population (Kinnett-Hopkins et al. 2017a). Our theme on *opinions on exercise associated with interventions* addressed that persons with MS who engage in exercise and physical activity experience and perceive the many benefits, yet, in general, many are not physical active. In this final theme, we discuss the relationship which persons with MS have with exercise, and, in particular, their motivations towards exercise and adherence towards exercise.

There is overlap between this theme and the theme *opinions on exercise associated with interventions*, and therefore some studies are discussed in both sections. Taking this into consideration, there are opinions from some 532 persons with MS, and these are described over 34 different studies.

The research was discussed globally and by several groups of researchers, research was conducted in North America (Kasser 2009; Schneider and Young 2010; Brown et al. 2012;

Dlugonski et al. 2012; Giacobbi et al. 2012; Horton et al. 2015; Learmonth et al. 2015, 2017a, 2017b, 2018b; Chiu et al. 2016; Hundza et al. 2016; Chard 2017; Dixon-Ibarra et al. 2017; Kinnett-Hopkins et al. 2017b; Ploughman 2017; Adamson et al. 2018; Fakolade et al. 2018; Fasczewski et al. 2018; Held Bradford et al. 2018), Europe (Borkoles et al. 2008; Elsworth et al. 2009; Kersten et al. 2014; Crank et al. 2017; Giunti et al. 2018), and Oceania (Kayes et al. 2011; Smith et al. 2011, 2013b, 2015; Hall-McMaster et al. 2016a, 2016b).

All of the studies were primarily qualitative in method and gathered data via interviews or focus groups. Table 18.4 provides study information, participant information, associated information, quality score, main thematic findings, and a summary of the authors main conclusions or relevant points.

To recruit participants, studies used convenience sampling (Brown et al. 2012; Giacobbi et al. 2012; Mulligan et al. 2013; Kersten et al. 2014; Horton et al. 2015; Hall-McMaster et al. 2016a, 2016b; Chard 2017; Dixon-Ibarra et al. 2017; Learmonth et al. 2017a, 2018b; Fasczewski et al. 2018), purposive sampling (Smith et al. 2011), purposive-convenience sampling (Kasser 2009; Crank et al. 2017), and purposeful sampling (Borkoles et al. 2008; Elsworth et al. 2009; Schneider and Young 2010; Kayes et al. 2011; Dlugonski et al. 2012; Sweet et al. 2013; VanRuymbeke and Schneider 2013; Learmonth et al. 2015, 2017b; Smith et al. 2015; Chiu et al. 2016; Hundza et al. 2016; Kinnett-Hopkins et al. 2017b; Ploughman 2017; Adamson et al. 2018; Fakolade et al. 2018; Giunti et al. 2018; Held Bradford et al. 2018). Data were collected via one-to-one interviews in 20 studies (Borkoles et al. 2008; Elsworth et al. 2009; Kasser 2009; Schneider and Young 2010; Kayes et al. 2011; Smith et al. 2011, 2015; Dlugonski et al. 2012; Mulligan et al. 2013; VanRuymbeke and Schneider 2013; Horton et al. 2015; Learmonth et al. 2015, 2017a, 2017b; Hall-McMaster et al. 2016a, 2016b; Hundza et al. 2016; Kinnett-Hopkins et al. 2017b; Ploughman 2017; Adamson et al. 2018), with some research groups adopting telephone interviews for some of their participants (Giacobbi et al. 2012; Chard 2017; Fasczewski et al. 2018; Held Bradford et al. 2018; Learmonth et al. 2018b). Research groups also conducted focus groups (Brown et al. 2012; Dixon-Ibarra et al. 2017; Fakolade et al. 2018) or a combination of focus groups and interviews (Smith et al. 2013b; Sweet et al. 2013; Chiu et al. 2016; Crank et al. 2017) to gather data from participants. Most studies described using a *content* or *content led thematic analysis*, although two studies described using *interpretative phenomenological analysis* (Borkoles et al. 2008; Adamson et al. 2018), with other studies using *semantic coding* (Chiu et al. 2016), *framework analysis* (Crank et al. 2017), or *grounded theory* (Kayes et al. 2011).

Participants

532 persons with MS took part in the interviews or focus groups. Demographic and clinical data were not always reported for participants and reported data can be seen in Table 18.4. For the 441 persons for whom age was reported, mean age of participants was 52.3 years, and of the 525 people for whom sex was reported, 400 (~75%) participants were female. Some studies reported time since diagnoses, type of MS, disability level (most commonly expressed via the EDSS or the self-reported EDSS and race). Of the 163 persons for whom mean time since diagnosis was recorded, this was 13.3 years, and of the of 361 persons for whom type of MS was reported, 228 had relapsing remitting MS, 70 had primary progressive MS, and 67 had secondary progressive MS. Of the 163 participants for whom EDSS was reported (some studies reported mean EDSS, some range of EDSS), the mean EDSS was 4.1, with EDSS between 1 and 6.5 and disability was more generally described for 227 participants in studies with 4 having no disability, 77 mild disability, 51 medium disability, and 26 high levels of disability.

Quality

For studies undertaken related to an exercise or physical activity intervention, quality assessment scores ranged from 10 to 20 (Table 18.4), suggesting a fairly wide range of quality. All of the studies reported the study purpose and provided a relevant review of the literature.

Thirteen studies identified a theoretical perspective (Elsworth et al. 2009; Kasser 2009; Brown et al. 2012; Dlugonski et al. 2012; Giacobbi et al. 2012; Smith et al. 2013b; Sweet et al. 2013; Chiu et al. 2016; Dixon-Ibarra et al. 2017; Learmonth et al. 2017a, 2018b; Fasczewski et al. 2018; Held Bradford et al. 2018), and these theoretical perspectives were social cognitive theory (Kasser 2009; Dlugonski et al. 2012; Dixon-Ibarra et al. 2017; Learmonth et al. 2017a, 2018b; Held Bradford et al. 2018), the Health Action Process Approach (Chiu et al. 2016), the health implementation model (Elsworth et al. 2009), Self-determination Theory (Fasczewski et al. 2018), Transtheoretical Model of Behaviour Change (Smith et al. 2013b), the people with disability model (Giacobbi et al. 2012), and the Comprehensive Model of Information Seeking (Sweet et al. 2013). The process of sampling was discussed in all studies, and sampling was continued until redundancy in nine studies (Schneider and Young 2010; Learmonth et al. 2015, 2017a, 2017b; Chiu et al. 2016; Chard 2017; Ploughman 2017; Giunti et al. 2018; Held Bradford et al. 2018). Seven studies did not clearly indicate that informed consent was taken from participants (Elsworth et al. 2009; Kasser 2009; Schneider and Young 2010; Mulligan et al. 2013; Smith et al. 2015; Hall-McMaster et al. 2016b; Dixon-Ibarra et al. 2017). In terms of data collection, seven studies provided a clear description of where the research took place (Elsworth et al. 2009; Giacobbi et al. 2012; Learmonth et al. 2015, 2017a, 2018b; Dixon-Ibarra et al. 2017; Kinnett-Hopkins et al. 2017b). Almost all studies gave a reasonably clear description of participants except for three studies (Elsworth et al. 2009; Hall-McMaster et al. 2016b; Giunti et al. 2018), and in nine studies, authors provided a clear description of the researchers credentials (Smith et al. 2009; Learmonth et al. 2015, 2017a, 2017b, 2018b; Crank et al. 2017; Dixon-Ibarra et al. 2017; Kinnett-Hopkins et al. 2017b; Adamson et al. 2018). Six studies provided a clear and complete description of the relationship between researchers and participants (Kasser 2009; Smith et al. 2011; Giacobbi et al. 2012; Adamson et al. 2018; Fakolade et al. 2018; Learmonth et al. 2018b), and five studies clearly provided researchers assumptions (Kasser 2009; Smith et al. 2011; Kersten et al. 2014; Dixon-Ibarra et al. 2017; Adamson et al. 2018; Fasczewski et al. 2018). Procedural rigour was described in 14 studies (Dodd et al. 2006; Kasser 2009; Plow et al. 2009; Aubrey and Demain 2012; Learmonth et al. 2013; Mulligan et al. 2013; Normann et al. 2013; Smith et al. 2013b; Kersten et al. 2014; Plow and Finlayson 2014; Salminen et al. 2014; Clarke and Coote 2015; Casey et al. 2016; Learmonth et al. 2018b).

For data analysis, almost all studies stated use of inductive analysis except for six (Elsworth et al. 2009; Brown et al. 2012; VanRuymbeke and Schneider 2013; Crank et al. 2017; Dixon-Ibarra et al. 2017; Kinnett-Hopkins et al. 2017b), all studies' findings reflected the data. Twenty of the studies reported following a decision trail to analyse data (Borkoles et al. 2008; Smith et al. 2011, 2013b, 2015; Dlugonski et al. 2012; Giacobbi et al. 2012; Learmonth et al. 2015, 2017b, 2018b; Chiu et al. 2016; Hall-McMaster et al. 2016b; Hundza et al. 2016; Crank et al. 2017; Dixon-Ibarra et al. 2017; Ploughman 2017; Adamson et al. 2018; Fakolade et al. 2018; Giunti et al. 2018; Held Bradford et al. 2018), most studies clearly indicated the process used for transforming data into themes except for five studies (Elsworth et al. 2009; VanRuymbeke and Schneider 2013; Kersten et al. 2014; Kinnett-Hopkins et al. 2017b; Learmonth et al. 2017a), and all studies resulted in a meaningful picture of the topic of interest. To ensure trustworthiness in the data, 13 studies reported triangulation of sources and methods (Elsworth et al. 2009; Schneider and Young 2010; Smith et al. 2011; Dlugonski et al. 2012; Giacobbi et al. 2012; VanRuymbeke and Schneider 2013; Horton et al. 2015; Dixon-Ibarra et al. 2017; Adamson et al. 2018; Fakolade et al. 2018; Giunti et al. 2018; Held Bradford et al. 2018; Learmonth et al. 2018b), and most studies clearly reported triangulation of researchers except for four studies (Kasser 2009; VanRuymbeke and Schneider 2013; Hall-McMaster et al. 2016b; Held Bradford et al. 2018), 11 studies showed apparent triangulation of theories (Elsworth et al. 2009; Kayes et al. 2011; Brown et al. 2012; Dlugonski et al. 2012; Giacobbi et al. 2012; Smith et al. 2013b; Horton et al. 2015; Learmonth et al. 2015; Chiu et al. 2016; Kinnett-Hopkins et al. 2017b; Fasczewski et al. 2018; Held Bradford et al. 2018), member checking was used to verify findings in 13 studies (Borkoles et al. 2008; Kasser 2009; Smith et al. 2011; Dlugonski et al. 2012; VanRuymbeke and Schneider 2013; Kersten et al. 2014; Horton et al. 2015; Chiu et al. 2016; Learmonth et al. 2017a, 2017b; Fakolade et al. 2018; Held Bradford et al. 2018). In relation to conclusions, all studies reported appropriate conclusions which are relevant to clinical and research practice for MS care.

Appraisal of Studies

The main findings and conclusion from the studies related to *moving when you have MS* are listed in Table 18.4. Between studies there were four emerging themes and these were: (1) balancing MS and exercise, (2) communication about exercise and physical activity, (3) harnessing inner strategies, and (4) health and physical activity/exercise services.

Balancing MS and Exercise

Studies have gathered information about the important balance and sometimes tentative relationship with persons with MS with exercise. This has included studies gathering data on the barriers to exercise and conflicting role exercise might play in persons with MS.

Barriers perceived by persons with MS in relation to exercise have previously been reported in review studies (Learmonth and Motl 2016; Ploughman 2017) (Table 18.3). Where barriers were identified as including access to facilities, advice from healthcare professionals, fatigue, and fear and apprehension, and more broadly in relation to the participants impairment, attitude and knowledge. Authors have begun to identify that where exercise is now considered beneficial and safe for persons with MS (Pilutti et al. 2014b), to some there is a tentative relationship beyond that of the identified barriers. Adamson et al. (2018) reported on the perceptions of the impact of physical activity in MS symptoms, relapse, and disability identity. These authors attempted to understand the present *exercise is medicine* agenda from the viewpoint of the person with MS, and, in doing so, capture the empowering role of exercise and the guilt related to exercise (or lack thereof) when MS symptoms fluctuate such as during times of relapse. These authors noted that their research participants felt the burden from healthcare professionals to follow an exercise prescription and when *life* prevented this, there were feelings of guilt when unable to exercise and concerns may escalate to increased feelings of depression.

Taking the barriers perceived by persons with MS and the tentative relationship some persons with MS may have, the qualitative research indicates that although we must continue to promote exercise as an effective treatment in persons with MS, this must be done in a manner respectful of each person's unique circumstances.

Communicating about Physical Activity and Exercise

The communication of physical activity and exercise to persons with MS is important. Communication may come from external sources (such as healthcare professionals, support groups, or Internet websites). Further, knowledge of what persons with MS already know about physical activity and exercise will help us better focus resources and interventions on physical activity.

There is evidence from these studies that persons with MS may be unsatisfied with the quality of the healthcare professional/patient relationship amongst persons with MS (Learmonth et al. 2017a), and so it is important to establish the current relationship and what aspects work well. There have been a number of studies that have considered the role of exercise leaders and healthcare professionals. Themes of interest range from the attitude of exercise facility staff (Brown et al. 2012), the importance of the carer (Horton et al. 2015; Fakolade et al. 2018), and the role of the healthcare professional. When the role of exercise leaders were a focus in studies (Brown et al. 2012; Learmonth et al. 2018b) staff knowledge (on MS, or neurological conditions) and positive attitude were perceived as important and thus must be considered when promoting exercise to persons with MS. This is similar to what persons with MS who participated in an exercise intervention told researchers about the exercise leaders (discussed in the theme on *opinions on exercise associated with interventions*). When exercise leaders are knowledgeable about MS, and have a positive attitude, they are important facilitators for persons with MS to exercise. Carers have been discussed in two studies, and from these works it is apparent that the carer might also need education and encouragement to promote (or undertake) physical activity and exercise. It is also apparent that the importance of collaboration between the carer and person with MS has a role in facilitating exercise, and there is a need for supportive external resources (e.g., healthcare providers to inform and direct about exercise) to guide the carer to encourage exercise.

The importance of the healthcare provider in the communication process regarding physical activity and exercise for persons with MS is beginning to be perceived as an important opportunity to change the behaviours of persons with MS. Researchers have established the importance of healthcare providers, particularly physiotherapists, when communicating, promoting, and prescribing exercise to persons with MS (Schneider and Young 2010; Smith et al. 2011; Held Bradford et al. 2018). Learmonth et al. (2017a, 2017b) have focused specifically on establishing from which healthcare providers, what type of information from those healthcare providers, and what format of information from healthcare providers persons with MS would like in relation to exercise promotion. They established that persons with MS were not receiving clear promotion on exercise from all their healthcare providers, and this included not receiving exercise promotion from their main health contact, their neurologist. Participants in this mid-United States-based study wanted to receive promotion on exercise from healthcare providers, and they almost unanimously wanted exercise to be promoted by their neurologist, as well as allied healthcare providers (e.g., physiotherapists and psychologists).

The type of information and the delivery of exercise information has been established (Sweet et al. 2013; Learmonth et al. 2017b), persons with MS want to receive exercise information from knowledgeable professionals with knowledge on both exercise and MS, and they want to receive this information via in-person consultations and reliable printed or online resources which they would like healthcare providers to advise upon.

In relation to providing information on and communicating about exercise, the understanding of these terminologies by persons with MS was established by the same United

States-based research group as discussed above (Kinnett-Hopkins et al. 2017b). The study established that less than half of participants had a consistent understanding of what physical activity is and what exercise is. It seemed that many of the participants defined physical activity in a manner more akin to the correct description of exercise (i.e., 'physical activity was defined as a structured or directed behaviour, which aligns more closely with the definition of exercise') (Kinnett-Hopkins et al. 2017b). The use of consistent messages about these terminologies is important when promoting physical activity and exercise behaviours in persons with MS.

Harnessing Inner Strategies

There is evidence indicating that psychological constructs have an important role in the exercise behaviour of persons with MS. For example, a review of the relevant literature suggests that psychosocial factors such as self-efficacy, outcome expectations, and goal setting are important strategies in facilitating positive changes in physical activity and exercise behaviour in persons with MS (Motl et al. 2011; Carter et al. 2014; Pilutti et al. 2014a), and that physical activity and exercise based on these constructs may increase overall participation (Sangelaji et al. 2016). In quantitative research, there has been a strong focus on the use of social cognitive theory (SCT) (Bandura 2004) to understand physical activity behaviours in MS, and this has also been the case in studies included in this review (Plow et al. 2009; Dlugonski et al. 2012; Dixon-Ibarra et al. 2017; Learmonth et al. 2017a, 2018a, 2018b; Thomas et al. 2017; Held Bradford et al. 2018). Recent research indicates that construct of SCT such as self-efficacy may have an important role in predicting physical activity behaviour in MS, but there are many other factors not yet fully investigated which may explain this behaviour.

Therefore it is important to acknowledge these psychological constructs in qualitative research. Doing so might hold informative information on constructs and strategies to better understand physical activity behaviour. To that end many of our included studies have established sociopsychological factors which persons with MS perceive to facilitate exercise (Kasser 2009; Dlugonski et al. 2012; VanRuymbeke and Schneider 2013; Chiu et al. 2016; Hall-McMaster et al. 2016a, 2016b; Crank et al. 2017; Dixon-Ibarra et al. 2017; Fasczewski et al. 2018). Two studies gathered participants views on the SCT constructs delivered in their interventions (Dixon-Ibarra et al. 2017; Learmonth et al. 2018b). Participants liked receiving knowledge about the consequences of, and the skills to complete, exercise (SCT construct of outcome expectations and behavioural learning), learning to acknowledge and overcome barriers, and use goal-setting techniques (SCT construct of self-efficacy), and reading about (Learmonth et al. 2018b) or interacting with others with MS who are participating in learning (SCT construct of vicarious learning). In other studies, participants discussed the importance of exercise self-monitoring, but this should be considered within the background of an external accountability source (e.g., a healthcare professional offering guidance at designated times or when requested by either party), further education on personal strengths, needs, and confidence capabilities with a focus on participants establishing exercise they enjoy.

Health and Physical Activity/Exercise Services

Poor accessibility to health and physical activity services has been acknowledged in review articles (Christensen et al. 2016; Learmonth and Motl 2016; Ploughman 2017) as important barriers or facilitators to exercise. A lack of a necessary or desired service might present a barrier to exercise, whilst availability of a service may act as a facilitator. Studies have heard from persons with MS that health and social services should be available that fit an individual's needs, and this might address disability, financial, social, and enjoyment needs (Borkoles et al. 2008; Elsworth et al. 2009; Sweet et al. 2013; Hundza et al. 2016; Chard 2017; Learmonth et al. 2017a, 2018b; Ploughman 2017). Researchers heard that many persons with MS do not necessarily have access to the physical activity and exercise support which they need in their local communities, and that if this were in place they would participate more (Borkoles et al. 2008; Chard 2017), further, researchers heard that participants weren't fully aware of what services were available to them in their own community, and this presented a barrier to attendance (Learmonth et al. 2017a). Studies also identified that persons with MS accept and use Internet/technology-based exercise programmes, and this offers a good alternative to local exercise options (Learmonth et al. 2017a, 2018b).

Summary

This final theme aims to learn from participants what their motivations and barriers towards exercise are, and what they currently have to act as exercise facilitators. Researchers, healthcare providers, and the general community must acknowledge that there is a careful balance to overcome for persons with MS, who want, in almost all cases, to exercise. Exercise should be enjoyable and not thought upon as a burden. As was discussed in the theme on *the wider MS community*, healthcare professionals and researchers play an important role in communicating the messages on physical activity and exercise activity in MS. We must aim to arm persons with MS with the knowledge on exercise, the skills to become motivated towards exercise, and finally access to physical activity and exercise services which are appropriate for them.

Discussion

There has been an increase in qualitative research undertaken with persons with MS in the last decade, and this has included a strong focus on physical activity and exercise participation. Within this chapter, we established that a number of review articles have been published based on qualitative work, and these reviews have focused upon some of the barriers and facilitators persons with MS have in term of increasing physical activity and participating in exercise (Christensen et al. 2016; Learmonth and Motl 2016; Ploughman 2017). In this chapter, we have expanded these reviews and added new themes not yet fully summarised from the literature. We have focused on three main themes and these are; *the wider MS community, opinions of exercise associated with exercise interventions*, and *moving when you have MS*.

We have established that the whole MS community is supportive of exercise as a management strategy in MS care, and, further, that the whole MS community of healthcare professionals and carers may play a pivotal role in MS care. Further, there is evidence from included studies and other work that persons with MS are not fully satisfied with the healthcare provider/patient relationship (Vickrey et al. 2000; Golla et al. 2001; Learmonth et al. 2017a). Thus, there is a need to develop exercise services delivered within a health setting for persons with MS. This is supported in quantitative research from various countries including America (Vickrey et al. 2000), Australia (McCabe et al. 2012), and the United Kingdom (Somerset et al. 2001), and in this research, it was established that patients and persons with MS want to receive physical activity and exercise promotion via their local healthcare system. The importance of the healthcare provider/patients relationship is further evidenced from qualitative research which has focused more broadly in other neurological conditions (Gladman et al. 2008) (including people with stroke, traumatic brain injury, Parkinson's disease, MS, and epilepsy) that exercise services should be provided within the health setting. The evidence to date suggests that healthcare providers are offering many physical activity and exercise programmes to research participants who have MS (İyigün et al. 2010; Haselkorn et al. 2015; Campbell et al. 2016; Learmonth et al. 2016), however, despite the research into these programmes, there may be rationale to increase awareness of promoting exercise amongst the wider MS community. Research is continuing to build upon the work of Learmonth and colleagues (2018a, 2017a) in establishing the promotion of exercise in MS via healthcare providers (Motl et al. 2018) and this work is developing conceptual models and driver diagrams to outline the next steps in research to optimise the promotion of exercise in MS care via healthcare providers. However, one important group which has not yet been asked about physical activity and exercise services within MS healthcare are the healthcare managers and commissioners, and these individuals may be the gatekeepers to unlocking more and better services. Thus, it is important to continue qualitative work in this area to not only gather the views on the person with MS, carers, and healthcare providers, but it is also important that we capture the opinions of healthcare managers and commissioners who may hold pivotal information to increase exercise promotion using this method.

The acceptance of exercise interventions which include group exercise classes and individual exercise programmes, and when delivered in-person and via the use of technology could be heard from the participants in the included studies. Reports from participants of the perceived benefits related to physical and psychological benefits have previously been established in quantitative research (Motl and Pilutti 2012; Latimer-Cheung et al. 2013b), and the qualitative findings underscore the established benefits which include improvements in aerobic and muscular fitness (Platta et al. 2016), fatigue (Pilutti et al. 2013), depression (Ensari et al. 2014; Adamson et al. 2015), walking (Pearson et al. 2015; Learmonth et al. 2016), balance (Paltamaa et al. 2012), cognition (Sandroff et al. 2016), and QOL (Motl and Gosney 2008). Furthermore, benefits may include improvements in CNS structure (Sandroff et al. 2017), sleep quality (Pilutti et al. 2014a)(16), and cardiovascular health (Wens et al. 2016) comorbidity (17,18). Exercise training has further been associated with reduced relapse rate (Pilutti et al. 2014b) and slowed disability progression (Motl et al.2012)(20). With the safety of exercise in MS being comparable to that of the general population (Pilutti et al. 2014b), the benefits established and the acceptance by persons with MS, then there seems no strong argument against exercise and increase physical activity in the management of persons with MS. In reviewing the opinions of persons with MS who have commented on exercise interventions, we are unable to make clear recommendations. The acceptance of the current physical activity guidelines for persons with MS (Latimer-Cheung et al. 2013a) should be established in more groups of participants, and it will further be important to include social interactions in interventions which should be grounded in exercise science and theories of behaviour change.

Within this chapter, we further established the barriers which persons with MS have in relation to physical activity and exercise, and the current findings are in line with previously published review studies (Learmonth and Motl 2016; Ploughman 2017). Common barriers included access to facilities, advice from healthcare professionals, fatigue, fear and apprehension, the participants impairment, attitude, and knowledge. This chapter expands on previous work by further acknowledging that communication about exercise must be improved to educate participants on the benefits or exercise and the *best* exercise for them. The important role of healthcare providers in this area has previously been discussed. Further, we acknowledge views of participants in relation to the use of *harnessing inner strength* to overcome barriers to exercise. The inclusion of strategies to help participants help themselves should include constructs of social cognitive theory as views from participants perceive their inclusion beneficial. Quantitative review indicates that inclusion of behaviour change theory will be beneficial to the end goal of improving overall exercise participation amongst persons with MS (Sangelaji et al. 2016).

In completing the systematic review for this review and content analysis, there are some areas of qualitative methodology which could be improved in future qualitative research. For example, studies should consistently report demographical and clinical data of participants. In doing so, readers will better apply the findings to their area of interest. Researchers should further adhere to qualitative methodology in, for example, reporting of data saturation, reporting of researchers reflexivity, and clear reporting of analysis and rigor.

There are some limitations associated with the review and discussion in this chapter. For example, we only included studies published in English, thus views reported in studies published in a foreign language are not included. In the main, we included studies which focused on physical activity and exercise, therefore we may not have captured studies where physical activity was discussed amongst a wider context of issues affecting persons with MS. Effort was made to include all relevant studies, however, we may still have failed to include all qualitative studies conducted amongst persons with MS and that met our inclusion criteria.

Conclusion

This chapter focuses on the qualitative research which has been conducted in persons with MS related to the topic of physical activity and exercise. Qualitative research seeks to determine and understand the behaviours of the MS community in relation to exercise and physical activity, and, in doing so, unlock missing information from quantitative inquiry which researchers and clinicians can use to improve the content of exercise interventions. Studies which engage directly with the patient, carer, or healthcare team offer opinions and expertise which cannot be gathered via quantitative research. Qualitative research offers true consumer-based participatory research, and this should be used to drive future research agendas.

We gather together views of over 1000 persons within the MS community and summarise that we now know the importance of the promotion of exercise via the healthcare system, the acceptance of exercise amongst persons with MS, and the common challenges persons with MS experience in relation to exercise. Research undertaken over the last 25 years highlights the importance of further encouraging persons with MS, and one important area of encouragement is appropriate use of physical activity and exercise to manage their health. The research gathered together in this chapter provides information on the lived experiences of the MS community and provides new information about the importance of the wider MS community and the power they (i.e., healthcare providers and carers) may have at influencing change in the behaviours of persons with MS. Furthermore, we learn from qualitative research what aspects of an exercise intervention engage persons with

MS, and this can be used to establish what elements of the intervention might increase retention. The views and opinions of the intervention participants further help us, as researchers and healthcare providers, to know what barriers we should help persons with MS overcome in relation to physical activity and exercise. Qualitative research in MS offers much insight into the experiences of the MS community, and we must continue capturing the views of the MS community to better future models of MS care.

Acknowledgements

I would like to thank Emily Stewart for her assistance in undertaking the literature search and review of study quality.

References

Adamson, B. C. et al. (2018) '"Move it or lose it": Perceptions of the impact of physical activity on multiple sclerosis symptoms, relapse and disability identity', *Qualitative Research in Sport, Exercise and Health*, 10(4), pp. 457–475. doi:10.1080/2159676X.2017.1415221.

Adamson, B. C., Ensari, I. and Motl, R. W. (2015) 'The effect of exercise on depressive symptoms in adults with neurological disorders: A systematic review and meta-analysis', *Archives of Physical Medicine and Rehabilitation*. doi:10.1016/j.apmr.2015.01.005.

American College of Sports Medicine. (2013) *ACSM's Guidelines for Exercise Testing and Prescription*. Philadelphia, PA: Lippincott Williams & Wilkins.

Anderson, C., Grant, R. L. and Hurley, M. V. (2017) 'Exercise facilities for neurologically disabled populations – Perceptions from the fitness industry', *Disability and Health Journal*, 10(1), pp. 157–162. doi:10.1016/j.dhjo.2016.09.006.

Aubrey, G. and Demain, S. (2012) 'Perceptions of group exercise in the management of multiple sclerosis', *International Journal of Therapy and Rehabilitation*, 19, pp. 557–565.

Bandura, A. (2004) 'Health promotion by social cognitive means', *Health Education and Behavior*, 31(2), pp. 143–164.

Baranowski, T. et al. (1997) 'Low validity of a seven-item fruit and vegetable food frequency questionnaire among third-grade students', *Journal of the American Dietetic Association*, 97(1), pp. 66–68. doi:10.1016/S0002-8223(97)00022-9.

Benito-León, J. (2011) 'Are the prevalence and incidence of multiple sclerosis changing?' *Neuroepidemiology*, 36(3), pp. 148–149. doi:10.1159/000325368.

Borkoles, E. et al. (2008) 'The lived experiences of people diagnosed with multiple sclerosis in relation to exercise', *Psychology & Health*, 23(4), pp. 427–441.

Brett, J. et al. (2014) 'Mapping the impact of patient and public involvement on health and social care research: A systematic review', *Health Expectations*, 17(5), pp. 637–650. doi:10.1111/j.1369-7625.2012.00795.x.

Brown, C., Kitchen, K. and Nicoll, K. (2012) 'Barriers and facilitators related to participation in aquafitness programs for people with multiple sclerosis: A pilot study', *International Journal of MS Care*, 14(3), pp. 132–141.

Campbell, E. et al. (2016) 'Physiotherapy rehabilitation for people with progressive multiple sclerosis: A systematic review', *Archives of Physical Medicine and Rehabilitation*, 97(1), pp. 141–151. e3. doi:10.1016/j.apmr.2015.07.022.

Carter, A. et al. (2014) 'Pragmatic intervention for increasing self-directed exercise behaviour and improving important health outcomes in people with multiple sclerosis: A randomised controlled trial', *Multiple Sclerosis*, 20(8), pp. 1112–1122. doi:10.1177/1352458513519354.

Casey, B. et al. (2016) 'What do people with MS want from a web-based resource to encourage increased physical activity behaviour?' *Disability and Rehabilitation*, 38(16), pp. 1557–1566. doi: 10.3109/09638288.2015.1106601.

Chard, S. (2017) 'Qualitative perspectives on aquatic exercise initiation and satisfaction among persons with multiple sclerosis', *Disability and Rehabilitation*, 39(13), pp. 1307–1312. doi:10.1080/09638288.2016.1194897.

Chenail, R. J. (2011) 'Learning to appraise the quality of qualitative research articles: A contextualized learning object for constructing knowledge', *The Qualitative Report*, 16(1), pp. 236–248.

Chiu, C.-Y. et al. (2016) 'Psychosocial factors influencing lifestyle physical activity engagement of African Americans with multiple sclerosis: A qualitative study', *Journal of Rehabilitation; Alexandria*, 82(2), pp. 25–30.

Christensen, M. et al. (2015) 'Important factors for the intention and execution of physical exercise in persons with multiple sclerosis: A qualitative metasynthesis', *Multiple Sclerosis Journal*, 21(4), pp. 509–510.

Christensen, M. E. et al. (2016) 'The intention to exercise and the execution of exercise among persons with multiple sclerosis--A qualitative metasynthesis', *Disability and Rehabilitation*, 38(11), pp. 1023–1033. doi:10.3109/09638288.2015.1091859.

Clarke, R. and Coote, S. (2015) 'Perceptions of participants in a group, community, exercise programme for people with multiple sclerosis', *Rehabilitation Research and Practice*, Article ID 123494. doi:10.1155/2015/123494.

Coote, S. (2014) 'Progressive resistance therapy is not the best way to rehabilitate deficits due to multiple sclerosis: Yes', *Multiple Sclerosis Journal*, 20(2), pp. 143–144. doi:10.1177/1352458513515087.

Crank, H. et al. (2017) 'Qualitative investigation of exercise perceptions and experiences in people with multiple sclerosis before, during, and after participation in a personally tailored exercise program', *Archives of Physical Medicine and Rehabilitation*, 98(12), pp. 2520–2525. doi:10.1016/j.apmr.2017.05.022.

Dennett, R. et al. (2016) 'Effectiveness and user experience of web-based interventions for increasing physical activity in people with multiple sclerosis: A comprehensive systematic review protocol', *JBI Database of Systematic Reviews and Implementation Reports*, 14(11), pp. 50–62. doi:10.11124/JBISRIR-2016-003174.

Dixon-Ibarra, A. et al. (2017) 'Using health promotion guidelines for persons with disabilities to develop and evaluate a physical activity program for individuals with multiple sclerosis: A feasibility study', *Evaluation and Program Planning*, 61, pp. 150–159. doi:10.1016/j.evalprogplan.2016.12.005.

Dlugonski, D., Joyce, R. and Motl, R. (2012) 'Meanings, motivations, and strategies for engaging in physical activity among women with multiple sclerosis', *Disability and Rehabilitation*, 34(25), pp. 2148–2157. doi:10.3109/09638288.2012.677935.

Doble, S. E. and Santha, J. C. (2008) 'Occupational well-being: Rethinking occupational therapy outcomes', *Canadian Journal of Occupational Therapy. Revue canadienne d'ergothérapie*, 75(3), pp. 184–190.

Dodd, D. K. J. et al. (2006) 'A qualitative analysis of a progressive resistance exercise programme for people with multiple sclerosis', *Disability and Rehabilitation*, 28(18), pp. 1127–1134. doi:10.1080/09638280500531842.

Elsworth, C. et al. (2009) 'A study of perceived facilitators to physical activity in neurological conditions...including commentary by Cup E, Pieterse A, Block P', *International Journal of Therapy & Rehabilitation*, 16(1), pp. 17–24.

Ensari, I., Motl R. W. and Pilutti, L. A. (2014) 'Exercise training improves depressive symptoms in people with multiple sclerosis: Results of a meta-analysis', *Journal of Psychosomatic Research*, 76(6), pp. 465–471.

Erwin, E. J., Brotherson, M. J. and Summers, J. A. (2011) 'Understanding qualitative metasynthesis issues and opportunities in early childhood intervention research', *Journal of Early Intervention*, 33(3), pp. 186–200. doi:10.1177/1053815111425493.

Fakolade, A. et al. (2018) 'Understanding leisure-time physical activity: Voices of people with MS who have moderate-to-severe disability and their family caregivers', *Health Expectations: An International Journal of Public Participation in Health Care and Health Policy*, 21(1), pp. 181–191. doi:10.1111/hex.12600.

Fasczewski, K. S., Gill, D. L. and Rothberger, S. M. (2018) 'Physical activity motivation and benefits in people with multiple sclerosis', *Disability and Rehabilitation*, 40(13), pp. 1517–1523. doi:10.1080/09638288.2017.1300946.

Forsberg, A., Nilsagård, Y. and Boström, K. (2015) 'Perceptions of using videogames in rehabilitation: A dual perspective of people with multiple sclerosis and physiotherapists', *Disability and Rehabilitation*, 37(4), pp. 338–344. doi:10.3109/09638288.2014.918196.

Giacobbi, P. R. et al. (2012) 'Exercise and quality of life in women with multiple sclerosis', *Adapted Physical Activity Quarterly*, 29(3), pp. 224–242. doi:10.1123/apaq.29.3.224.

Giunti, G. et al. (2018) 'Exploring the specific needs of persons with multiple sclerosis for mHealth Solutions for physical activity: Mixed-methods study', *JMIR mHealth and uHealth*, 6(2), p. e37. doi:10.2196/mhealth.8996.

Gladman, J. et al. (2008) *Specialist Rehabilitation for Neurological Conditions: Literature Review and Mapping Study*. London, UK: National Co-ordinating Centre for NHS Service Delivery and Organisation R & D.

Golla, H. et al. (2001) 'Unmet needs of severely affected multiple sclerosis patients: The health professionals' view', *Palliative Medicine*, 26(2), pp. 139–151.

Hale, L. A. et al. (2012) '"Tell me what you want, what you really really want....": Asking people with multiple sclerosis about enhancing their participation in physical activity', *Disability and Rehabilitation*, 34(22), pp. 1887–1893. doi:10.3109/09638288.2012.670037.

Hall-McMaster, S. M., Treharne, G. J. and Smith, C. M. (2016a) 'Positive thinking and physical activity motivation for one individual with multiple sclerosis: A qualitative case-study', *New Zealand Journal of Physiotherapy*, 44(1), pp. 26–32. doi:10.15619/NZJP/44.1.04.

Hall-McMaster, S. M., Treharne, G. J. and Smith, C. M. (2016b) '"The positive feel": Unpacking the role of positive thinking in people with multiple sclerosis's thinking aloud about staying physically active', *Journal of Health Psychology*, 21(12), pp. 3026–3036. doi:10.1177/1359105315592047.

Haselkorn, J. K. et al. (2015) 'Summary of comprehensive systematic review: Rehabilitation in multiple sclerosis: Report of the Guideline Development, Dissemination, and Implementation Subcommittee of the American Academy of Neurology', *Neurology*, 85(21), pp. 1896–1903. doi:10.1212/WNL.0000000000002146.

Hedström, A. K., Alfredsson, L. and Olsson, T. (2016a) 'Environmental factors and their interactions with risk genotypes in MS susceptibility', *Current Opinion in Neurology*, 29(3), pp. 293–298. doi:10.1097/WCO.0000000000000329.

Hedström, A. K., Olsson, T. and Alfredsson, L. (2016b) 'Smoking is a major preventable risk factor for multiple sclerosis', *Multiple Sclerosis Journal*, 22(8), pp. 1021–1026.

Held Bradford, E. H. et al. (2018) 'Maximizing gait and balance: Behaviors and decision-making processes of persons with multiple sclerosis and physical therapists', *Disability and Rehabilitation*, 40(9), pp. 1014–1025. doi:10.1080/09638288.2017.1283448.

Horton, S. et al. (2015) 'A qualitative investigation of exercising with MS and the impact on the spousal relationship', *European Review of Aging and Physical Activity*, 12. doi:10.1186/s11556-015-0148-5.

Hundza, S. et al. (2016) 'Similar barriers and facilitators to physical activity across different clinical groups experiencing lower limb spasticity', *Disability and Rehabilitation*, 38(14), pp. 1370–1381. doi:10.3109/09638288.2015.1101789.

İyigün, G., Yildirim, S. A. and Snowdon, N. (2010) 'Is physiotherapy effective in improving balance and gait in patients with multiple sclerosis?: A systematic review', *Turkiye Klinikleri Journal of Medical Sciences*, 30(2), pp. 482–493.

Kasser, S. (2009) 'Exercising with multiple sclerosis: Insights into meaning and motivation', *Adapted Physical Activity Quarterly*, 26(3), pp. 274–289. doi:10.1123/apaq.26.3.274.

Kayes, N. M. et al. (2011) 'Facilitators and barriers to engagement in physical activity for people with multiple sclerosis: A qualitative investigation', *Disability and Rehabilitation*, 33(8), pp. 625–642. doi:10.3109/09638288.2010.505992.

Kersten, P. et al. (2015) 'Bridging the goal intention-action gap in rehabilitation: A study of if-then implementation intentions in neurorehabilitation', *Disability and Rehabilitation*, 37(12), pp. 1073–1081. doi:10.3109/09638288.2014.955137.

Kersten, S. et al. (2014) 'A pilot study of an exercise-based patient education program in people with multiple sclerosis', *Multiple Sclerosis International*, 2014. doi:10.1155/2014/306878.

Kinnett-Hopkins, D. et al. (2017a) 'People with MS are less physically active than healthy controls but as active as those with other chronic diseases: An updated meta-analysis', *Multiple Sclerosis and Related Disorders*, 13, pp. 38–43. doi:10.1016/j.msard.2017.01.016.

Kinnett-Hopkins, D. et al. (2017b) 'The interpretation of physical activity, exercise, and sedentary behaviours by persons with multiple sclerosis', *Disability and Rehabilitation*, pp. 1–6. doi:10.1080/09638288.2017.1383519.

Kraft, G. H. (1999) 'Rehabilitation still the only way to improve function in multiple sclerosis', *Lancet*, 354(9195), pp. 2016–2017. doi:10.1016/S0140-6736(99)90035-1.

Kurtzke, J. F. (1983) 'Rating neurologic impairment in multiple sclerosis an expanded disability status scale (EDSS)', *Neurology*, 33(11), pp. 1444–1452.

Latimer-Cheung, A. E. et al. (2013a) 'Development of evidence-informed physical activity guidelines for adults with multiple sclerosis', *Archives of Physical Medicine and Rehabilitation*, 94(9), pp. 1829–1836.

Latimer-Cheung, A. E. et al. (2013b) 'The effects of exercise training on fitness, mobility, fatigue, and health related quality of life among adults with multiple sclerosis: A systematic review to inform guideline development', *Archives of Physical Medicine and Rehabilitation*, 94(9), pp. 1800–1828.

Learmonth, Y. C. et al. (2013) 'A qualitative exploration of the impact of a 12-week group exercise class for those moderately affected with multiple sclerosis', *Disability and Rehabilitation*, 35(1), pp. 81–88. doi:10.3109/09638288.2012.688922.

Learmonth, Y. C. et al. (2015) 'Perspectives on physical activity among people with multiple sclerosis who are wheelchair users', *International Journal of MS Care*, 17(3), pp. 109–119. doi:10.7224/1537-2073.2014-018.

Learmonth, Y. C. et al. (2017a) 'Multiple sclerosis patients need and want information on exercise promotion from healthcare providers: A qualitative study', *Health Expectations*, 20(4), pp. 574–583. doi:10.1111/hex.12482.

Learmonth, Y. C. et al. (2017b) 'Identifying exercise promotion strategies for individuals with MS that can be delivered through healthcare providers', *Health Expectations*, 20(5), pp. 1001–1010.

Learmonth, Y. C. et al. (2018a) 'Investigating the needs and wants of healthcare providers for promoting exercise in persons with multiple sclerosis: A qualitative study', *Disability and Rehabilitation*, 40(18), pp. 2172–2180. doi:10.1080/09638288.2017.1327989.

Learmonth, Y. C., Ensari, I. and Motl, R. W. (2016) 'Physiotherapy and walking outcomes in adults with multiple sclerosis: Systematic review and meta-analysis', *Physical Therapy Reviews*, 21(3–6), pp. 160–172.

Learmonth, Y. C., Kinnett-Hopkins, D. and Motl, R. W. (2018b) 'Capitalising on the opinions of persons with multiple sclerosis to inform the main trial – Participant opinions from participation in a feasibility study, a qualitative extension study', *Disability and Rehabilitation*.

Learmonth, Y. C. and Motl, R. W. (2016) 'Physical activity and exercise training in multiple sclerosis: A review and content analysis of qualitative research identifying perceived determinants and consequences', *Disability and Rehabilitation*, 38(13), pp. 1227–1242. doi:10.3109/09638288.2015.1077397.

Letts, L. et al. (2007a) *Critical Review Form - Qualitative Studies (Version 2.0)*. Hamilton, Canada: McMaster University.

Letts, L. et al. (2007b) *Guidelines for Critical Review Form: Qualitative Studies (Version 2.0)*. McMaster University, Hamilton, Canada.

McCabe, M. et al. (2012) 'A needs analysis of Australians with MS', *AMSLS Survey and Report commissioned by MS Research Australia*. Available at: https://www.ms.asn.au/assets/documents/National-MS-Needs-Analysis-2012.pdf (Accessed 9 November 2016).

Moher, D. et al. (2009) 'Preferred reporting items for systematic reviews and meta-analyses: The PRISMA statement', *PLoS Med*, 151(4).

Motl, R. W. et al. (2011) 'Internet intervention for increasing physical activity in persons with multiple sclerosis', *Multiple Sclerosis*, 17(1), pp. 116–128.

Motl, R. W. et al. (2012) 'Premorbid physical activity predicts disability progression in relapsing-remitting multiple sclerosis', *Journal of the Neurological Sciences*, 15(323 [1–2]), pp. 123–127.

Motl, R. W. et al. (2018) 'Promotion of exercise in multiple sclerosis through healthcare providers', *Exercise and Sport Sciences Reviews*, 46(2), pp. 105–111. doi:10.1249/JES.0000000000000140.

Motl, R. W. and Gosney, J. L. (2008) 'Effect of exercise training on quality of life in multiple sclerosis: A meta-analysis', *Multiple Sclerosis*, 14(1), pp. 129–135.

Motl, R. W. and Pilutti, L. A. (2012) 'The benefits of exercise training in multiple sclerosis', *Nature Reviews. Neurology*, 8(9), pp. 487–497.

Motl, R. W. and Sandroff, B. M. (2018) 'Exercise as a countermeasure to declining central nervous system function in multiple sclerosis', *Clinical Therapeutics*, 40(1), pp. 16–25.

Mulligan, H. et al. (2013) 'Combining self-help and professional help to minimize barriers to physical activity in persons with multiple sclerosis: A trial of the "blue prescription" approach in New Zealand', *Journal of Neurologic Physical Therapy*, 37(2), pp. 51–57. doi:10.1097/NPT.0b013e318292799e.

Newitt, R., Barnett, F. and Crowe, M. (2016) 'Understanding factors that influence participation in physical activity among people with a neuromusculoskeletal condition: A review of qualitative studies', *Disability and Rehabilitation*, 38(1), pp. 1–10. doi:10.3109/09638288.2014.996676.

Normann, B. et al. (2013) 'Contextualized perceptions of movement as a source of expanded insight: People with multiple sclerosis' experience with physiotherapy', *Physiotherapy Theory and Practice*, 29(1), pp. 19–30.

Olsson, T., Barcellos, L. F. and Alfredsson, L. (2017) 'Interactions between genetic, lifestyle and environmental risk factors for multiple sclerosis', *Nature Reviews Neurology*, 13(1), p. 25.

Palacios-Ceña, D. et al. (2016) 'Multiple sclerosis patients' experiences in relation to the impact of the kinect virtual home-exercise programme: A qualitative study', *European Journal of Physical and Rehabilitation Medicine*, 52(3), pp. 347–355.

Paltamaa, J. et al. (2012) 'Effects of physiotherapy interventions on balance in multiple sclerosis: A systematic review and meta-analysis of randomized controlled trials', *Journal of Rehabilitation Medicine*, 44(10), pp. 811–823. doi:10.2340/16501977-1047.

Paul, L. et al. (2014) 'Web-based physiotherapy for people moderately affected with multiple sclerosis; Quantitative and qualitative data from a randomized, controlled pilot study', *Clinical Rehabilitation; London*, 28(9), pp. 924–935. doi:10.1177/0269215514527995.

Pearson, M., Dieberg, G. and Smart, N. (2015) 'Exercise as a therapy for improvement of walking ability in adults with multiple sclerosis: A meta-analysis', *Archives of Physical Medicine and Rehabilitation*, 96(7), pp. 1339–1348.e7. doi:10.1016/j.apmr.2015.02.011.

Pilutti, L. A. et al. (2013) 'Effects of exercise training on fatigue in multiple sclerosis: A meta-analysis', *Psychosomatic Medicine*, 75(6), pp. 575–580.

Pilutti, L. A. et al. (2014a) 'Randomized controlled trial of a behavioral intervention targeting symptoms and physical activity in multiple sclerosis', *Multiple Sclerosis (Houndmills, Basingstoke, England)*, 20(5), pp. 594–601. doi:10.1177/1352458513503391.

Pilutti, L. A. et al. (2014b) 'The safety of exercise training in multiple sclerosis: A systematic review', *Journal of the Neurological Sciences*, 343(1–2), pp. 3–7.

Platta, M. E. et al. (2016) 'Effect of exercise training on fitness in multiple sclerosis: A meta-analysis', *Archives of Physical Medicine and Rehabilitation*, 97(9), pp. 1564–1572. doi:10.1016/j.apmr.2016.01.023.

Ploughman, M. (2017) 'Breaking down the barriers to physical activity among people with multiple sclerosis – A narrative review', *Physical Therapy Reviews*, 22(3–4), pp. 124–132. doi:10.1080/10833196.2017.1315212.

Plow, M. et al. (2014) 'A formative evaluation of customized pamphlets to promote physical activity and symptom self-management in women with multiple sclerosis', *Health Education Research*, 29(5), pp. 883–896. doi:10.1093/her/cyu034.

Plow, M. A. and Finlayson, M. (2014) 'A qualitative study exploring the usability of Nintendo Wii Fit among persons with multiple sclerosis', *Occupational Therapy International*, 21(1), pp. 21–32. doi:10.1002/oti.1345.

Plow, M. A., Resnik, L. and Allen, S. M. (2009) 'Exploring physical activity behaviour of persons with multiple sclerosis: A qualitative pilot study', *Disability and Rehabilitation*, 31(20), pp. 1652–1665. doi:10.1080/09638280902738375.

Prochaska, J. O. and Velicer, W. F. (1997) 'The transtheoretical model of health behavior change', *American Journal of Health Promotion: AJHP*, 12(1), pp. 38–48.

Ratzker, P. K. et al. (1997) 'Self-assessment of neurologic impairment in multiple sclerosis', *Neurorehabil and Neural Repair*, 11(4), pp. 207–211.

Rhead, B. et al. (2016) 'Mendelian randomization shows a causal effect of low vitamin D on multiple sclerosis risk', *Neurology Genetics*, 2(5), p. e97.

Salminen, A.-L., Kanelisto, K. J. and Karhula, M. E. (2014) 'What components of rehabilitation are helpful from the perspective of individuals with multiple sclerosis?' *Disability and Rehabilitation*, 36(23), pp. 1983–1989. doi:10.3109/09638288.2014.885092.

Sandroff, B. M. et al. (2016) 'Systematic, evidence-based review of exercise, physical activity, and physical fitness effects on cognition in persons with multiple sclerosis', *Neuropsychology Review*, 26(3), pp. 271–294. doi:10.1007/s11065-016-9324-2.

Sandroff, B. M., Johnson, C. L. and Motl, R. W. (2017) 'Exercise training effects on memory and hippocampal viscoelasticity in multiple sclerosis: A novel application of magnetic resonance elastography', *Neuroradiology*, 59(1), pp. 61–67. doi:10.1007/s00234-016-1767-x.

Sangelaji, B. et al. (2016) 'The effectiveness of behaviour change interventions to increase physical activity participation in people with multiple sclerosis: A systematic review and meta-analysis', *Clinical Rehabilitation*, 30(6), pp. 559–576.

Schneider, M. and Young, N. (2010) '"So this is my new life": A qualitative examination of women living with multiple sclerosis and the coping strategies they use when accessing physical activity', *Disability Studies Quarterly*, 30(3/4), pp. 1–8.

Sellner, J. et al. (2011) 'The increasing incidence and prevalence of female multiple sclerosis—A critical analysis of potential environmental factors', *Autoimmunity Reviews*, 10(8), pp. 495–502.

Smith, C. et al. (2011) 'How does fatigue influence community-based exercise participation in people with multiple sclerosis?' *Disability and Rehabilitation*, 33(22–23), pp. 2362–2371. doi:10.3109/09638288.2011.573054.

Smith, C. M. et al. (2009) 'How does exercise influence fatigue in people with multiple sclerosis?' *Disability & Rehabilitation*, 31(9), pp. 685–692.

Smith, C. M. et al. (2013a) 'Healthcare provider beliefs about exercise and fatigue in people with multiple sclerosis', *Journal of Rehabilitation Research and Development; Washington*, 50(5), pp. 733–744.

Smith, C. M. et al. (2013b) 'Participant perceptions of a novel physiotherapy approach ("Blue Prescription") for increasing levels of physical activity in people with multiple sclerosis: A qualitative study following intervention', *Disability and Rehabilitation*, 35(14), pp. 1174–1181. doi:10.3109/09638288.2012.723792.

Smith, C. M., Fitzgerald, H. J. M. and Whitehead, L. (2015) 'How fatigue influences exercise participation in men with multiple sclerosis', *Qualitative Health Research*, 25(2), pp. 179–188. doi:10.1177/1049732314551989.

Somerset, M. et al. (2001) 'What do people with MS want and expect from health-care services?' *Health Expectations: An International Journal of Public Participation in Health Care and Health Policy*, 4(1), pp. 29–37.

Strong, S. et al. (1999) 'Application of the person-environment-occupation model: A practical tool', *Canadian Journal of Occupational Therapy*, 66(3), pp. 122–133.

Sweet, S. N. et al. (2013) 'Identifying physical activity information needs and preferred methods of delivery of people with multiple sclerosis', *Disability and Rehabilitation*, 35(24), pp. 2056–2063. doi:10.3109/09638288.2013.800915.

Thomas, S. et al. (2017) 'Mii-vitaliSe: A pilot randomised controlled trial of a home gaming system (Nintendo Wii) to increase activity levels, vitality and well-being in people with multiple sclerosis', *BMJ Open*, 7(9). doi:10.1136/bmjopen-2017-016966.

Thorpe, O., Johnston, K. and Kumar, S. (2012) 'Barriers and enablers to physical activity participation in patients with COPD: A systematic review', *Journal of Cardiopulmonary Rehabilitation and Prevention*, 32(6), pp. 359–369.

Toomey, E. and Coote, S. (2013) 'Exploring the use of "Exercise Buddies" to augment physiotherapy in the community for people with multiple sclerosis', *Physiotherapy Practice & Research*, 34(2), pp. 67–74. doi:10.3233/PPR-130019.

van der Linden, M. L. et al. (2014) 'Pilates for people with multiple sclerosis who use a wheelchair: Feasibility, efficacy and participant experiences', *Disability & Rehabilitation*, 13(11), pp. 932–939.

VanRuymbeke, B. and Schneider, M. A. (2013) 'The perceived influence of a targeted group exercise program on the well-being of women living with multiple sclerosis: A qualitative study', *Critical Reviews in Physical and Rehabilitation Medicine*, 25(1–2), pp. 23–43. doi:10.1615/CritRevPhysRehabilMed.2013007713.

Vickrey, B. G. et al. (2000) 'Management of multiple sclerosis across managed care and fee-for-service systems', *Neurology*, 55(9), pp. 1341–1349.

Vollmer, T. et al. (2012) 'Exercise as prescriptive therapy in multiple sclerosis. A consensus conference white paper', *International Journal of MS Care*, 14(S3), pp. 2–14.

Walsh, D. and Downe, S. (2005) 'Meta-synthesis method for qualitative research: A literature review', *Journal of Advanced Nursing*, 50(2), pp. 204–211.

Wens, I., Eijnde, B. O. and Hansen, D. (2016) 'Muscular, cardiac, ventilatory and metabolic dysfunction in patients with multiple sclerosis: Implications for screening, clinical care and endurance and resistance exercise therapy, a scoping review', *Journal of the Neurological Sciences*, 367, pp. 107–121. doi:10.1016/j.jns.2016.05.050.

Williams, T. L., Ma, J. K. and Ginis, K. A. M. (2017) 'Participant experiences and perceptions of physical activity-enhancing interventions for people with physical impairments and mobility limitations: A meta-synthesis of qualitative research evidence', *Health Psychology Review*, 11(2), pp. 179–196. doi:10.1080/17437199.2017.1299027.

Section III

Methodological Considerations for Qualitative Researchers

19

Designing Qualitative Research to Have an Impact on Healthcare from the Outset

Sally Thorne

CONTENTS

Introduction

Much as with nursing, rehabilitation exists as a distinct professional practice for the explicit purpose of making a difference in the real world of people. Each of our applied practices derives from an academic discipline that, whilst sharing a great deal of common scientific, theoretical, and factual material with other disciplines, also represents a unique 'angle of vision' on the problems of health and healthcare in our society. In each case, knowledge generation traditions have evolved in order to advance the profession's capacity for impact on the health of people and populations and to bring a disciplinary perspective to the wider arena of clinical wisdom.

Until the late 1970s, the common understanding of health research was generally limited to quantification and measurement. For some kinds of applied disciplinary questions, the available scientific methods were reasonably adequate. However, in nursing, and ultimately in rehabilitation as well, clinicians were often preoccupied with problems of a more 'complex and messy' nature that were not easily amenable to measurement and were curious about how the more subjective, experiential, and contextual factors that characterise real world healthcare might be brought into the equation. I attribute nursing's early entry into qualitative inquiry to its philosophical commitment to particularising general knowledge in the clinical context (Thorne & Sawatzky 2014) – applying a critically reflective lens to all generalised knowledge so that the distinctive circumstances of each new patient or family might be either integrated into or prioritised over standardised procedure. From a social justice perspective, nursing was not only interested in what approaches to care might have proven effectiveness for the majority, but also in who might be disadvantaged by those approaches, how we would anticipate or notice that, and what other considerations might be applied to a decision as to whether and how to use them. This relentless commitment towards individualised (or personalised) care meant that nursing was quite hungry for alternative approaches to the available quantitative methods.

When nursing 'discovered' qualitative methods, it faced a considerable challenge in arguing that they constituted a legitimate scientific approach. Biomedical science methods were serving much of the spectrum of healthcare disciplines fairly well, and scholars in many fields had found reasonable ways to work within the confines of measurement to advance their understandings of human health experience and intervention towards optimising health. To those with a conventional understanding of science, qualitative research was a major departure, and not an easy fit within the spectrum of scholarly work. In an attempt to confirm the credibility of these intriguing new approaches, nursing located them within the domain of 'social science' and borrowed methodological technique from that which had been developed in such fields as sociology and anthropology. Methods such as phenomenology, grounded theory, and ethnography were popularised as health research resources during those early years. Framing the work as established social science technique helped position it with the biomedical science community as a legitimate practice, but brought with it a new problem in trying to adhere to the disciplinary rule structures of the methodological traditions it was deploying.

Over time, a number of researchers in the applied health practice disciplines began to feel overly constrained by the design conditions inherent in the available social science methodological options. Paradoxically, they could follow what seemed to be good methodology or they could do meaningful research, but not both at the same time (Chamberlain 2000). When they prioritised careful conformity to some of the methodological expectations of the social science traditions, they found that steered them towards generating findings that only partially answered their own disciplinary research questions or produced what we might call 'bloodless findings'. Alternatively, when they creatively bent and adapted those methodological traditions to align with the kind of knowledge their disciplinary logic told them would best answer their research question in a manner that spoke to their applied practice discipline, they risked censure from funding panels, manuscript reviewers, and sectors within the health science community for supposed methodological infractions. Thus, as the philosophical thinkers within the applied disciplines were increasingly appreciating the implications of complexity, the tenets of quality assessment were often steering applied scholars in the direction of tight designs within well-established method. In the context of these evolving conditions, I found myself amongst the members of the qualitative health research community who were pushing at the edges of what constituted quality criteria in applied health research and came to appreciate how differently the social and applied sciences engage with their understanding of the world and what constitutes relevant, meaningful work – or 'good science'.

What Is a 'Disciplinary Lens'?

The term 'disciplinary lens' refers to the fundamental values, beliefs, and assumptions that underpin our understanding of how the world works according to the knowledge structure of our various health professions – the kind of material that might be contained in the typical academic course on 'theoretical foundations of ...' nursing, physical therapy, medicine, social work, and so on. We all learned these ideas as an inherent part of our socialisation into the applied professional discipline we represent, and they were reinforced throughout our enculturation into professional practice standards and ideals. For most of us, they become second nature and, as we carry them into the world of our practice, we extend, diversify, and expand on them so that they reside somewhere in the background, rather than necessarily at the foreground of our everyday practice world. They become the self-evident ideas upon which we are trying to build an increasing understanding of how to do the thing we do better for the benefit of those we serve.

In modern times, as we have come to recognise the disciplinary cultural barriers to team-based healthcare, we have seen considerable focus placed on interdisciplinarity and striving to practice in an interprofessional manner. Across many of our care institutions, there have been conscious attempts to break down the disciplinary infrastructures of our practice settings so as to incentivise better teamwork and discourage intra-professional siloing. Although the academic world has retained a structure characterised by disciplinary distinctions, there is widespread interest in expanding our curricula towards increasing levels of interprofessional learning amongst the healthcare disciplines who will be working together in the practice fields. Further, in the research context, we are increasingly prioritising interdisciplinary research as a preferred approach to addressing the complex challenges of healthcare. Thus, we might argue that a wider environment in healthcare education and practice seems increasingly to be silencing the voice of our distinctive disciplines.

What Is a Disciplinary Lens in the Qualitative Health Research Context?

In the expanding industry of health research, our knowledge generation traditions evolved within the philosophical aspirations of the distinct disciplines. Researchers within the applied health practice disciplines (i.e., the health professions) understand themselves not simply as technicians of health science, but as professionals who have expanded their practice to engage in addressing the knowledge challenges that face their discipline. Thus, in an increasingly interdisciplinary world of practice and research, it becomes important to reflect on what that means with respect to knowledge generation. Top quality graduate (higher degree) programs within the health professional fields often place considerable focus on the philosophical underpinnings of the discipline, ensuring that those who go on to become health researchers are well grounded in that disciplinary knowledge as they add on new skill sets in research technique. They engage students in considering, from a disciplinary perspective, questions such as: How does our discipline relate to the world of ideas? And what are the ideas that our discipline stands for? What is the role of ideas in shaping the expectations, understandings, and constraints upon our practices? And what does it mean to interpret quality claims within our science?

Beyond the graduate seminar context, fringe conferences, and occasional discussion papers in our scholarly journals, most health professionals rarely encounter occasions in which they are explicitly called upon to critically reflect on the ideas underpinning their disciplinary hardwiring. As a consequence, their capacity to call up and articulate their disciplinary lens can become somewhat elusive. They might 'know' that there is a difference in how they think in contrast to how their colleagues from other health disciplines think, but find that the nature of that difference does not easily find its way into expression. It seems that we often forget the language of our differences in our attempt to bridge the gaps in our interprofessional understanding. And this becomes important because it helps explain why that disciplinary lens is so often ignored when we set down the ideas upon which we will build our study design.

Interestingly, despite the extensive investment our educational programs makes in socialising us to think like a member of our profession, the ideas we have been encouraged to take with us as intellectual scaffolding into our qualitative research studies are those that are entirely theoretical. In the world of qualitative research, we seem to have uncritically taken up the assumption that all studies must be grounded on an explicit 'theoretical framework', meaning that we name the theoretical lens we will be applying as we enter into a study. A study that is 'atheoretical' is considered to be lacking an essential element (Neergaard, Olesen, Andersen, & Sondergaard 2009). That theoretical framework is expected to influence the way we position our research question, the design decisions we make, often our sampling and data collection technique, perhaps the analytic framework with which we display our data, and may even predetermine the kinds of interpretations we will ultimately make on the basis of our findings. In other words, although the qualitative health research community has taken up the assumption that a theoretical framework is essential to the integrity of a qualitative study, it understands the role of that theoretical framework as being fulfilled by ideas that have been articulated by other theorists and often that explicitly means social theorists within the social science traditions from whence the methods derived (Sandelowski 1993).

Bringing a disciplinary lens into our qualitative inquiries as applied health professional researchers means that we afford at least as much respect to the intellectual foundations and knowledge traditions of our own discipline as we do to the theoretical ideas that may have been generated within disciplines that exist within society for some other purpose than our own. It means that I as a nurse (or you as an occupational therapist or pharmacist, for example), explicitly recognise and illuminate that disciplinary understanding within our explanation of the rationale for a study, our decisions with respect to design choices, and our ultimate rendering of findings and interpretation of those findings. As such, it calls for a consciousness throughout a research endeavour of why we are engaging in the work that we do, an appreciation for the world out there that needs this knowledge, and the social and ideational context within which that knowledge has the potential to make a difference. Thus, it is not atheoretical as much as it is drawing upon the discipline as its theoretical base. A disciplinary lens honours the ontological core of our different disciplines and ensures that their epistemological structure informs the process and ultimately the product of our research. In that our disciplines are inherently applied disciplines, it helps ensure that the choices we make about what to study and the ways in which we engage with those studies can yield research findings that are as meaningful and useful to the applied world as possible. In this sense, the disciplinary lens serves as our relevance factor. If we embrace it as an inherent component of the way we engage in the knowledge development enterprise, we increase our likelihood of producing research outcomes that matter. If we attempt to push it aside and build our studies on the basis of conformity to the research rules of other knowledge traditions, we run the risk of adding to the already problematic body of somewhat meaningless and irrelevant study findings.

How Might a Disciplinary Lens Influence Identification of Researchable Problems?

In the conventional social science world, a researchable problem comes at the edges of prior theorising and builds upon something theoretical to add application to a new context or explore a phenomenon within a wider theoretical structure. It is motivated by theorising and expects the outcome of a good study to have advanced that theorising.

In the applied health disciplinary world, a researchable problem would more properly be derived from a deep understanding of the limitations of knowledge in the practice context: Why is it that not all patients benefit from the way we are delivering care? What further factors ought we to be considering when we try to improve our practices in relation to a specific population group or health context? What else might there be to know that might help us imagine better ways to do what we do for those who are in need of our services? Knowledge that is relevant to the applied disciplines is knowledge that is (or at least seems to be) helpful in moving our collective capacities forward in the direction the discipline envisions as an ideal world (optimal health, equitable access to health services, holistic care, etc). Research questions derived in this way sit squarely in disciplinary relevance and speak to our appreciation for the role our discipline was derived to fulfil within the larger scheme of society and health.

Remembering the historic context within which the modern phenomenon of qualitative health research derived, the idea of a 'researchable problem' had to do with an acknowledgement that, whilst our practice interests might be complex and messy, only a small subset of that practice was amenable to measurement. And so when our only science tools were quantitative, we focused on trying to find aspects of our disciplinary problems that could be measured. The rapid uptake of qualitative approaches into our disciplines once they were 'discovered' in the late 1970s/early 1980s was testament to the hunger amongst those who sought to advance knowledge for the health professions for which quantitative research was insufficient and there were many intriguing aspects to what we do that required alternatives. Qualitative methods in the social science tradition seemed much closer to allowing for the kinds of knowledge we were seeking. However, in embracing them, and trying hard to adhere to their rule structures in order to ensure our work was seen to be credible, we all too often struggled with the embedded understandings within them as to how research problems ought to be identified and positioned within a theoretical context. For example, drawing on phenomenological tradition, many nurses have framed their research questions using language such as: 'What is *the* lived experience of [name of disease or health context]?', even as their disciplinary epistemological hardwiring ought to be telling them that there will be no essential or unitary experience, and that excellent practice will require an increasingly sophisticated appreciation for variations within experience. Breaking free of those ideas about what the methods tell us are researchable problems, we can prioritise that which our disciplinary understandings lead us to 'see' in a particular manner and begin to think about relevant research questions from that perspective. We might as a result consider reframing that question into a recognition that patient perspectives in the collective will have something to teach us about how we conceptualise and deliver care, even as each patient will come with his or her own distinctive perspective. In this manner, the question we ask and the study we design to answer it will reflect that explicit appreciation for how the knowledge we create will be used in the real world. A research question such as: 'What can be learned from the perspectives of a diversity of patients about effective and equitable [context] care?', can therefore launch us on a path of inquiry that will depart from the more theoretical 'lived experience' question in all aspects of design and implementation.

How Could a Disciplinary Lens Shape the Components of Research Design?

Whilst many of the conventional qualitative methods were developed with the goal of tight and coherent theorising, the kind of knowledge we require in the applied health fields is rarely of that nature. We are comfortable operating in a world of incomplete knowledge, and it is inherent in all of our professions that we anticipate knowledge to continue to grow and evolve. We are not seeking truth, grand theories, or ultimate answers, but better ideas to apply to the problems of our practice and more useful understandings to help us figure out how to do things more effectively. Therefore, we don't need our qualitative studies to conclude with coherent theorising or complete answers, but rather we need them to usefully add to the body of knowledge we already have available in the service of doing what we do. Sometimes we hope they will disrupt those ideas and uncover their unintended consequences. And sometimes they will confirm their general direction, but add a new twist, a new insight, or a new context in which they might be applied. What we need most of all is interpretation of the new elements that have arisen in the course of a study back into the contextual world from which the question arose. We want the 'so what' that takes us beyond description and into the domain of reflecting on practice.

In order to conduct qualitative studies that will ensure continual movement in the direction of better care or professional healthcare practice, we need to consider our intended audience from the outset. As we make decisions about where and how we will recruit a study sample, what we will do with them when we get them, and how we interpret what they tell us, our most important guidance should come from what makes best sense from the perspective of the world that might need the knowledge we create. For example, rather than adhering to the strict inclusion/exclusion criteria qualitative research convention seems to prefer, we may find it entirely reasonable to include 'outliers' or expand the reach of our sample recruitment along the course of our study as the intriguing dimensions of the phenomenon in question start to become apparent in our preliminary analysis. We might quite reasonably shift our course based on the evolving data set, realising that an enhanced data collection strategy or a broader set of data inputs will enhance our capacity to have confidence in the interpretations we are starting to form about the phenomenon.

Notwithstanding the practical realities of what is available to us in our research endeavours (time, resources, etc.), the natural intellectual inclination of our applied health disciplines is to follow new and emerging leads in our inquiry, to use research as a form of detective work towards deeper understandings of things, appreciation for more nuances in that which we already understand, or digging deeper into discoveries of possible alternative explanations of aspects we understand in particular ways. The natural course of the fine minds of our applied health disciplines would not be to compartmentalise our thinking into discrete and disconnected fundable pieces, but rather to continue to search, explore, reflect, and examine the phenomena of our interest in a lifetime of thinking about the problems we see in our world. Thus, we learn to conduct our research in a world in which funding and publication infrastructures are designed for the purposes of research as piecework. And we may forget, as we do that, that there ought to be an ultimate purpose and coherent driver behind all of those discrete studies. Instead of uncritically adopting the design elements that are available to us through conventional methods, an understanding of what we are doing as applied health professional detective work allows us to be creative and purposeful in our design choices. For example, increasingly we are seeing qualitative health researchers recognise that, because any one data collection method will have its inherent limitations, a more robust set of findings with the capacity to get at complexity is more likely to come from a study design that includes multiple data collection strategies. Instead of relying entirely on patient interviews as a singular data source, which is a recognisable proclivity in nursing (Nunkoosing 2005; Sandelowski 2002), a researcher using a disciplinary lens might add in a few focus groups, harvest some collateral or contextual data (such as health records, stakeholder inputs), and test the emerging ideas of the research against strategically selected practice thought leaders or decision makers. Knowing the intended audience, and being able to anticipate the places of hesitation or questioning, it becomes possible to pre-empt the predictable resistance and produce a set of findings in which the audience can have a more comfortable confidence. In knowing your audience, you are understanding not simply the people, but also the knowledge traditions and contexts within which the fruits of your research are intended to have meaning and drawing upon that insight as you develop and implement study design.

What Does the Disciplinary Lens Have to Do with Quality Criteria?

In the qualitative world, the 'holy trinity' of reliability, validity, and generalisability of the quantitative world have been generally dealt with through alternative 'trustworthiness' mechanisms: dependability (are the findings stable over time?), credibility (are the findings plausible?), transferability (could the results have relevance elsewhere?), and confirmability (could the results be confirmed or corroborated by another researcher?) (Anney 2014; Guba 1981; Lincoln & Guba 1985). Interestingly, these quality criteria favour the more simplistic sorts of findings, such as common patterns, or self-evident aspects of a phenomenon, rather than the complex renderings that might more usefully characterise the kinds of qualitatively derived knowledge products that are most likely to have impact upon the field. It's not that they are irrelevant, but rather that we are more likely to find 'fit' (for example) if we are working within a theoretical tradition and have used it to guide study design, than if we are exploring what might lie beyond our usual ways of thinking about a practice phenomenon. So the very best qualitative research, the kind that uncovers a new insight, proposes a new way of thinking about something, or even just organises our thinking about a phenomenon in a new way in order to allow us to see it through fresh eyes, may not fare as well on standard quality criteria than will the more mundane studies (Sandelowski 2014).

Further complicating this problem is the relatively recent advent of champions of the quality checklist. In our enthusiasm to demonstrate credibility and quality in the evidence-based practice environment, and strengthen our capacity to synthesise findings across multiple studies, we have tended to revert to standardised reporting mechanisms in the expectation that all study reports ought to contain equivalent information. Commonly referenced examples include the Consolidated Criteria for Reporting Qualitative Research (Tong, Sainsbury, & Craig 2007) and Standards for Reporting Qualitative Research (O'Brien, Harris, Beckman, Reed, & Cook 2014). The assumption underlying these checklists is that the presence or absence of certain design element claims constitutes a quality index. However, by limiting the gaze to design elements, and not attending to the relevance of the results in the context of the purpose for which the study was designed, as Pawson (2007) reminds us, great new insights can derive from applied studies of a phenomenon that don't quite fit our conventional sense of methodological application technique.

In the world of applied health research, arguably the quality criteria applied to an estimation of the worth of our qualitative products ought to have more to do with the alignment of the study elements with the need for knowledge to advance the work of our professional disciplines. For example, applied health professionals tend not to respond well to assertions of fact, but rather they need to understand the basis upon which that factual claim is being made. Therefore, epistemological credibility within the discipline, or the sense that there is a defensible line of reasoning from foundational assumptions on which the study is grounded through to the methodological decisions from which the findings are made and the conclusions that are derived from those decisions (Thorne 2016a), ought to be an essential quality criterion against which we assess a study's worth. Similarly, we must demonstrate a transparent analytic logic that allows our audience to see our reasoning process throughout rather than accepting our interpretive assertions as a leap of faith (Morse 1994) and choose sample populations that reasonably reflect the type of population towards which the findings, if implemented, would be directed, or guide us to understand their limits with respect to that population. Further, in order to be convincing to our intended applied audience, we need to demonstrate an interpretive authority. In other words, we need to sound like we know what we are talking about within the discipline and provide a plausible reflexive accounting for how we got to where we interpretively arrived (Altheide & Johnson 1994).

Beyond an epistemological integrity to the knowledge traditions of our applied health disciplines, quality interpretations justifiably should consider such issues as the disciplinary relevance of the way we frame our conclusions, the moral and ethical defensibility of how we put forth our interpretations, our capacity to demonstrate awareness of the impact of context on our study findings and outcomes, and the pragmatics of the practice world that might shape the discipline's capacity to use our study findings. Further, given the nature of their understandings of the knowledge they depend upon, the forms in which we convey our findings must be consistent with the level of certainty that our disciplines will tolerate. We deal in the world of provisional or probable truths that may be the best we can do for now, but with the full expectation that they will not stand the test of time because we will have inspired others to take the insights forward and continue to advance knowledge in the field. As a result, we don't own (or cling to, or protect) our findings as much as we offer them to our disciplinary audiences to see if they help solve problems and add value to the practice knowledge base – for now.

Can a Disciplinary Lens Pose Limitations?

If we accept that the disciplinary lens functions as a powerful theoretical scaffolding shaping all aspects of our reasoning around qualitative study design and implementation when we engage in it within our applied fields, then we also need to consider the manner in which it might actually create blind spots. Just as every theoretical framework we might draw upon will illuminate some aspects of a complex clinical phenomenon and obscure others, it is quite reasonable to consider the manner in which our allegiance to a disciplinary understanding might lead us to recreate established beliefs, assumptions and ideas that underpin our practice realities, and miss some of the insights that would actually allow us to advance our discipline's knowledge base.

An example of this might be when healthcare professionals privilege patient-centredness, they can sometimes have difficulty appreciating the wider societal or relational context within which most patients actually want to experience their lives. It might become easy to slip from respecting the victim narrative with which a patient might explain his or her perspective to an assumption that the patient has been victimised. In my discipline of nursing, the pervasive conviction that a nursing disciplinary lens inherently reflects a holistic view of patient experience, including all components of the bio-psycho-social world, might sometimes blind nurse researchers from seeing specific economic or political dimensions of a patient's circumstance. In family practice medicine, it might be difficult to see beyond disease management as the priority and understand chronic illness self-care as primarily about living a life as well as possible. So it behooves us in our disciplinary circles to strive to understand our disciplines – warts and all – in order that we don't inadvertently recreate disciplinary biases that could be limiting our ability to advance the work of our professions. The kind of qualitative inquiry work that allows for, even encourages, continuous critical reflection – an intellectual stance that ought to be consistent with all of our professional practices is our best defence against seeing only what our discipline is accustomed to seeing.

Arguably, the reason we have a robust body of literature from which to critically reflect on our design decisions (such as what we might differently expect from focus group data in comparison to individual interviews) is because we have been expected to make our design decisions transparent in our study proposals and reports. However, it remains relatively rare that we see explicit mention of discipline as a theoretical grounding within a published study report, and, therefore, we have not yet built up a tradition around what it looks like to examine its implications and potential limitations. We seem to need a literature that can guide us to think more clearly about the influence of our disciplinary lens on the shape and texture of our studies, as well as the nature and form of our findings. Possibly some of these insights may emerge from the evolving project of qualitative meta-study – systematically reviewing and deconstructing what has been qualitatively studied in a field in order to expose the ways in which our various disciplinary, theoretical, and methodological positionings have shaped what we think we know over the evolution of knowledge in a particular field of interest. By encouraging applied health professional scholars to 'own' their underpinnings and try to account for the way their disciplinary lens may have shaped their qualitative inquiries, we increase the probability that this issue will attract the attention of those who are fascinated by these evolving methodological developments. From my perspective, a disciplinary lens is often discernible just below the surface of the report of a great applied qualitative study. And conversely, when an applied researcher has gone through the exercise of doing a qualitative study, and the results leave us wondering what was the point, then it is likely that the disciplinary lens was bracketed out or set aside in favour of other drivers.

How Would Disciplinary Lens Work in the Interdisciplinary Context?

To this point in the discussion, we have been considering the disciplinary lens within qualitative research as if it operates as a coherent and self-sufficient orientation. But as we know, applied health researchers often prefer to do their work within interdisciplinary teams, and even if our teams only reflect a single health discipline, they may aspire to generate knowledge that transcends disciplinary boundaries. Rather than seeing this as a contradiction, however, I would argue that the disciplinary lens that an applied health researcher operates from is quite capable of incorporating an infinite number of additional ideas and perspectives. Once a practitioner is out there in the practice domain, for example, we would never set an arbitrary limit on the number of theoretical perspectives and possibilities that he or she might have in the clinical toolbox for use on appropriate occasions. Similarly, my nursing lens does not preclude my capacity to try to see the world through the lens of my physical therapy or radiation oncology research collaborators. In fact, when I listen to what they 'see' in the data or how they instinctively draw connections between patterns in the analysis, I expand my own ability to consider possibilities beyond what seems self-evident. In other words, my disciplinary lens resides as a constant in the background of all that I do, even as I engage in thinking beyond it.

Said differently, my disciplinary lens is not the only theoretical framework I bring with me. It is just one that I never let go of as one component of my research engagement. Although I don't need it to dominate the research team's deliberations as to analytic structure or the framing of findings, for example, it would assert itself if there was any aspect of the team's intended direction or application within the research that violated a fundamental value of my discipline. For example, I could envision the possibility of a study that used methodology in a technically elegant manner to generate findings that could cause harm to sub-groups of patients if they were taken up in practice. Such a study might reflect excellent social theorising, but problematic interpretations from the moral and ethical perspectives of my discipline. Thus, the disciplinary lenses each team member brings, and to some extent the manner in which each team member understands the role of his or her disciplinary lens, will determine whether an interdisciplinary team can or cannot become a crucible for bigger and better ideas informed by the wisdom of the multiplicity of perspectives.

How Can We Design Qualitative Studies for Maximal Impact?

In the world of the applied health disciplines, we engage in research not for the thing itself, but for what it can do to advance the work of our professions and address the problems of the world that our professions were designed to address. Thus, it seems to me that our conventional style of qualitative research – interest driven and guided by methodological rulesets that are often quite inconsistent with our professional practice disciplinary logic – has sometimes led us to design and conduct studies that are not particularly relevant for or amenable to translation into practice. Conversely, if we foreground our disciplinary lens in the process of designing and conducting our qualitative inquiries, we can build that knowledge translation potential from the outset.

Interpretive description (Thorne 2016a) is amongst the many applied qualitative methodologies that has entered the field in recent years in an attempt to try to correct the problems associated with over-reliance on social science traditions in our study designs and to emancipate qualitative researchers in the applied health fields to draw more strongly on their disciplinary epistemology in building design logic that aligns with why they are doing the research and what it is meant to accomplish when it is done (Thorne 2011). As such, it avoids prescribing a particular way to enact method in favour of encouraging the researcher to think through and articulate the approach to any study that will suit the disciplinary purpose – to generate knowledge not for the primary purpose of social theorising, but to generate knowledge that is 'of use' to our applied practice world (Sandelowski 1997). For those who are generally comfortable working within one or another of the established qualitative methodological traditions, but recognise that they are exposing themselves to critique when they depart from the original design rule requirement in trying to shape a study towards meeting the knowledge needs of their intended audience, interpretive description provides a resource with which to logically justify the departures. Such departures might involve sidestepping the usual requirement to name a theoretical framework (Sandelowski 2000), using alternative ways to justify sufficiency other than data or theoretical 'saturation' (Malterud, Siersma, & Guassora 2015), using techniques other than formal coding to work data (Thorne 2016a), or drawing on methodological elements that are more usually associated with distinct traditions – phenomenological style interviewing within an institutional ethnographic style of study, for instance (Kahlke 2014). The key is to stay true to the purpose of the study within an applied disciplinary knowledge generation context and to find ways of moving through the research process that make sense within that logic, regardless of whether or not they conform to an established formalised method.

Elsewhere, we have articulated what we think qualitative research might look like if explicitly informed by a nursing epistemological orientation (Thorne, Stephens, & Truant 2016). We would encourage qualitative researchers in other applied health disciplines to engage in a similar kind of exercise, exploring where the disciplinary logic that so powerfully shapes the practice and general knowledge generation of the professions can also be applied to the enterprise of qualitative method. We firmly believe that this is key to the challenge of impact – of ensuring that as much of our research has utility for the work that needs to be done in the field, and that we can advance practice on the basis of the kinds of insights that qualitative methods are capable of producing.

Integrating knowledge translation from the outset of a study means that we try to ask the kinds of questions for which there is a practice community that wants the answers (Thorne 2016b). We frame our research question in a manner that highlights that knowledge need and sets out to find those answers using methods selected for their capacity to do justice to the task. When we understand the need for that knowledge, we also recognise the complex context within which any answers will ring true and make sense to our intended audience or not. Thus we engage in our research in a manner that engages with those layers of complexity so that our findings, whatever they may be, are seen to have relevance. Instead of approaching the problem of knowledge translation as an afterthought, or assuming the evidence uptake problem is a deficiency of the clinical world, we make it our business to weave a relevance consideration through all phases of our studies.

Concluding Comments

All researchers hope that their studies will have impact and make a difference in some aspect of their field of interest. Researchers in the applied health professions hope that the impact of their studies will be in the direction of the betterment of someone's life or the improvement in some aspect of professional practice. By consciously aligning the coherent and robust intellectual structures of our applied heath disciplinary epistemologies with the infinite range of methodological design options that have evolved in the qualitative health universe, and creatively building our projects in a manner that makes sense within an applied disciplinary logic, we can expand our capacity to tackle real problems, engage with the complexities of our real world, and nudge forward our societal capacity to serve. When we name our disciplinary lens, and demonstrate the manner in which it informs our qualitative work, we increase our chance of doing studies that contribute meaningfully to the world and make a difference for something that matters. The point, after all, is the doing of good research – and optimising the possibility of a relevant return on the investment that entails.

References

Altheide, D. L., & Johnson, J. M. (1994). Criteria for assessing validity in qualitative research. In N. K. Denzin & Y. S. Lincoln (Eds.), *Handbook of Qualitative Research*. Thousand Oaks, CA: Sage, pp. 485–499.

Anney, V. N. (2014). Ensuring the quality of the findings of qualitative research: Looking at trustworthiness criteria. *Journal of Emerging Trends in Educational Research and Policy Studies*, 5(2), pp. 272–281.

Chamberlain, K. (2000). Methodolatry and qualitative health research. *Journal of Health Psychology*, 5(3), pp. 285–296.

Guba, E. G. (1981). Criteria for assessing the trustworthiness of naturalistic inquiries. *Educational Communication and Technology Journal*, 29(2), pp. 75–91.

Kahlke, R. (2014). Generic qualitative approaches: Pitfalls and benefits of methodological mixology. *International Journal of Qualitative Methods*, 13(1), pp. 37–52.

Lincoln, Y. S., & Guba, E. G. (1985). *Naturalistic Inquiry*. Newbury Park, CA: Sage.

Malterud, K., Siersma, V. D., & Guassora, A. D. (2015). Sample size in qualitative interview studies: Guided by information power. *Qualitative Health Research*, 26(13), pp. 1753–1760.

Morse, J. M. (1994). 'Emerging from the data': The cognitive process of analysis in qualitative inquiry. In J. M. Morse (Ed.), *Critical Issues in Qualitative Research Methods*. Thousand Oaks, CA: Sage, pp. 23–43.

Neergaard, M. A., Olesen, F., Andersen, R. S., & Sondergaard J. (2009). Qualitative description: The poor cousin of health research? *BMC Medical Research Methodology*, 9(1), pp. 52–56.

Nunkoosing, K. (2005). The problem with interviews. *Qualitative Health Research*, 15(4), pp. 698–706.

O'Brien, B. C., Harris, I. B., Beckman, T. J., Reed, D. A., & Cook, D. A. (2014). Standards for reporting qualitative research: A synthesis of recommendations. *Academic Medicine*, 89, pp. 1245–1251.

Pawson, R. (2007). Digging for nuggets: How 'bad' research can yield 'good' evidence. *International Journal of Social Research Methodology*, 9, pp. 127–142.

Sandelowski, M. (1993). Theory unmasked: The uses and guises of theory in qualitative research. *Research in Nursing & Health*, 16(3), pp. 213–218.

Sandelowski, M. (1997). 'To be of use': Enhancing the utility of qualitative research. *Nursing Outlook*, 45(3), pp. 125–132.

Sandelowski, M. (2000). Whatever happened to qualitative description? *Research in Nursing & Health*, 23, pp. 334–340.

Sandelowski, M. (2002). Reembodying qualitative inquiry. *Qualitative Health Research*, 12(1), pp. 104–115.

Sandelowski, M. (2014). A matter of taste: Evaluating the quality of qualitative research. *Nursing Inquiry*, 22, pp. 86–94.

Thorne, S. (2011). Toward methodological emancipation in applied health research. *Qualitative Health Research*, 21(4), pp. 443–453.

Thorne, S. (2016a). *Interpretive Description: Qualitative Research for Applied Practice* (2nd edn.). New York: Routledge.

Thorne, S. (2016b). The status and use value of qualitative research findings: New ways to make sense of qualitative work. In M. Lipscomb (Ed.), *Exploring Evidence-Based Practice: Debates and Challenges in Nursing*. London, UK: Routledge, pp. 151–164.

Thorne, S., & Sawatzky, R. (2014). Particularizing the general: Sustaining theoretical integrity in the context of an evidence-based practice agenda. *Advances in Nursing Science*, 27(1), pp. 5–18.

Thorne, S., Stephens, J., & Truant, T. (2016). Building qualitative study design using nursing's disciplinary epistemology. *Journal of Advanced Nursing*, 72(2), pp. 451–460.

Tong, A., Sainsbury, P., & Craig, J. (2007). Consolidated criteria for reporting research (COREQ): A 32-item checklist for interviews and focus groups. *International Journal for Quality in Health Care*, 19, pp. 349–357.

20

Ethnography and Emotions: New Directions for Critical Reflexivity within Contemporary Qualitative Health Care Research

Shane Blackman, Adele Phillips and Rajeeb Sah

CONTENTS

Introduction

In this chapter, we look at the potential of ethnographic research to enhance healthcare policy and practice, through placing a greater emphasis on the emotional dimension of health. This chapter aims to explore the role of emotional relationships between researchers and research participants to develop an understanding of healthcare beyond that of the predominantly clinical focus on physical functioning, to incorporate the social and cultural contexts of healthcare on a holistic basis.

Qualitative research approaches build on an exchange relationship shaped by emotions, which can enable researchers and research participants to engage in a deep understanding of sensitive topics to co-construct their lived experience. Drawing on several fieldwork examples of ethnographic studies, we demonstrate the importance of the research participants' voice in understanding their healthcare provision. Firstly, we address the positivist nature of medical disciplines and the rise of ethnography within healthcare research. Secondly, we explore the place of emotion, reflexivity, and autoethnography linked to researcher positionality and commitment in qualitative health research.

Conservative Disciplines, the Biomedical Model and the Chicago School

The clinical model of medicine based on an objective science is referred to as the dominant biomedical explanation. Sarah Nettleton (1995: 3) argues that whilst health disciplines have been subject to contemporary social changes, the legacy of the biomedical model is that: 'Secure in its approach, medicine has scribed its own history'. On the nature of disciplines, Basil Bernstein (1977: 168) makes it clear that the processes of what is legitimate within a discipline is based on power, coercion, and struggle: 'New legitimations are socially constructed'. For early health career researchers, Bernstein's thoughts are particularly relevant where he suggests that: 'We are told and socialised into what to reject, but rarely told how to create' (167). In this chapter, we base our ideas, theories, and methods on an interpretive approach within healthcare founded on Weber's idea of verstehen, where the emphasis is placed on understanding the meaning and feeling of experience from those involved (Weber 1964). At the same time, we recognised that our approach towards emotions is sometimes positioned in opposition to the dominant positivist models operated within health (Weber 1964). Recently, in terms of sexuality and health, in the United Kingdom in 2018 there was a re-emergence of the opposition between the biomedical model and contemporary social and cultural change with regard to conversion therapy in relation to homosexual men. For example, the *Daily Mail* July 3rd, 2018 reports that: 'Gay cure' therapy will be outlawed: Prime Minister Theresa May tackles 'burning injustices' faced by homosexuals. The roots of conversion therapy go back to the beginning of the twentieth century, these were advocated by authorities and religious organisations as medical interventions to cure homosexuality based on the notion of disease, because homosexuality was considered to be not only a perversion, but incurable. Practices such as transplanting heterosexual testicles on to homosexual men and chemical castration with hormonal treatment serve as a reminder of Foucault's (1977) notion that moral assumptions have formed a foundation for certain medical practices which have a major impact on people's mental health and subjective experience.

For us, it is the central position of the person, not merely the body that shapes the ethnographic approach which is based on sharing and co-operation. Crucially, we assert that health professions research explores caring behaviours empathically underpinned by emotions made explicit through physical touch. Within health research, Kathleen Gilbert (2001: 10) critically questions the place of rationality because for her, there has been a suppression and rejection of the place of emotion in research. Epistemology, as Alison Jaggar (1989: 159) demonstrates is not based on reason, because the dominant paradigms of knowledge assess emotion negatively through 'suspicion' and 'hostility'. Qualitative researchers have historically been criticised for 'contaminating' the research process with their emotions (McKenzie 2017). We see Thomas Kuhn's (1970) idea about the conservative nature of dominant paradigms as relevant, through its construction of barriers to creative development and innovation. As Holliday and MacDonald (2019) point out, the dominant paradigm not only protects the old scientific orders, but 'established careers'. We argue that there are degrees of sustained recidivism within old paradigms which serve to protect previous ideas from change, through what Deanna Kuhn (1991: 68) has argued is a form of 'pseudo evidence' where existing explanations are restated as evidence. Thomas Kuhn (1970: 146) states: 'No theory ever solves all the puzzles which it is confronted at a given time; nor are the solutions already achieved often perfect. On the contrary, it is just the incompleteness and imperfection of the existing data-theory fit that, at any time define many of the puzzles that characterise normal science'. In Kuhn's terms, the biomedical model is the established paradigm, and we argue that its power requires critical reassessment because the biomedical model is not able to capture, explain, or fully understand healthcare.

According to George Engel (1977: 129): 'The dominant model of disease today is biomedical, and it leaves no room within this framework for the social, psychological, and behavioural dimensions of illness'. In the United Kingdom, Engel (1960) first developed his critique, but in the United States the challenge to the positivist model began in the 1950s with Renne Fox's (1957) 'Training for Uncertainty' in the collection *The Student Physician* edited by Merton, Reader, and Kendall and subsequently in Fox's *Experiment Perilous* (1959), alongside *Boys in White* by Becker, Geer, Hughes, and Strauss (1961). These are landmark studies in establishing the initial insights into the value of understanding everyday sensitivities within medical spaces through participant observation. These were followed by Julios Roth's (1963) *Timetables Structuring the Passage of Time in Hospital Treatment*, who studied at the University of Chicago and was mentored by Everett Hughes of the Chicago School, who also championed participation observation. Joseph Gusfield (1963, 1967: 231, 1968: 61), who did his PhD at the University of Chicago, builds on Howard Becker's et al. (1961) approach to argue that illness is not merely socially constructed or only a 'medical fact' it is 'a political issue'. The symbolic interaction tradition at Chicago focusing on health includes the work of Irving Goffman (1961, 1963), alongside Glaser and Strauss's (1965) *Awareness of Dying*, which was the foundation upon which they subsequently built and developed the ideas of grounded theory within qualitative research (Blackman 2010). The impact of this early work is described by Paul Atkinson and Lesley Pugsley (2005: 231) in terms of the: '...methodological commitment to investigation of everyday social life in situ'. They identify this Chicago School approach focused on the systematic observation of detail and context through participatory sensitivity as the beginning of contemporary ethnographic commitment to healthcare.

The dominant paradigm within healthcare is positivist, its epistemological position is defined through the methodological principle of replicability. Quantitative research offers reliability, enables generalisation, and enhances the status of biomedical science and supports its hegemonic position. This epistemological construction of medicine has been transferred to healthcare and consequently held in check insights from ethnographic approaches. For us, the continued processes of objectification, reductionism, or dehumanisation which feature within the clinical gaze, demonstrate the urgent necessity to bring together the social and cultural world of the patient as a resource to enable more diversity and sensitivity to the biomedical world where agency could be seen as an interactive feature within health studies. The challenge for contemporary ethnography is to embrace its biographical and empathic foundation of urban ethnography within the Chicago School of Sociology and take up the challenge of subjectivity, emotion, and interpretation to develop a more fit for purpose ethnography where reflexivity rests at the heart of qualitative approaches (Merrill and West 2009).

The Rise of Ethnography with Healthcare Research

Goodson and Vassar (2011) maintain that whilst: 'Ethnography has been used in medical education for more than 50 years', it has been kept on the periphery and criticised for being too vague, difficult to measure, not replicable, and too subjective. Within health professions research, it has now become increasingly recognised that qualitative and in particular ethnographic research has been identified as contributing to an increased understanding of healthcare. The recent rise of ethnography has also been integrally related to the slow growth of acceptance towards the role that emotions can play within qualitative fieldwork. Jones and Hunter (1995), Pope et al. (2000), Meyer (2000), Caprara and Landim (2008), Morgan-Trimmer and Wood (2016), and McGarrol (2017) detail the value of fieldwork and emotion to access culture and beliefs to enhance a more sensitive and responsive delivery of healthcare. It is in this sense that Jan Savage (2000: 1402) argues that the clinical world has everything to gain because: 'Ethnography can help healthcare professionals to solve problems beyond the reach of many research approaches'. Within radiography, for Hayre (2016: 195), the value of ethnographic method is: '…to capture and understand naturally occurring world activities in real-world settings'. The rise of qualitative research is not surprising, according to Janice Jones and Joanna Smith (2017: 100) who argue that: 'The value of focused ethnographic studies in healthcare is essential to develop an in-depth understanding of healthcare cultures and explore complex phenomenon in real world contexts'. In contrast, Rashid et al. (2015:11) argue that: 'Researchers in health disciplines do not divulge much about their fieldwork'. They further add that: 'Health researchers conducting ethnographic research rarely discuss ethical concerns that they might have encountered during the conduct of their research'. This serves as a warning to ethnographers that increased recognition does not equate with increased acceptance or understanding. This accusation, however, does not square with Atkinson and Pugsley's (2005: 232) understanding of ethnography as defined through a clear and open 'commitment to reflexivity'.

The paradigm of positivism within healthcare according to Goodson and Vassar (2011) should be placed within a historical, social, and cultural context. For them, ethnography within health is not about testing theory or value neutrality, it is about how: '…knowledge is socially constructed and situated within a particular context'. This is the real value of ethnography within health studies for Draper (2015: 36) who focuses on 'real-life contexts' and 'culturally shared' experiences to maintain that ethnography can: '…provide rich, contextual and valuable insights uncovering meaning and experience … . of both giving and receiving care' (41). Our argument in this chapter is that doing fieldwork within health studies is a messy business, it is emotional labour, but also highly effective and can offer new knowledge for healthcare within a context of rigor and responsive sensitivity. The heart of ethnographic research is to capture people's real-life encounters and experiences within everyday contexts through the development of relationships based on emotion.

It is the methodological integration of ethnography and emotion which we identify as the strength of the method, not its weakness. A key factor about ethnography is its focuses on presence, being live in the field through observation, and this in turn supports the validity of the data through 'being there'. Hayre et al. (2016: 2) argue that participant observation created the opportunity for immersion to: '…provide original insight into radiographic practices underexplored within the UK offering original insight by exploring PCC practices within the X-ray room using advanced technology'. On this basis of immersion within the culture of the everyday, the researchers embrace the diverse worlds of the participants, and the method calls forth for the researcher to recognise their own place within that world through researcher positionality. Our argument highlights the necessary value of fieldwork and emotion within health studies. The benefit of ethnography within healthcare is that it offers, according to Dixon-Woods (2003: 327): '…probing into areas where measurement is not easy, where issues are sensitive and multifaceted'. We see ethnography as of value to address issues of causality to offer contextually relevant data that can offer support, imagination, and sensitivity within person-centred healthcare (Draper 2015). It is not our endeavour to advance the case for ethnographic approaches in health studies by dismissing the positivist biomedical model of medicine, we want to open up the paradigm to increase its responsiveness.

Researcher Positionality, the Discipline and the Profession

The development of researcher positionality within qualitative fieldwork studies has enabled methodological accounts to be more honest and informed about how the data are not only collected and managed, but also to show how interpretation takes place and theory is constructed from data (Blackman 2007). This 'reflexive turn' has demonstrated the importance of subjectivity in the formal process of data collection. Bourdieu (1990) asks us to think about our 'situatedness', the personal meaning of our research within a critical context (Blommaert 2005). In response to the challenge of the 'crisis of representation' in ethnography, reflexivity established the opportunity for researchers to describe, assess, and theorise the practice of doing and writing research. Reflexivity in healthcare is about dialogue to explain that your research is not about disclosure or a confession, it reflects back on researchers to describe what they do and how they did it.

Initially, we want to highlight the difference between making a critical stance within the discipline and how this critical position may be understood by PhD researchers and early career researchers. From within healthcare I shall highlight two different examples, the first relates to health and drug workers as researcher participants who were concerned that their critical perspective may have an impact on their organisation, and the second example relates to two PhD research students, one focused on an ethnography of X-ray units and the other focused on an ethnographic study on operating theatres. Both doctoral students through their findings began to develop a critical stance towards their profession. As professional practitioners, they were personally concerned that their fieldwork evidence could be seen in a negative light against their profession. This made them feel uncomfortable and was identified as: 'I could be undermining my own profession. Showing weaknesses! I didn't think that was the aim of my research'.

The first example involved ethnographic interviewing and participant observation over a 9-month period with health and drug practitioners (Blackman et al. 2018). The ethics of the research project stipulated that the research participants could read what they had said during data collection and how the initial report was draft. The work was read by the professionals, two initially stated: 'I was shocked at what I read. Collectively we are all supposed to take the same position, but we weren't. We can't let this go out!' Another stated: 'Who said that? You have got to be joking! Hold on! I have an idea. How did you get that out of them!' The healthcare professionals were reflecting on the meaning of the ethnographic data. Through conversational interviewing as an ethnographic technique, the use of empathy and common ground enabled direct intimate data and real emotions based on experience to emerge. The consequent issue was that being a professional in a recognisable organisation or institution made some of the research participants wary of their critical comments because it looked bad on the organisation or 'the comment might be traced to me'. This made them concerned about their employment status. On this basis, it became essential to reaffirm the ethical consent and work with professional healthcare workers to ensure that their consent was agreed, but also to guarantee that their data released, i.e., their comments could not be traced to them, or their organisation. On this basis, the individuals and administrative identities of the participating organisations and professionals were anonymised so that each person felt confident and gave their consent. Subsequently, all professional practitioners were positive about the research experience enabling them to reflect on and to develop more effective work within their organisation and the holistic delivery of healthcare provision.

The second example relates to supervision of two PhD research students who were undertaking ethnographies within hospital environments, one which focused on X-ray units and the other on operating theatres. During the fieldwork, there came a point where both PhD students observed critical moments which either demanded their intervention in the research setting or made them aware that medical practitioners and patients were coming at the issues of healthcare from different perspectives.

Both PhD researchers experienced contact with other medical professionals where a language of objectivity defined patients as passive. There was a domination of the physical body to such an extent that the person appeared superfluous, they were reduced to the physical bit part, for example, 'the knee'. The medicalisation of patients that defines them in terms of their illness, disease, or body part can intensify patient feelings of reductionism to a medical problem. In contrast, within these medical settings it was found that patients sometimes sought humour and irony to deflect their health condition, whereas the medical practitioners seemed unaware of how personal and intimate their interventions were in the lives of ordinary people. Initially, both researchers were reluctant to speak of these incidents because such observations may look badly on their research methods and also their respective professions. Here, the patient does not have a name, but is labelled as the illness. Only after considerable reflection, did both researchers realise that the diagnostic application to reduce the human being to a medical label had an impact on patients as well as their own researcher positionality, as they felt uncomfortable in the manner that the patient was addressed by senior medical professionals.

Further, the PhD students found that during a series of fieldwork observation they were being asked questions by other professionals within the health setting that demonstrated other professionals lack of knowledge or skill. The specific intervention by the PhD students offered support, but at the same time revealed weaknesses within the profession. Thus, qualitative fieldwork enabled these researchers to assist fellow professional practitioners with patient care, but brought serious reflection because they were aware of how other professional practitioners were engaged in interventions which had shortcomings. It is at this moment that both PhD research students were excited that they had gained new knowledge of how medical professionals' interact with patients, but at the same time the data showed the professional as wanting. Their researcher positionality made them concerned about how much they should reveal, how much to tell, so rather than promote agency, here, reflexivity heightened personal tension for both health researchers. On this basis, reflexivity was experienced as a worry and concern rather than an experience of agency.

The basis of ethnographic research lies in the empathetic interaction between the researcher and the research participants to develop a relationship of trust to explore lived experiences, which has the potential to impact upon health conditions. Patients perceive their behaviour, health, and well-being as private and confidential, and the sensitivity attached with health conditions makes them feel vulnerable and emotional to share their experiences. Talking to people about their feelings and experiences towards health and well-being is emotional and sensitive. Although healthcare workers are backed by their professional competence making patients relatively comfortable and confident to share their health experiences, it also creates barriers amongst patients about the details of the information that are required to be shared with a professional. Patients often are reluctant to uncover their feelings beyond the health and illness because of the fear that judgements might be made about them (Råheim et al. 2016). The challenge for the patient is an attempt to balance the information that they want to share with a professional and/or a researcher, which has the potential to create further distress and concerns about their well-being. Therefore, the role of health professionals as researchers becomes more challenging, as they are required to avoid any additional distress or concerns to their participants because of the research and negotiate the access to the patient ensuring that they are dedicated to the care and welfare of their patients.

Managing Emotions and Researcher Commitment

Qualitative research explores social processes and practices by examining people's attitudes, perceptions, and thoughts within specific contexts to understand experiences of service users and service providers to improve the quality of healthcare. There is a growing awareness that qualitative research is an embodied experience for the researcher and the research participant and emotions play a key role throughout the research process (Dickson-Swift et al. 2009). Burkitt (2012: 469) suggests that feelings and emotions are central to the reflexive processes during the qualitative research. The emotions here incorporate thinking as well as feeling aspects of people's experiences. The role of emotions in understanding the social world through qualitative, and in particular ethnographic research, within healthcare can be understood at two levels. Firstly, we need to reflect on the patient's emotions whilst thinking and sharing their feelings and experiences about health and well-being issues with an unknown or relatively less known person who comes as a researcher to collect information. Secondly, we also need to reflect on the researcher's emotions who navigates through the process of accessing patients or research participants, building rapport, trust, and relationships and eventually having to exit the fieldwork to complete the research project, leaving all the feelings and affections behind.

The dual roles and responsibilities of a health professional researcher have a potential impact on the researcher's positionality when participating with research participants or being with people during the research process. An understanding about researcher's positionality helps researcher to recognise their experiences, beliefs, research interests, and personal stance in the context of the given research study, so that they may acknowledge how these factors influence the research (Savin-Baden and Major 2013). For a health professional researcher, it may be appropriate to separate the professional role whilst acting as a researcher, but this is not always possible, and health professional researchers need to manage their emotions to make conducive decisions that assist patients in the best possible way. For example, during my ethnographic research (Sah 2017), once I had initial contacts with a group of young people, the challenge was to build rapport that would facilitate the discussions around sensitive topics of sexual lifestyles and relationships. Although my professional identity and competence made my research participants relatively comfortable and confident, they were unwilling to provide detailed information about their sexual lifestyle experiences because of the fear that the information might not remain confidential and judgments would be made about them. I had to consistently remind them about my professional roles and responsibilities, which included ensuring confidentiality, but at the same time I had to restrain myself from providing sexual health advices. I had to negotiate around my positioning between a health professional and a researcher, which meant I had to constantly balance my emotional engagement during the process of the in-depth interviews, and reflexivity was a key research tool that helped me to navigate through this emotional process.

To pursue a career in the health professions involves making a commitment to engaging in everyday working practices which are underpinned by duties of caring for others. Pulcini (2017) emphasises that caring is a moral and practical activity, which is motivated by emotions of love, compassion, and generosity. Qualitative researchers frequently reflect on their motivations for their research interests and highlight the emotional attachment to their topic of study. When researching controversial areas such as sexuality and health, we found that even being a medical doctor may not facilitate access and present hurdles. For example, for my ethnographic research exploring sexual lifestyles and relationships of Nepalese young people in the United Kingdom (Sah 2017), I found comparatively easy access to the field because of my professional background of being a doctor, which is a widely respected profession within the Nepalese community. I started my fieldwork by talking to everyone and anyone with an aim to build support and gain trust from the close-knit Nepalese community, where discussing sexual health topics are taboo. I expected this would build a relationship and parents would introduce me to their sons and daughters, which would help me to understand the multiple field realities of young people and their family, with whom they live. However, the sensitiveness of the topic meant Nepalese parents and community leaders were not comfortable to relate themselves with such research.

In another example focused on emotion and commitment, my own motivations for conducting research into drug and alcohol using behaviours were driven by my experiences as a harm reduction practitioner in a community-based drug and alcohol service. I was emotionally attached to the work I did and to the service users with whom I worked. I cared about what had happened to them during the course of their lives leading up to them accessing the service and wanted the best possible treatment outcomes for them so that they could lead healthier, happier lives. There is increasing recognition that qualitative researchers who are investigating emotionally sensitive topics can be at risk of feelings of guilt, vulnerability, and exhaustion (Dickson-Swift et al. 2007). Reflecting on her experiences conducting research with women who were awaiting trial, Wincup (2000) recalls that when the participants in her research became upset or cried, she instinctively attempted to avoid the situation by steering the conversation into another direction. She reports that she felt guilty and anxious in instances where her questioning had caused the upset. Further guilty feelings were experienced by this researcher at the notion of an exploitative aspect to this kind of research, that researchers may enjoy the rich learning experience involved and potentially build a career on the basis of the emotional fatigue experienced by the participants. However, Wincup (2000) expressed that she was able to reconcile some of her guilty feelings through considering the potential benefits for the research participants. Despite the expressions of sadness, the participants reported that they had actually enjoyed taking part in the research and had found it beneficial to voice their emotional distress.

It is argued that emotional distress in the field does not necessarily result in damage (Watts 2008). It has been shown that confronting negative emotions can actually benefit health and attenuate the advancement of chronic illness through the promotion of resilience and the development of approach coping (Hershfield et al. 2013). Whilst research protocol and ethics processes should seek to protect both researchers and the researched from dangerous practices, this should not be at the expense of enabling the clear benefits that ethnographic work can convey. Ethical processes and supervision should adequately prepare researchers and participants for the emotional experiences which result from entering the field, the data collection itself, and exiting the field, arguably, these processes frequently neglect the emotional dimensions of the research. For example, in my own research experience looking at the alcohol-related life experiences of older people through qualitative interviews which took place in their homes, the ethics process very much focused on my personal safety at the prospect of entering people's homes, and the research that I had read emphasised the importance of quickly developing a sense of rapport with my participants upon entry to the field. To my relief, I was able to do these things without difficulty, however, the processes had not prepared me for exiting the field. Whilst interviewing one male participant, a widower aged 74 years, it became apparent to me that he felt sad that I would have to leave his home once the interview had drawn to a close. I felt that he was devising strategies for keeping me in his home for a longer period, such as talking for longer than we had agreed, expressing sadness that his family did not visit him often enough, showing me personal possessions in the house, and touring the garden. This evoked a strong sense of guilt in me, particularly as it made me wonder about my own older family members, and I felt guilty that perhaps I had not visited them enough when they were alive! Eventually, I managed to draw the conversation to a close and explained that I needed to be elsewhere. As I left, he insisted on giving me a pot plant from his garden, which I think was of comfort to us both, as it represented that in some small way, the researcher-participant relationship would continue. I left his home feeling that the research process should better prepare both researchers and participants for ending the emotional connection and exiting the field with an understanding of the benefits that the research can bring.

Taking part in the research can legitimise the recounting of personal experiences and normalise conventionally unacceptable emotions, which Jaggar (1989) describes as 'outlaw emotions', such as anger or embarrassment in the face of discrimination. It is suggested that policies, practices, and discourse concerning chronic health conditions construct people with these conditions as 'the other' (Walton and Lazzaro-Salazar 2015), so it is beneficial when participants can gain a sense of catharsis through the telling of marginalised experiences. Watts' (2008) ethnographic study examining how health professionals learn on a medical ward, found that clinical artefacts such as paper-based drug charts and clinical equipment created physical spaces within which participants clustered and interacted (Sheehan et al. 2016). It was found that these artefacts reinforced hierarchies and positions of power within medical teams. As Conrad and Barker (2010: 71) argue, '…the patient experience is not the same as the illness'. Understanding how patients connect through observing and examining the physical environment are under-explored areas within ethnographic work, and it is suggested that further research seeks to incorporate other ways of knowing.

Autoethnography: Writing, Rapport, and Trust

Autoethnography enables us to reconstruct both others and ourselves through an understanding of the self in relation to the research participants. In this way, our personal history is integrated into our professional research practice. These ideas were first explored by C.W. Mills' (1959) *The Sociological Imagination*, where he urged us to examine individual biographies and histories within the social structure, to re-set our ambition and reimagining research methodologies. Autoethnography as a qualitative research method is another way of furthering our understanding of the emotional relationship between the researcher and the researched. Heewon Chang (2016: 444) argues that autoethnographic research methods aim to 'connect the personal with the social'. Importantly, Deborah Reed-Danahay (2001: 410) demonstrates that autoethnographic approaches are not only focused on exploring the relevance of life history and subjectivity, but also the relationship between the narrator and the research participants through the creation of writing. The dominant voice in autoethnography Holliday (2016: 122) argues '...in the written form of research, the only narrative is that of the researcher', but at the same time he admits that interactivity and dialogue shape the creation of the text. The tension in all ethnographic work stems from the researcher being both the subject and object of the fieldwork and aims to elicit the author's voice through the exploration and analysis of their personal experiences (Ellis and Bochner 2000).

Although, autoethnography has been contested for its 'confessional basis' and an over preoccupation with the personal as 'navel gazing' (Delamont 2007; Allen-Collinson and Hockey 2008). We support Sonyini Madison's (2012: 198) argument that autoethnography can form part of a critical reflexive ethnography to '...deepen, extend and complicate the world around and beyond the researcher's grasp'. The recalling of often intense experiences as they are remembered by the author, through a critical lens, invokes deep emotional responses. In addition to autoethnographic work being valid data in itself, it can also be used to elucidate richer data concerning the emotional experiences of others, through training research participants to analyse their own emotional experiences (Buckley 2015). In Langhout's (2006) research on community garden projects with African American women, she found that although she viewed her relationship with the participants through the lens of gender and class, her research collaborator, who was an African American woman, viewed this through the lens of race and white privilege. This challenged Langhout's (2006) assumptions concerning her positionality as a researcher, she had not considered how being a white woman from an academic community oriented her into a position of privilege. Boyd (2008) argues that autoethnography can enable transformational learning, as positions of social power such as white privilege may remain largely invisible to the researcher themselves. Researchers need to initiate appropriate spaces for narratives, whereby the discourse is not constrained by oppressive forces, which may reinforce the internalisation of such oppression. Allowing the research participants to speak also enables the researcher to integrate their own voice and experience. Where participants experience marginality, they may feel their voice or experience is unwelcome. It is here that autoethnography can prioritise participants through sharing, making interaction live and personal (Blackman 1997). However, following an analysis of pregnant and postpartum women's narratives concerning drug treatment, Radcliffe (2011) suggests that drug-using women who are participants in qualitative research frame their stories within a 'moral transformation' guise, so, in essence, the research encounter serves to provides a space in which the participants locate themselves within a frame of subordination. Ethnographic studies can develop our understanding of professional identities and challenge the feasibility of assumed hierarchies within healthcare organisations, thus invoking change at the institutional level (Kielmann 2012). Therefore, considering how researcher identity shapes the emotional connections with participants can cast a critical light on how positions of privilege operate and work towards the decolonisation of research (Datta 2017).

The emotional experiences of research participants are widely reported during and after the research, whereas the discussion about researcher's emotions has less attention or there is an ambiguity in acknowledging it publicly (Gilbert 2001; Blackman 2007). Even when discussed, the focus is often on managing, rather than integrating, emotions into the research process. In the chapter, we have raised some issues about the researcher's own turmoil in understanding, managing, and integrating their emotions during building relationship with participants, identifying positionality, and experiencing reflexivity during the research process. Auto and ethnographic research require researchers to enter into the subjective world of the research participants to understand them and their wider culture by exploring their experiences, feelings, perceptions, and thoughts. In order to achieve this, the researcher acts as a 'human instrument' (Fetterman 2010: 33) in the field and relies on all their senses, thoughts, and feelings, including emotions, to connect with research participants to examine the sociocultural landscape of the research topic in the particular context. Davis (2001) argues that healthcare researchers experience a constant interplay between personal, emotional, and intellectual work (Mills 1959). The first step for initiating research is talking to the people, and the opening conversations and communications are acts of negotiation to build relationships, rapport, and support to gain access to the sites and potential research participants for the research fieldwork. Many health professional researchers will probably have straightforward access to the healthcare settings and other health researchers may gain access to the community through rapport building with initial conversations, however, it is challenging for them to be with people everywhere in their everyday lives. Nevertheless, the aim of being with people is to achieve social and cultural immersion in a constructed research site, which has the sense of cultural boundedness and where researchers are able to talk, participate, and observe patients for the purpose of health research.

Health professionals have empathy towards their patients that generates intense emotions on both sides to help establish rapport with research participants, which is key whilst talking to the people in an initial stage of ethnographic research. However, there is a need to find a balance of emotional engagement since researchers are expected to be responsible and careful to avoid preconceptions influencing the research data because of the close relationships with patients, which becomes burdensome for health professional researcher. The challenges lie in a successful negotiation with the patients to gain a sufficient level of trust, which would ensure the deep exploration of experiences, feelings, perceptions, and thoughts, maintaining the emotional sensitiveness attached to the healthcare topics.

However, there are instances when researchers are so emotionally overwhelmed during the research that they are not able to or do not try to hold back or manage their emotions during the interviews, instead prefer to be part of that experience (Dickson-Swift et al. 2009). This works well, as qualitative research requires an immersion from the researcher to be with people or participate with research participants during the fieldwork to infer their viewpoints, feelings, perceptions, and thoughts. Gilbert (2001) maintains that the emotions expressed from the researcher during the research process can be positive as well as negative. The effective use of emotions during research processes can provide rich narratives of patient's perspectives and interpretations, whereas mismanagement and ineffective use of emotions may increase the vulnerability of the research participants. For example, during my ethnographic research (Sah 2017), the discussions around perceptions and experiences of research participants about the topics such as secrecy in dating and romantic relationships, importance of parental consent for marriage, transformation, and expectations from love and arranged marriage were so relational that I ended up sharing my perceptions and experiences on those topics. From an autoethnographic position, this generated intense emotions on both sides that helped to establish rapport and build trusting relationships to motivate young people to uncover their hidden experiences and feelings through the mutual emotional conversations, which would have remained unexplored through general conversations. The key aspects of autoethnography are to be flexible and adapt to the context and exercise the roles and responsibilities based on the requirements of the time and space, rather than trying to have a distinctive position.

Conclusion

We have argued that the conservative nature of the biomedical paradigm can set limits on the contribution of ethnographic methods to demonstrate the value of emotions to an improved understanding of healthcare. Within healthcare, a major obstacle to overcome has been the idea that the physical determines health and this deterministic force also shapes our emotion that responds to health conditions. In short, we challenge the hegemony of the physical over the emotional, and this is shown through our ethnographic studies and people's relationship to their well-being. From the fieldwork examples, we found that emotional contact brought forward a range of contradictory, oppositional, and pleasurable experiences through encounters with anger, frustration, guilt, irony, and humour. Recognition of these different and diverse emotions and experiences enabled us to address healthcare issues from different perspectives where emotion and ethnography are positive assets in understanding and sharing. Researchers' initial motivations for undertaking research can involve close engagement with people's everyday lives and are also emotionally driven.

Ethnographic work involves a shared emotional relationship between the researcher and participants, which can convey a number of benefits to research participants. These include enabling an exploration of the meaning attached to health status and conditions, providing a space to develop an empowered voice, and initiating mechanisms for reducing societal marginalisation. This chapter has explored the researcher-participant relationship within qualitative research and argued that ethnographic research is underpinned by emotions throughout the whole research process.

References

Allen-Collinson, J. and Hockey, J. (2008) Autoethnography as 'valid' methodology? A study of disrupted identity narratives, *International Journal of Interdisciplinary Social Sciences*, 3, 6: 209–217.

Atkinson, P. and Pugsley, L. (2005) Making sense of ethnography and medical education, *Medical Education*, 39, 2: 228–234.

Becker, H., Geer, B., Hughes, E. and Strauss, A. (1961) *Boys in White: Student Culture in Medical School*. Chicago: University of Chicago Press.

Bernstein, B. (1977) *Class, Codes and Control: Towards a Theory of Educational Transmission*. London, UK: Routledge.

Blackman, S. (1997) 'Destructing a Giro': A critical and ethnographic study of the youth 'underclass', in MacDonald, R. (Ed.) *Youth, the 'Underclass' and Social Exclusion*. London, UK: Routledge: 113–129.

Blackman, S. (2007) 'Hidden Ethnography': Crossing emotional borders in qualitative accounts of young people's lives, *Sociology*, 41, 4: 699–716.

Blackman, S. (2010) 'The ethnographic mosaic' of the Chicago School: Critically locating Vivien Palmer, Clifford Shaw and Frederic Thrasher's research methods in contemporary reflexive sociological interpretation, in Hart, C. (Ed.) *The Legacy of the Chicago School of Sociology*. Kingswinsford: Midrash Publishing: 195–215.

Blackman, S., Bradley, R., Fagg, M. and Hickmott, N. (2018) Towards sensible drug information: A critical exploration of one drug service response to shifting attitudes toward drug trends and acceptable advice, *Drugs: Education, Prevention & Policy: Special Issue: Intersections in New Drug Research*: 1–9. doi:10.1080/09687637.2017.1397100.

Blommaert, J. (2005) Bourdieu the ethnographer. The ethnographic grounding of habitus and voice, *The Translator*, 11, 2: 219–236.

Bourdieu, P. (1990) *The Logic of Practice*, Cambridge, UK: Polity Press.

Boyd, D. (2008) Autoethnography as a tool for transformative learning about white privilege, *Journal of Transformative Education*, 6, 3: 212–225.

Buckley, R. (2015) Autoethnography helps analyse emotions, *Frontiers in Psychology*, 209, 6: 1–3. https://www.ncbi.nlm.nih.gov/pmc/articles/PMC4340136/pdf/fpsyg-06-00209.pdf. (Accessed 10 April 2018).

Burkitt, I. (2012) Emotional reflexivity: Feeling, emotion and imagination in reflexive dialogues, *Sociology*, 46, 3: 458–472.

Caprara, A. and Landim, L. (2008) Ethnography: Use, potentialities and limits in health research, Interface – Comunicação, Saúde, Educação, 4(se), http://socialsciences.scielo.org/scielo.php?script=sci_arttext&pid=S1414-32832008000100010&lng=en&tlng=en. (Accessed 10 April 2018).

Chang, H. (2016) Autoethnography in health research: Growing pains. *Qualitative Health Research*, 26, 4: 443–451.

Conrad, P. and Barker, K. (2010) The social construction of illness: Key insights and policy implications, *Journal of Health and Social Behavior*, 51: 67–79.

Daily Mail, July 3rd (2018) 'Gay cure' therapy will be outlawed: Prime Minister Theresa May tackles 'burning injustices' faced by homosexuals. http://www.dailymail.co.uk/news/article-5911469/Gay-cure-therapy-outlawed.html (Accessed 10 April 2018).

Datta, R. (2017) Decolonizing both researcher and research and its effectiveness on Indigenous research, *Research Ethics*, doi:10.1177/1747016117733296.

Davis, H. (2001) The management of self: Practical and emotional implications of ethnographic work in a public hospital setting, in K.R. Gilbert (Ed.) *The Emotional Nature of Qualitative Research*, London, UK: CRC Press: 37–61.

Delamont, S. (2007) Arguments against auto-ethnography, *Qualitative Researcher*, 4: 2–4., http://www.cardiff.ac.uk/socsi/qualiti/QualitativeResearcher/QR_Issue4_Feb07.pdf. (Accessed 10 April 2018).

Dickson-Swift, V. et al. (2007) Doing sensitive research: What challenges do qualitative researchers face? *Qualitative Research*, 7, 3: 327–353.

Dickson-Swift, V., James, E. L., Kippen, S. and Liamputtong, P. (2009) Researching sensitive topics: Qualitative research as emotion work, *Qualitative Research*, 9, 1: 61–79.

Dixon-Woods, M. (2003) What can ethnography do for quality and safety in health care, *Quality and Safety in Health Care*, 12, 5: 326–327.

Draper, J. (2015) Ethnography: Principles, practice and potential, *Nursing Standard*, 29, 36: 36–41.

Ellis, C. and Bochner, A. P. (2000) Autoethnography, personal narrative, reflexivity, in Denzin, N. K. and Lincoln, Y. S. (Eds.) *Handbook of Qualitative Research*. 2nd ed. Thousand Oaks, CA: Sage: 733–768.

Engel, G. L. (1960) A unified concept of health and disease, *Perspectives in Biology and Medicine*, 3, 459–485.

Engel, G. L. (1977) The need for a new medical model: A challenge for biomedicine, *Science*, 196: 129–136.

Fetterman, D. (2010) *Ethnography: Step by Step*. 3rd ed. London, UK: Sage Publications.
Foucault, M. (1977) *Discipline and Punish: The Birth of the Prison*. New York: Pantheon Books.
Fox, R. (1957) Training for uncertainty, in Merton, R. K., Reader, G. and Kendall, P. (Eds.) *The Student-Physician: Introductory Studies in the Sociology of Medical Education*. Cambridge, MA: Harvard University Press: 207–241.
Fox, R. (1959) *Experiment Perilous*. Glencoe, IL: The Free Press.
Gilbert, K. R. (2001) Introduction: Why are we interested in emotions?, in Gilbert, K. R. (Ed.) *The Emotional Nature of Qualitative Research*. London, UK: CRC Press: 3–15.
Glaser, B. G. and Strauss, A. L. (1965) *Awareness of Dying*. Chicago, IL: Aldine Publishing.
Goffman, E. (1961) *Asylums: Essays on the Social Situation of Mental Patients and Other Inmates*. New York: Doubleday Anchor.
Goffman, E. (1963) *Stigma: Notes on the Management of Spoiled Identity*. Englewood Cliffs, NJ: Prentice Hall.
Goodson, L. and Vassar, M. (2011) An overview of ethnography in healthcare and medical education research, *Journal of Education Evaluation for Health Professions*, 8, 4: 4. doi:10.3352/jeehp.2011.8.4.
Gusfield, J. (1963) *Symbolic Crusade. Status Politics and the American Temperance Movement*. Urbana, IL: University of Illinois Press.
Gusfield, J. (1967) Moral passage: The symbolic process in public designations of deviance, *Social Problems*, 15, 2: 175–188.
Gusfield, J. (1968) On legislating morals: The symbolic process of designating deviance, *California Law Review*, 56, 1: 54–73.
Hayre, C. M. (2016) 'Cranking up', 'whacking up' and 'bumping up': X-ray exposures in contemporary radiographic practice. *Radiography*, 22: 194–198.
Hayre, C. M., Blackman, S. and Eyden, A. (2016) Do general radiographic examinations resemble a person-centred environment? *Radiography*, 22, 4: 245–251.
Hershfield, H. E. et al. (2013) When feeling bad can be good: Mixed emotions benefit physical health across adulthood, *Social Psychology and Personality Science*, 4, 54–61.
Holliday, A. (2016) *Doing & Writing Qualitative Research*. London, UK: Sage.
Holliday, A. R. and MacDonald, M. N. (2019) Researching the intercultural: Intersubjectivity and the problem with postpositivism. *Applied Linguistics*. (Forthcoming).
Jaggar, A. (1989) Love and knowledge: Emotion in feminist epistemology, *Inquiry*, 32, 2: 151–176.
Jones, J. and Hunter, D. (1995) Qualitative research: Consensus methods for medical and health services research, *British Medical Journal*, 311: 376.
Jones, J. and Smith, J. (2017) Ethnography: Challenges and opportunities, *Evidence-Based Nursing*, 20, 4: 98–100.
Kielmann, K. (2012) The ethnographic lens, in Gilson, L. (Ed.) *Health Policy and Systems Research: A Methodology Reader*. Geneva, Switzerland: World Health Organization: 235–252.
Kuhn, D. (1991) *The Skills of Argument*. Cambridge, UK: Cambridge University Press.
Kuhn, T. (1970) *The Structure of Scientific Revolutions*. Chicago, IL: University of Chicago Press.
Langhout, R. D. (2006) Who am I? Locating myself and its implications for collaborative research, *American Journal of Community Psychology*, 37: 267–274.
McGarrol, S. (2017) The emotional challenges of conducting in-depth research into significant health issues in health geography: Reflections on emotional labour, fieldwork and life course, *Area*, 49, 4: 436–442.
McKenzie, S. (2017) Emotional reflexivity and the guiding principle of objectivity in an inter-disciplinary, multi-method, longitudinal research project, The Open University in Scotland. Sociological Research Online, 22, 1: 8. www.socresonline.org.uk/22/1/8.html (Accessed 10 April 2018).
Merrill, B. and West, L. (2009) *Using Biographical Methods in Social Research*. London, UK: Sage.
Merton, R., Reader, G. and Kendall, P. (1957) (Eds.) *Introductory Studies in the Sociology of Medical Education*. Cambridge, MA: Harvard University Press.
Meyer, J. (2000) Using qualitative methods in health-related action research, *British Medical Journal*, 320: 178.

Mills, C. W. (1959) *The Sociological Imagination*. New York: Oxford University Press.
Morgan-Trimmer, S. and Wood, F. (2016) Ethnographic methods for process evaluations of complex health behaviour interventions, *Trials*, 17: 232. doi:10.1186/s13063-016-1340-2.
Nettleton, S. (1995) *The Sociology of Health and Illness*. Cambridge, UK: Polity Press.
Pope, C., Ziebland, S. and Mays, N. (2000) Analysing qualitative data, *British Medical Journal*, 320: 114.
Pulcini, E. (2017) What emotions motivate care? *Emotion Review*, 9: 64–71.
Radcliffe, P. (2011) Motherhood, pregnancy and the negotiation of identity: The moral career of drug treatment, *Social Science and Medicine*, 72: 984–991.
Råheim, M., Magnussen, L. H., Sekse, R. J. T., Lunde, Å., Jacobsen, T. and Blystad, A. (2016) Researcher–researched relationship in qualitative research: Shifts in positions and researcher vulnerability. *International Journal of Qualitative Studies on Health and Well-Being*, 11, 1. doi:10.3402/qhw.v11.30996.
Rashid, M., Caine, V. and Goez, H. (2015) The encounters and challenges of ethnography as a methodology in health research, *International Journal of Qualitative Methods*, 14: 1–16.
Reed-Danahay, D. E. (2001) Auto-biography, intimacy and ethnography, in Atkinson, P. et al. (Eds.) *Handbook of Ethnography*, London, UK: Sage: 407–425.
Roth, J. (1963) *Timetables: Structuring the passage of time in hospital treatment and other careers*, Indianapolis, IN: Bobbs-Merrill.
Sah, R. K. (2017). Positive Sexual Health: An Ethnographic Exploration of Social and Cultural Factors Affecting Sexual Lifestyles and Relationships of Nepalese Young People in the UK. Doctoral Dissertation, Canterbury Christ Church University, UK.
Savage, J. (2000) Ethnography and health care, *British Medical Journal*, 321, 7273: 1400–1402.
Savin-Baden, M. and Major, C. H. (2013) *Qualitative Research: The Essential Guide to Theory and Practice*. London, UK: Routledge.
Sheehan, D. et al. (2016) Clinical learning environments: Place, artefacts and rhythm, *Medical Education*, 51: 1049–1060.
Sonyini Madison, D. (2012) *Critical Ethnography*. London, UK: Sage.
Walton, J. and Lazzaro-Salazar, M. (2015) Othering the chronically ill: A discourse analysis of New Zealand health policy documents, *Health Communication*, 31, 4: 460–467.
Watts, J. H. (2008) Emotion, empathy and exit: Reflections on doing ethnographic qualitative research on sensitive topics, *Medical Sociology Online*, 2, 3: 3–14. http://oro.open.ac.uk/10901/1/jhwatts.pdf.
Weber, M. (1964) *The Theory of Social and Economic Organisation*. New York: The Free Press. (Originally published as *Wirtschaft und gesellschaft*, 1922).
Wincup, E. (2000) Feminist research with women awaiting trial: The effects on participants in the qualitative research process, in Gilbert, K. R. (Ed.) *The Emotional Nature of Qualitative Research*. London, UK: CRC Press: 17–35.

[illegible] (19[illegible]) [illegible]. New York: Columbia University Press.
[illegible] and Wong [illegible] (20[illegible]) [illegible] methods [illegible] cases [illegible] [illegible].
[illegible]. Thousand Oaks [illegible]: [illegible] Press.
[illegible] and [illegible] (20[illegible]) [illegible] and [illegible] [illegible].
[illegible] (19[illegible]) [illegible] and the [illegible] [illegible] of [illegible]. [illegible], [illegible].
[illegible] (2010). [illegible] of [illegible] with [illegible] [illegible] [illegible]. [illegible], [illegible]: [illegible].
[illegible] (19[illegible]) [illegible] [illegible] [illegible] [illegible] [illegible].
[illegible] (20[illegible]) [illegible] [illegible] [illegible] ethnography [illegible] [illegible].
[illegible] (19[illegible]) [illegible] [illegible]. [illegible] [illegible] [illegible].
[illegible] (20[illegible]) [illegible] [illegible] [illegible] Sexual [illegible] [illegible] [illegible] [illegible] and [illegible] [illegible] [illegible] [illegible] [illegible]. Doctoral Dissertation [illegible] [illegible].
[illegible] (19[illegible]) [illegible] [illegible] [illegible].
[illegible] (20[illegible]) [illegible] [illegible] [illegible] [illegible] [illegible].
[illegible] (20[illegible]) [illegible] [illegible] [illegible] [illegible].
[illegible] (20[illegible]) [illegible] [illegible] [illegible] [illegible] [illegible] [illegible] [illegible].
[illegible] (20[illegible]) [illegible] [illegible] [illegible] [illegible] [illegible]. [illegible], [illegible] (20[illegible]).
[illegible] (19[illegible]) [illegible] [illegible]. New York: [illegible] [illegible].
[illegible] (20[illegible]) [illegible] [illegible] [illegible] [illegible]. [illegible] [illegible] [illegible] [illegible] [illegible] [illegible] [illegible] [illegible].

Index